Case St

This book is written as a system-based clinical–radiological review providing images from the latest available imaging modalities and covers all major diseases that are encountered in everyday clinical practice. A problem-orientated approach is used. Each chapter contains a collection of clinical cases each with a short clinical description and initial imaging followed by pertinent questions regarding the imaging findings (colour coded in red outline). The second part of each chapter contains the case diagnosis, a discussion of the role of imaging in the presenting problem, a recommended sequence for further imaging evaluation, and illustrative examples of the same disease using different imaging modalities for further investigation. Images of conditions in the differential diagnosis are also provided (colour coded in blue outline).

This book is written by experienced radiologists currently working in undergraduate and postgraduate medical education. The cases are a collection of their illustrative teaching material.

Professor Anil T. Ahuja is currently Professor and Chairman in the Department of Diagnostic Radiology and Organ Imaging at The Chinese University of Hong Kong

Dr Gregory E. Antonio is Associate Professor in the Department of Diagnostic Radiology and Organ Imaging at The Chinese University of Hong Kong

Dr K. T. Wong is an Honorary Clinical Assistant Professor in the Department of Diagnostic Radiology and Organ Imaging at The Chinese University of Hong Kong

Dr Edmund H. Y. Yuen is a former Honorary Clinical Assistant Professor in the Department of Diagnostic Radiology and Organ Imaging at The Chinese University of Hong Kong

Case Studies in Medical Imaging

Radiology for Students and Trainees

A. T. Ahuja

The Chinese University of Hong Kong

G. E. Antonio, K. T. Wong, and H. Y. Yuen

The Chinese University of Hong Kong

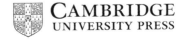

CAMBRIDGE UNIVERSITY PRESS
Cambridge, New York, Melbourne, Madrid, Cape Town, Singapore, São Paulo

CAMBRIDGE UNIVERSITY PRESS
The Edinburgh Building, Cambridge CB2 2RU, UK

Published in the United States of America by Cambridge University Press, New York

www.cambridge.org
Information on this title: www.cambridge.org/9780521682947

© Cambridge University Press 2006

First published 2006

Printed in the United Kingdom at the University Press, Cambridge

A catalogue record for this publication is available from the British Library

ISBN-13 978-0-521-68294-7 paperback
ISBN-10 0-521-68294-0 paperback

Contents

Contributors   vi

Preface   viii

01 CHEST   1
K.T. Wong, Edmund H.Y. Yuen, Anil T. Ahuja

02 CENTRAL NERVOUS SYSTEM   57
Edmund H.Y. Yuen, Ann D. King, Anil T. Ahuja

03 VASCULAR   123
Simon S.M. Ho, Gregory E. Antonio, Simon C.H. Yu, Stella S.Y. Ho

04 MUSCULOSKELETAL   169
Gregory E. Antonio, James F. Griffith, Simon S.M. Ho, Anil T. Ahuja

05 TRAUMA   227
Gregory E. Antonio, James F. Griffith, Anil T. Ahuja

06 GASTROINTESTINAL SYSTEM   261
Alex W.H. Ng, David P.N. Chan, K.T. Wong, Gregory E. Antonio,
Edmund H.Y. Yuen, Anil T. Ahuja

07 GENITOURINARY SYSTEM   305
K.K. Shing, K.T. Wong, Gregory E. Antonio, Shlok J. Lolge,
Anil T. Ahuja

08 HEPATOBILIARY SYSTEM   359
David P.N. Chan, Alex W.H. Ng, K.T. Wong, Gregory E. Antonio,
Edmund H.Y. Yuen, Anil T. Ahuja

09 HEAD & NECK   395
K.T. Wong, Edmund H.Y. Yuen, Ann D. King, Anil T. Ahuja

10 PAEDIATRIC   425
Monica S.M. Chan, K.T. Wong

11 BREAST   457
Edmund H.Y. Yuen, Alice Tang

12 FOREIGN BODIES   471
Simon S.H. Ho, K.T. Wong, Edmund H.Y. Yuen, Gavin M. Joynt, Anil
T. Ahuja

Contributors

Anil T. Ahuja
MBBS(Bom), MD(Bom), FRCR, FHKCR,
FHKAM(Radiology)
Professor
Department of Diagnostic Radiology and
Organ Imaging
The Chinese University of Hong Kong
Prince of Wales Hospital
Shatin
Hong Kong
China

Gregory E. Antonio
MD(CUHK), MBBS(UNSW), BSc(Med),
FRANZCR, FHKCR, FHKAM(Radiology)
Associate Professor
Department of Diagnostic Radiology and
Organ Imaging
The Chinese University of Hong Kong
Prince of Wales Hospital
Shatin
Hong Kong
China

David P.N. Chan
MBChB, FRCR, FHKCR, FHKAM(Radiology)
Honorary Clinical Assistant Professor
Department of Diagnostic Radiology and
Organ Imaging
The Chinese University of Hong Kong
Prince of Wales Hospital
Shatin
Hong Kong
China

Monica S.M. Chan
MBChB, FRCR, FHKCR, FHKAM(Radiology)
Honorary Clinical Assistant Professor
Department of Diagnostic Radiology and
Organ Imaging
The Chinese University of Hong Kong
Prince of Wales Hospital
Shatin
Hong Kong
China

James F. Griffith
MBCh, BAO, MRCP(UK),FRCR, FHKCR,
FHKAM(Radiology)
Professor
Department of Diagnostic Radiology and
Organ Imaging
The Chinese University of Hong Kong
Prince of Wales Hospital
Shatin
Hong Kong
China

Simon S.M. Ho
BSc, MBBS(London), MRCP(UK), FRCR
Assistant Professor
Department of Diagnostic Radiology and
Organ Imaging
The Chinese University of Hong Kong
Prince of Wales Hospital
Shatin
Hong Kong
China

Stella S.Y. Ho
PhD, MPhil, BSc(Hon),PDDR, RDMS, RVT
Adjunct Assistant Professor
Department of Diagnostic Radiology and
Organ Imaging
The Chinese University of Hong Kong
Prince of Wales Hospital
Shatin
Hong Kong
China

Gavin M. Joynt
MBBCh(Witwatersrand), FFA(SA)
(CritCare), FHKCA,FHKCA(IC),
FHKAM(Anaesthesiology), FEICANZCA,
FJFICM, FCCP
Professor
Department of Anaesthesia and Intensive Care
The Chinese University of Hong Kong
Prince of Wales Hospital
Shatin
Hong Kong
China

Contributors

Ann D. King
MBCh, MRCP, FRCR, FHKCR,
FHKAM(Radiology)
Professor
Department of Diagnostic Radiology and
Organ Imaging
The Chinese University of Hong Kong
Prince of Wales Hospital
Shatin
Hong Kong
China

Shlok J. Lolge
MBBS, MD(Radiology)
Lecturer
Department of Radiology
King Edward Memorial Hospital
Parel
Mumbai
India

Alex W.H. Ng
MBChB, FRCR, FHKCR, FHKAM(Radiology)
Honorary Clinical Assistant Professor
Department of Diagnostic Radiology and
Organ Imaging
The Chinese University of Hong Kong
Prince of Wales Hospital
Shatin
Hong Kong
China

K.K. Shing
MBChB, FRCR, FHKCR, FHKAM(Radiology)
Medical Officer
Department of Diagnostic Radiology and
Organ Imaging
Prince of Wales Hospital
Shatin
Hong Kong
China

Alice Tang
MBBS, FRCR, FHKCR, FHKAM(Radiology)
Consultant
Department of Diagnostic Radiology
Alice Ho Mui Ling Nethersole Hospital
Taipo
Hong Kong
China

K.T. Wong
MBChB, FRCR, FHKCR,
FHKAM(Radiology)
Honorary Clinical Assistant Professor
Department of Diagnostic Radiology and
Organ Imaging
The Chinese University of Hong Kong
Prince of Wales Hospital
Shatin
Hong Kong
China

Simon C.H. Yu
MBBS, FRCR, FHKCR, FHKAM(Radiology)
Honorary Clinical Associate Professor
Department of Diagnostic Radiology and
Organ Imaging
The Chinese University of Hong Kong
Prince of Wales Hospital
Shatin
Hong Kong
China

Edmund H.Y. Yuen
MBChB, FRCR, FHKCR, FHKAM(Radiology)
Honorary Clinical Assistant Professor
Department of Diagnostic Radiology and
Organ Imaging
The Chinese University of Hong Kong
Prince of Wales Hospital
Shatin
Hong Kong
China

Preface

Radiology (Medical Imaging) now plays a pivotal role in modern medical practice. Clinical decision making depends on timely and accurate interpretation of imaging studies particularly in acute situations. Its importance in daily clinical practice is reflected by the fact that almost no patient leaves the hospital without undergoing an imaging study. Many clinicians now need to interpret images themselves and the information provided is particularly useful for minimally invasive treatment. It is therefore essential that imaging take its rightful place in the Medical School Core Curriculum so that future doctors have the necessary knowledge and skills to provide high quality medical care to the community they serve.

Radiology is a 'visual' science and is best taught and learnt viewing images rather than text alone. These images can be used to demonstrate anatomy, physiology, pathology (in cross-section, real time, 3D, multi-planar and virtual reality) and are a powerful tool when combined with relevant clinical information. Its applications cover every aspect of medicine and across all specialties making radiology the key to prompt diagnosis and management. Future doctors must therefore be familiar with all aspects of Radiology (diagnostic and interventional). It is with this in mind that 'Case Studies in Medical Imaging: Radiology for Students and Trainees' is written.

Radiology is constantly being revolutionized by rapidly advancing technology. There is a wealth of encyclopedic radiology textbooks (some of which have been used in the preparation for this book) available in the market for residents undergoing specialist training. However, they may be too exhaustive for medical students and trainees to squeeze into their already overwhelmed curriculum. There exist student textbooks on radiology but they are didactic and tend to focus on text rather than images.

In this book, knowledge is conveyed predominantly through case studies using images and supplemented with brief text in a question and answer format. The core knowledge in Radiology that a medical graduate 'must know' is covered in these cases. This book does not discuss the physical principles of the various imaging modalities, as these have been adequately covered in other 'textbooks', but focuses on imaging information for common cases medical student and young residents must be familiar with.

In the preparation of this book two other books have been extensively referred to. These are Wolfgang Dahnert: Radiology Review Manual and Chapman S, Nakielny R: Aids to Radiological Differential Diagnosis. They have distilled the basic facts regarding imaging and clinical information and have become essential reading material for most radiology residents and trainees. The facts stated in these books are clear, indisputable and have themselves been obtained with the help of many other reputable radiology texts. This is a legacy that is passed on from teachers, colleagues, collaborators which continues to benefit medical education.

All the authors and co-editors in this book are teachers in academic departments and have a wealth of teaching experience. They are strongly committed to medical teaching and their efforts are appreciated by students and colleagues alike. They have put to paper knowledge and skills acquired over many years of teaching with the aim of improving Radiology teaching in the Medical Curriculum.

Preface

I owe a large debt of gratitude to colleagues and staff in The Department of Diagnostic Radiology & Organ Imaging, The Chinese University of Hong Kong, without whose help none of this would have been possible. They have shared their knowledge, images, time, patience and expertise and for this I remain grateful. I would also like to thank Professor Ravi Ramakantan, Head of Department, Radiology Department, Seth G.S Medical College, K.E.M Hospital, Mumbai, India for his support and contributing teaching material from his department (where I originally trained!). His efforts are much appreciated.

On a personal note, for me, this book is for my late father, Dr T.S Ahuja, who taught Histology and Anatomy to medical students (including myself) in their preclinical years at The Seth G.S Medical College, K.E.M Hospital, Mumbai, India. He is still fondly remembered by all his students for his hard work and dedication towards teaching. Finally, I remain forever grateful for the close help and support of my mother Mrs Laj Ahuja, wife Chu Wai Po and daughters Sanjali and Tiana (who have helped me maintain my sanity).

Anil Ahuja

CHEST

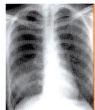

Contributors:

K.T. Wong, Edmund H.Y. Yuen, Anil T. Ahuja

Chapter 01

Questions

Case 1 - 21   2 - 22

Discussion

Pneumonia   23 - 24

Lung collapse   25 - 26

Pneumothorax   27

Pneumomediastinum   28 - 29

Primary lung carcinoma   30 - 31

Pancoast tumour   32

Pulmonary metastases   33 - 34

Pleural effusion   35

Empyema   36

Lung abscess   37

Post-primary pulmonary tuberculosis   38 - 39

Cystic bronchiectasis   40 - 41

Chronic obstructive airways disease   42

Lymphoma   43 - 44

Silicosis   45

Pulmonary embolism   46 - 47

Re-expansion pulmonary oedema   48

Trauma   49 - 50

Heart failure   51 - 52

Mitral stenosis   53 - 55

Tetralogy of Fallot   56

Case 1

A 35-year-old man presented with fever and productive cough for 3 days. He was febrile, hypoxic and physical examination showed focal decrease in air entry and coarse crepitations over the right lower chest. Laboratory investigations revealed leukocytosis and a CXR was performed (Fig. 1a).

Questions

(1) What abnormalities do you see on this CXR ?
   - Area of increased opacity with ill-defined borders
   - Faint air bronchogram within the area of opacification
(2) What is the most likely diagnosis ?

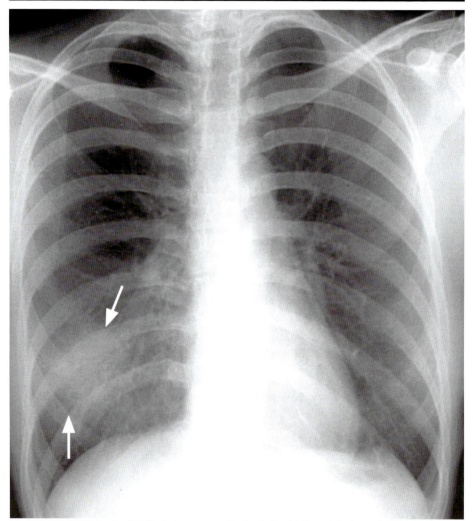

Fig.1a *Frontal CXR showing ill-defined air space opacification in the right lower lobe (arrows) due to consolidation from pneumonia.*

Case 2

A 70-year-old chronic smoker presented with haemoptysis and weight loss for 2 months. He had no fever, chills or rigor and a physical examination of both hands showed finger clubbing. There was decreased chest wall expansion and air entry over right upper chest.

Laboratory investigations were essentially unremarkable and WCC was within normal limits.

A CXR was performed for further evaluation (Fig. 2a).

Questions

(1) What abnormality can you see on this CXR ?
   - Opacity with a sharp well-demarcated lateral border (arrows) in right upper zone with lack of air within the abnormality.
   - Focal convex bulge at the apex of the abnormality.
   - Hyperinflation of the right lower lobe.
   - Elevated right hemidiaphragm.
(2) What is the radiological diagnosis ?

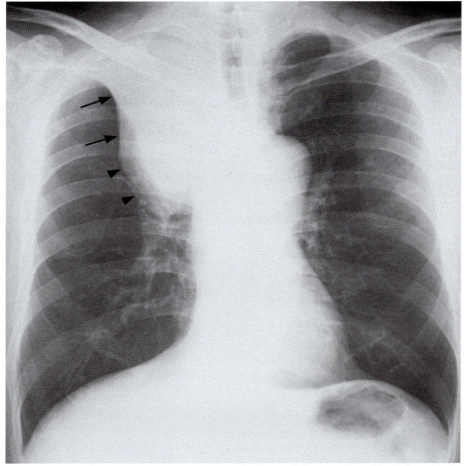

Fig.2a The 'Golden S sign' – collapse of the right upper lobe with a well demarcated lateral border formed by the elevated horizontal fissure (arrows), and a focal convex bulge at the apex due to the centrally located bronchogenic carcinoma (arrowheads).

Case 3

A 23-year-old man with good past health, presented with sudden onset left sided chest pain and shortness of breath. The pain was sharp in nature and more severe on inspiration. Physical examination showed decreased air entry in the left upper chest which was hyperresonant on percussion. Laboratory investigations were essentially normal. A CXR was performed for further evaluation (Fig. 3a).

Questions

(1) What radiological abnormality can you identify ?
- Hyperlucent zone devoid of vascular marking in periphery of left hemithorax.
- Shift of midline to the right.

(2) <u>What is the most likely diagnosis ?</u>

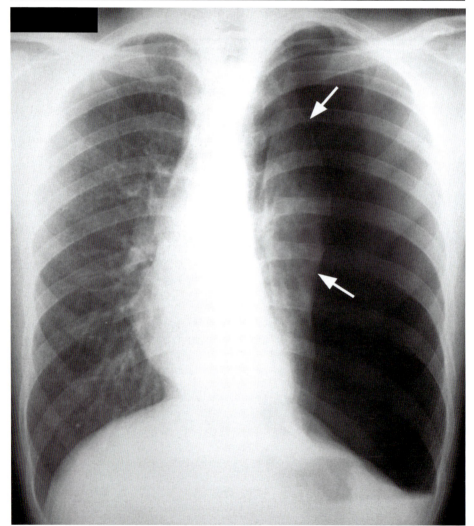

Fig.3a *Large left pneumothorax with mediastinal shift to the right. Note the collapsed left lung (arrows) and the hyperlucent left hemithorax.*

Case 4

A 30-year-old lady presented with severe retrosternal pain, and pain on swallowing, shortly after accidental ingestion of fish bone 2 days earlier. Physical examination showed the patient was afebrile, haemodynamically stable and examination of respiratory and cardiovascular systems were unremarkable. Blood tests were essentially normal and a CXR was performed for further assessment (Fig. 4a).

Questions

(1) What radiologic abnormality can you identify ?
- Air lucency in mediastinum outlining the left heart border and aortic knuckle
- Subcutaneous emphysema in the lower neck

(2) <u>What is the radiological diagnosis ?</u>

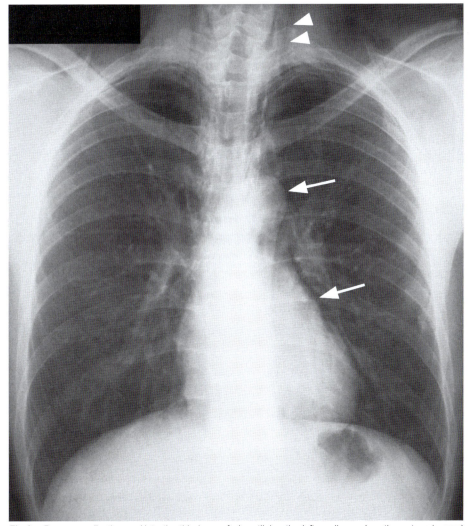

Fig.4a *Pneumomediastinum. Note the thin layer of air outlining the left cardiac and aortic contour (arrows) and subcutaneous emphysema in the lower neck (arrowheads).*

Case 5

A 75-year-old chronic smoker complained of chronic cough and weight loss of 20 pounds over recent 3 months. On physical examination, he was cachectic with little subcutaneous fat and a 2 cm hard mass was palpable in the right supraclavicular fossa. Examination of respiratory system was essentially normal. Laboratory investigations showed normochromic normocytic anaemia and raised erythrocyte sedimentation rate. White cell count was not raised. A CXR was performed (Fig. 5a).

Questions

(1) What radiologic abnormalities do you see ?
- Soft tissue mass with ill-defined irregular border projected over the right upper zone.
- Enlarged and bulging right hilum.
- Thickened right paratracheal stripe.

(2) What is the radiological diagnosis ?

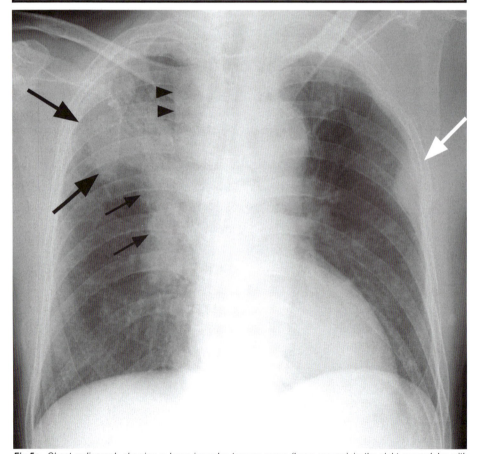

Fig.5a *Chest radiograph showing a large irregular tumour mass (large arrows) in the right upper lobe with right hilar lymphadenopathy (small arrows). The thickened right paratracheal stripe (arrowheads) also indicates enlarged paratracheal nodes. Note the presence of a pleural metastasis in the left mid zone (white arrow).*

Case 6

A 66-year-old chronic smoker presented with one-month history of cough with blood-stained sputum and right upper chest and arm pain. General examination showed signs of Horner's syndrome on the right and muscle wasting of right hand. Examination of the respiratory system was unremarkable. Laboratory investigations revealed normochromic normocytic anaemia and suspicious malignant cells were detected on sputum cytology. A CXR was performed (Fig. 6a).

Questions

(1) What radiological abnormality can you identify ?
- Mass in right lung apex
- Bony invasion of right upper ribs

(2) What is the working diagnosis ?

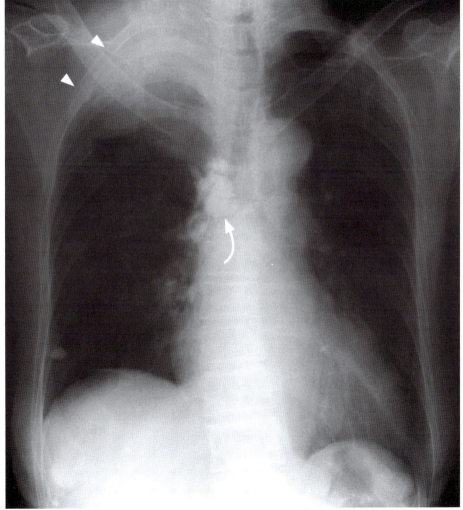

Fig.6a *Chest radiograph showing right apical lung opacity with rib infiltration (arrowheads) and destruction (absent anterior first rib, compare with left side). The trachea is deviated to the left side. There is evidence of previous TB with calcified lymph nodes and granuloma (curved arrow).*

Case 7

A 50-year-old man with a known history of colonic carcinoma, complained of cough with occasional blood-streaked sputum for 2 months, and recent loss of appetite and weight. Physical examination of the respiratory system was normal and abdominal examination revealed hepatomegaly with multinodular edges. Laboratory investigations showed elevated alkaline phosphatase, bilirubin level and markedly elevated CEA. A chest x-ray followed by CT of the thorax (Fig. 7a, b) and abdomen was performed.

Questions

(1) What radiological abnormality is present on this CXR and CT of the thorax ?
  - Multiple round well-defined soft tissue masses in both lungs.
(2) <u>What is the working diagnosis ?</u>

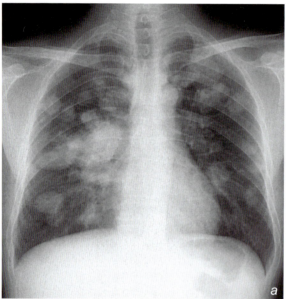

Fig.7a,b
Frontal chest radiograph and axial CT thorax showing multiple round metastases in both lungs.

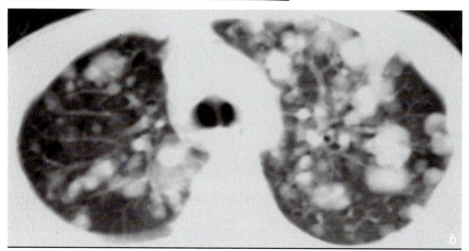

Case 8

A 53-year-old non-smoker presented with fever, dyspnoea and productive cough for 3 days. A physical examination of the respiratory system revealed decreased air entry over the right chest where the percussion note was stony dull in nature. Laboratory investigations showed leukocytosis, sputum culture grew Haemophilus influenzae and a CXR was performed (Fig. 8a).

Questions

(1) What radiological abnormality can you identify ?
- Complete opacification of the right mid and lower zones effacing the right heart border and right hemidiaphragm
- Blunting of the right costophrenic angle
- No evidence of mediastinal shift

(2) What is the radiological diagnosis ?

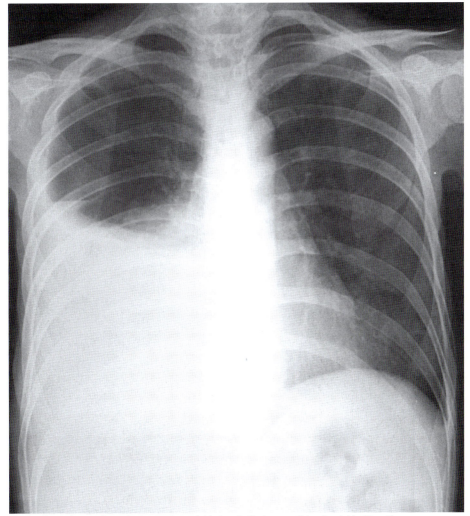

Fig.8a *Erect chest radiograph showing large right pleural effusion opacifying the right mid and lower zone.*

Case 9

A 75-year-old man presented with productive cough and high swinging fever for 3 days. Physical examination showed he was febrile and there was decreased air entry in right lower chest where the percussion note was stony dull. Laboratory investigations revealed marked leucocytosis and CXR was performed (Fig. 9a).

Questions

(1) What radiological abnormality is identified on the CXR ?
   - Complete opacification of the right hemithorax with mediastinal shift to the left
(2) What is the radiological diagnosis ?

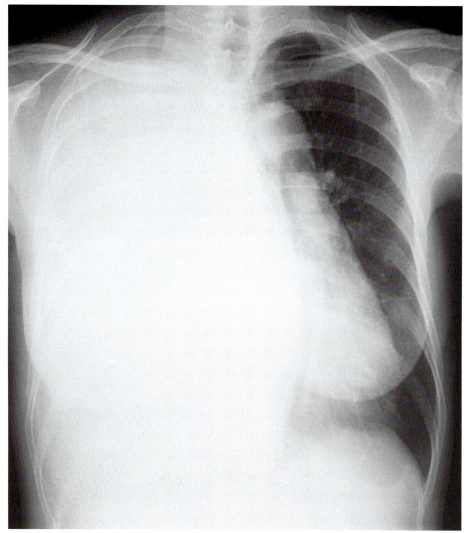

Fig.9a *Frontal CXR showing complete opacification of the right hemithorax, blunting of the right costo-phrenic angle with mediastinal shift to the left due to a large pleural collection.*

Case 10

A 53-year-old diabetic presented with fever, chills and rigor, cough and purulent sputum for 5 days. He was febrile and examination of the respiratory system was unremarkable apart from increased respiratory rate. Laboratory investigations showed marked leukocytosis and raised ESR and sputum and blood culture grew Klebsiella. A CXR was performed as the initial investigation (Fig. 10a). As the patient's condition did not improve after 3 days of antibiotics treatment a contrast CT thorax was performed (Fig. 10b).

Questions

(1) What radiological abnormalities are seen on the frontal CXR ?
 - Cavitating lung lesion in right upper zone with thick irregular walls
 - Air-fluid level within the lesion
 - Adjacent air-space opacification
(2) What abnormality can you identify on CT thorax ?
 - Thick walled cavitating lesion containing both fluid and air
 - Consolidative changes in adjacent lung parenchyma
(3) What is the likely diagnosis ?

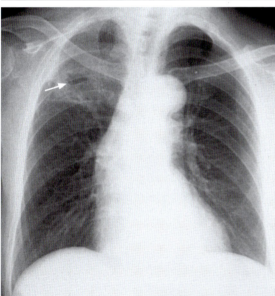

Fig.10a Chest radiograph showing a right upper lobe abscess. Note the cavitation (arrow) with thick irregular walls and an air-fluid level within, and the adjacent pneumonia.

Fig.10b Contrast enhanced axial CT thorax showing the thick walled cavitating abscess (arrows) containing both pus and air, and consolidative changes in the adjacent lung parenchyma.

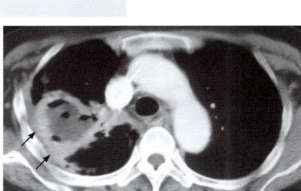

Case 11

A 45-year-old woman with poorly controlled diabetes mellitus, presented with productive cough for 1 month. She also noticed low grade fever, night sweating and weight loss during this period. Examination of the chest showed a dull percussion note, decreased air entry and coarse crepitations in the right upper zone. Laboratory investigations revealed raised ESR, normal white cell count and a CXR was performed (Fig. 11a).

Questions
(1) What radiological abnormalities can you identify ?
 - Multiple areas of air-space opacification in the right lung also involving the apex
 - Cavitation and air-fluid level within the opacified areas
 - Blunting of right CP angle due to exudative effusion
(2) What is the radiological diagnosis ?

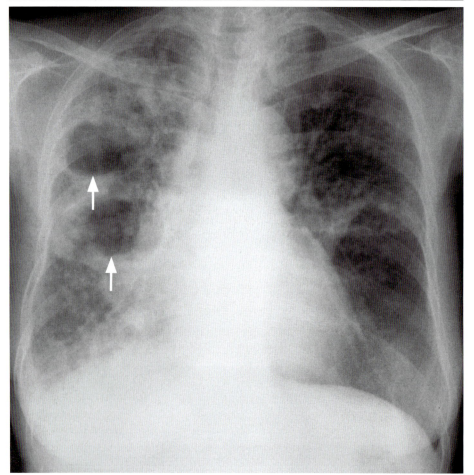

Fig.11a *Frontal chest radiograph showing air-space opacification in the right lung with cavitating lesions (arrows) due to caseous necrosis in tuberculosis.*

Case 12

A 55-year-old non-smoker presented with on and off haemoptysis and purulent sputum for 1 year. There was no fever or constitutional symptoms. Physical examination showed finger clubbing and coarse crepitations over the lung base. Blood tests were essentially normal and an initial CXR (Fig. 12a) was performed.

Questions

(1) What abnormality can you see on CXR ?
   - Clusters of cystic spaces with air-fluid levels involving multiple zones bilaterally.
(2) <u>What is the most likely diagnosis ?</u>

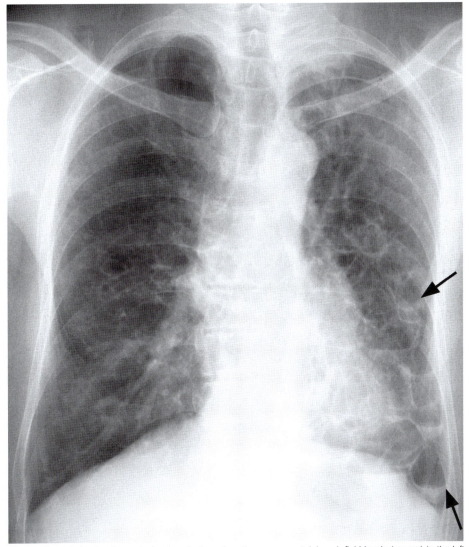

Fig.12a *Frontal chest radiograph showing clusters of cystic spaces containing air-fluid levels (arrows) in the left mid and lower zones due to retained secretions in dilated bronchioles in bronchiectasis.*

Case 13

A 70-year-old chronic smoker for 50 years presented with exertional shortness of breath for 1 year. His exercise tolerance was limited to 1 flight of stairs and he remained largely home-bound for recent 6 months. Physical examination showed he was tachypnoeic with central cyanosis. Examination of respiratory system revealed use of accessory muscles of respiration and hyperinflated chest on both sides. Air entry was globally decreased in both lungs. A CXR was performed for further evaluation (Fig. 13a).

Questions
(1) What abnormality can you identify on CXR ?
- Hyperinflated, hyperlucent lungs
- Flat diaphragm
(2) What is the clinical diagnosis ?

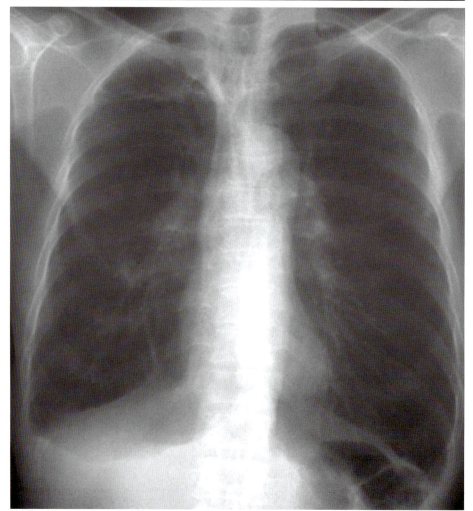

Fig.13a *Frontal chest radiograph showing bilateral hyperlucent, hyperinflated lungs of chronic obstructive airway disease. There is some minor fibrosis in the right upper zone from previous TB.*

Case 14

An 18-year-old Asian man with good past health, presented with weight loss, night sweats, cough and generalized malaise for 1 month. Physical examination revealed palpable enlarged lymph nodes in cervical, axillary and groin regions. Examination of the respiratory system was essentially normal. Laboratory investigations showed normochromic normocytic anaemia and raised LDH. A CXR (Fig.14a) was performed, followed by contrast CT thorax (Fig. 14b).

Questions

(1) What radiological abnormality can you identify on CXR ?
   - Enlarged hila with rounded contours.
   - Widened upper mediastinum with lobulated outline. The aortic knuckle is clearly seen suggesting the mass is in the anterior mediastinum.
(2) What abnormality can you identify on the CT thorax ?
   - Extensive mass of matted nodes in the anterior mediastinum.
(3) What is the most likely diagnosis ?

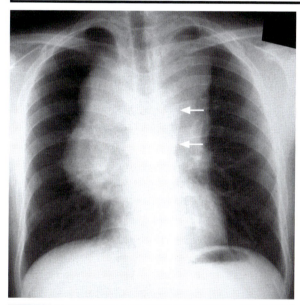

Fig.14a Frontal chest radiograph showing widened mediastinal contour and enlarged hila with lobulated contours suggestive of enlarged lymphadenopathy. Note the clearly seen aortic knuckle (arrows) suggesting the lesion is in the anterior mediastinum.

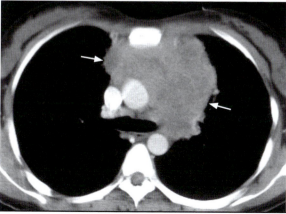

Fig.14b Contrast enhanced axial CT thorax confirms extensive matted mass of lymph nodes (white arrows) in the anterior mediastinum.

Case 15

A 55-year-old non-smoker presented with progressive exertional shortness of breath for 3 years. He was previously a construction site worker for more than 20 years. Physical examination was unremarkable except that the patient was tachypnoeic. Laboratory investigations were essentially normal and lung function test revealed a constrictive pattern. A CXR was performed (Fig. 15).

Questions

(1) What radiological abnormality can you identify ?
- Multiple small dense nodular opacities in both lungs
- Egg-shell calcification of hilar lymph nodes

(2) What is the working diagnosis ?

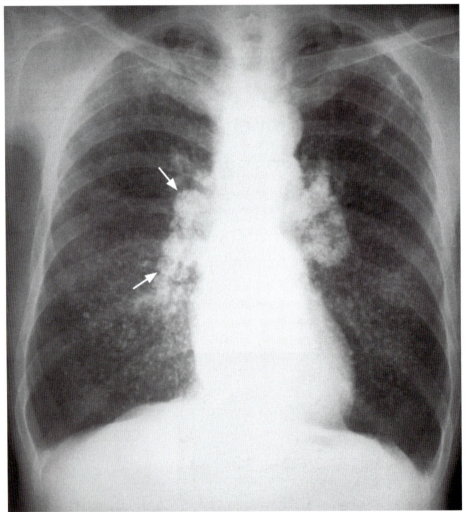

Fig.15 *Chest radiograph showing multiple small dense nodules in both lungs in silicosis. Note the 'egg-shell' calcification of hilar lymph nodes (arrows).*

Case 16

A 47-year-old woman who had pelvic surgery 5 days earlier presented with sudden onset shortness of breath and bilateral chest pain. Physical examination showed she was in respiratory distress and tachycardic. Examination of the chest was essentially normal. Laboratory investigations showed hypoxia and hypocapnia. A preliminary CXR was unremarkable and a CT examination was performed (Fig. 16a, b).

Questions

(1) What is the preliminary diagnosis ?
   - Pulmonary embolism
(2) What type of CT examination has been performed ?
   - CT Pulmonary Angiogram (CTPA)
(3) What abnormality do you see on this CTPA ?
   - Multiple filling defects within the pulmonary arteries
(4) What is the radiological diagnosis ?

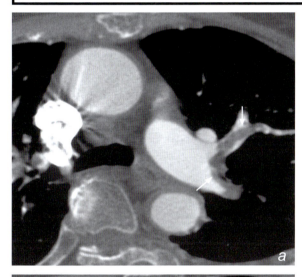

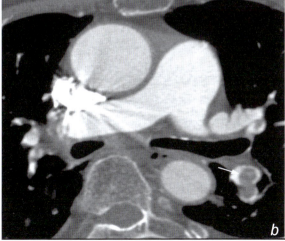

Fig.16 a,b CT pulmonary angiogram showing filling defects (arrows) of emboli within the branches of the left pulmonary artery confirming the diagnosis of pulmonary embolism.

Case 17

A 66-year-old with good past health presented to the Emergency Department complaining of acute onset of right chest pain and shortness of breath, increasing in severity for the past 36 hours. He was afebrile but tachypnoeic and on physical examination the right lung showed hyper-resonance on percussion and decreased air entry on auscultation. A chest X-ray was performed (Fig. 17a).

Questions

(1) What abnormality is demonstrated on the CXR ?
   - Right hydropneumothorax (note the fluid level) with almost complete collapse of the right lung.

A chest drain was inserted and a follow-up chest radiograph was performed 6 hours later for reassessment (Fig. 17b).

(2) What abnormality is demonstrated on the second chest radiograph and what is the likely cause ?
   - The right chest drain is noted in a satisfactory position. However, there is extensive diffuse air-space shadowing involving the entire right lung. The left lung appears normal.

(3) <u>What is the cause for the right lung haziness ?</u>

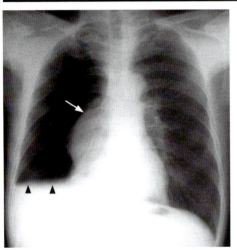

Fig.17a Frontal chest radiograph showing a large right hydropneumothorax (arrowheads) and collapse of the right lung (arrows).

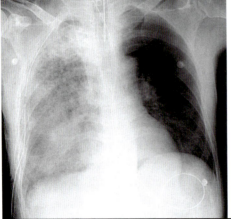

Fig.17b Chest radiograph showing re-expansion pulmonary oedema of the right lung, after rapid evacuation of the right pneumothorax. Note the chest drain. Note the diffuse opacification of the right lung.

Case 18

A 23-year-old man was transferred to the resuscitation room after sustaining a road traffic accident. He was comatose and haemodynamically unstable on arrival. On initial clinical assessment there was bruising and deformity over the right chest wall. Chest expansion and air entry were markedly diminished on the right side and the percussion note was hyper-resonant. A right pneumothorax was clinically diagnosed and a chest drain was inserted immediately. A CXR was then performed as a part of trauma series (Fig. 18a).

Questions

(1) What abnormalities can you identify on this CXR ?
- - The right lung has re-expanded after insertion of the chest drain
- - Lucent line lateral to and outlining the right heart border and the right side of the mediastinal contour, elevating the mediastinal pleura - pneumomediastinum
- - Abnormal gas within soft tissues of axillae and right lower neck - surgical emphysema
- - Air-space opacification at the right upper zone probably due to lung contusion

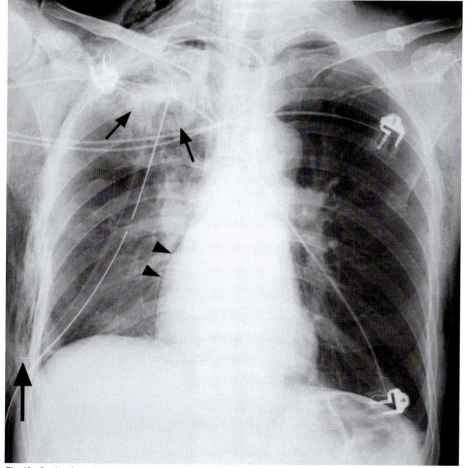

Fig.18a *Supine frontal chest radiograph of a patient with multiple sites of trauma. Note the pneumomediastinum (arrowheads), surgical emphysema (large arrow) and air-space opacification in the right upper zone (small arrows) possibly due to contusion. The right lung has re-expanded after the chest drain insertion for pneumothorax.*

Case 19

A 65-year-old man presented to the Accident and Emergency Department with crushing chest pain and shortness of breath and a CXR was performed (Fig. 19a).

Questions

(1) What are the chest radiograph findings ?
- Cardiomegaly
- Upper lobe venous diversion
- Septal lines (Kerley B lines) best seen in the right lower zone
- Sharply outlined haziness in the right upper zone with no evidence of an air bronchogram suggestive of fluid in the right horizontal fissure

(2) What is the diagnosis?

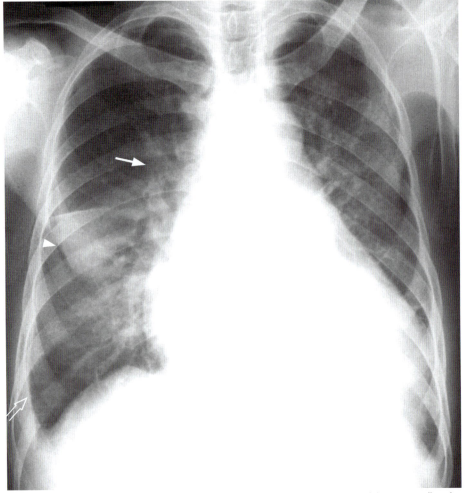

Fig.19a Congestive cardiac failure. Chest radiograph showing cardiomegaly, upper lobe venous diversion (arrow), septal lines (Kerley B lines) best seen in the right lower zone (open arrow) and thickening/fluid in the horizontal fissure (arrowhead). The fluid in the right horizontal fissure is sometimes called the 'Phantom tumour' as it may disappear on subsequent radiographs as the patient's condition improves (Image courtesy of Radiology Department, KEM Hospital, Mumbai, India).

Case 20

A 25-year-old woman with a history of rheumatic fever in childhood presented with repeated episodes of respiratory tract infections and shortness of breath. On physical examination the patient was acyanotic and a diastolic murmur was detected. A CXR (Fig. 20a) was performed as a preliminary investigation.

Questions

(1) What are the CXR findings ?
   - Cardiomegaly
   - Enlarged left atrium seen as a double density through the right upper cardiac border
   - Prominent pulmonary artery
   - No obvious upper lobe blood diversion or signs of cardiac failure
(2) What is the diagnosis ?

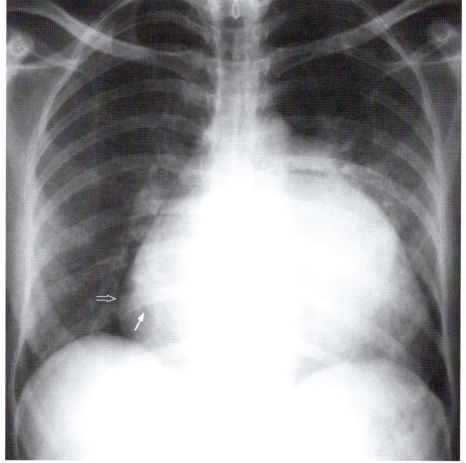

Fig.20a *Mitral stenosis. Chest radiograph showing enlarged left atrium with double density (arrow) seen through the right heart border (open arrow) and prominent central pulmonary artery (arrowhead). No radiographic evidence of cardiac failure (Image courtesy of Radiology Department, KEM Hospital, Mumbai, India).*

Case 21

A 2-year-old child presented with shortness of breath on playing and multiple short episodes of loss of consciousness. On examination the child was cyanotic and a heart murmur was noted. A CXR (Fig. 21a) was performed as an initial examination.

Questions
(1) What are the CXR findings ?
  - The cardiac apex is rounded and elevated off the left hemidiaphragm (suggestive of right ventricular hypertrophy)
  - The pulmonary bay is concave
  - There is pulmonary oligaemia
  - No evidence of cardiac failure
(2) What is the most likely diagnosis ?

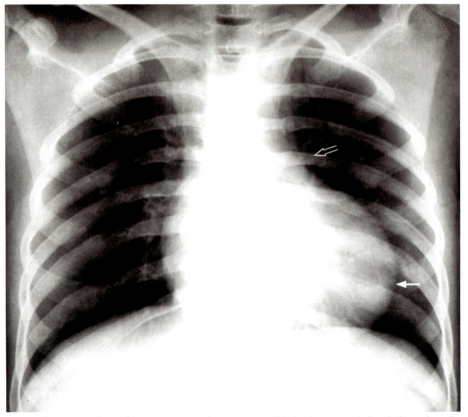

Fig.21a *Tetralogy of Fallot. Chest radiograph of a cyanosed child showing a rounded and elevated cardiac apex (arrow) suggestive of right ventricular hypertrophy, a concave pulmonary bay (open arrow) and pulmonary oligaemia (Image courtesy of Radiology Department, KEM Hospital, Mumbai, India).*

Pneumonia

Pneumonia (Fig. 1a)
- The inflammatory exudate within air-spaces and interstitium of the affected lung causes the opacification and air-filled bronchioles outlined by adjacent fluid-filled alveoli in affected lung produce the air bronchogram.

Discussion
- Pneumonia is a common disease and is usually caused by bacterial infection.
- Apart from the typical features of lobar pneumonia, *other probable radiological findings not seen on this CXR* include:
  1. Pleural effusion – seen as blunting of lateral costophrenic angle
  2. Cavitation – more common in staphylococcus pneumonia or pulmonary tuberculosis

- Pneumonia caused by certain organisms may produce characteristic radiologic features
  1. Unilateral lobar involvement in streptococcus infection
  2. Bilateral patchy involvement (Fig. 1b), sometimes with cavitation in staphylococcus pneumonia (Fig. 1c)
  3. Upper lobe involvement with cavitation in pulmonary TB (Fig. 1d)
  4. Bilateral symmetrical perihilar distribution which progresses rapidly over 3-5 days in PCP pneumonia in immune-compromised patients (Fig. 1e)
- In most cases imaging cannot accurately predict the causative organism.

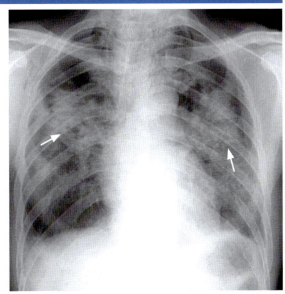

Fig.1b *Frontal CXR showing Staphylococcal pneumonia with bilateral ill-defined air space opacification (arrows).*

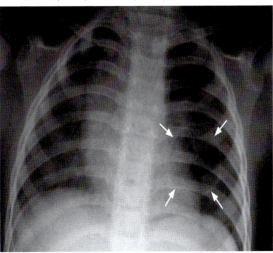

Fig.1c *Frontal radiograph of a child recovering from Staphylococcal pneumonia showing a pneumatocele in the left lung (arrows) (Image courtesy Dr. W.T. Fung, North District Hospital, Hong Kong).*

Discussion Case 1
Pneumonia

Role of imaging in patients with pneumonia

1. Confirm the clinical diagnosis
2. Detect possible complications such as pleural effusion / empyema or lung abscess if clinically not responsive to appropriate antibiotic treatment
3. Follow-up CXR to monitor response to treatment
   - may take 4-6 weeks for consolidative changes to resolve
   - Radiologic improvement usually lags behind clinical improvement
   - If radiologic signs still present after adequate treatment, underlying predisposing factors have to be excluded (e.g. central obstructive carcinoma in elderly patients)

Note:
(1) Diagnosis of pneumonia is based on a combination of clinical and radiological findings.
(2) Radiological finding of air-space opacity with ill-defined borders and air-bronchogram in the appropriate clinical setting helps to make the diagnosis.

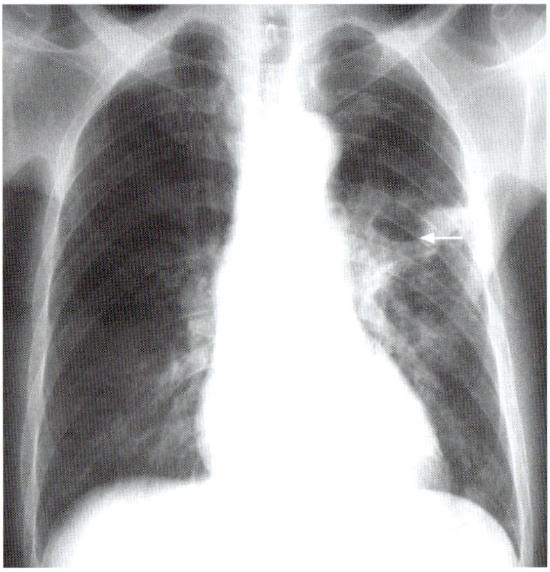

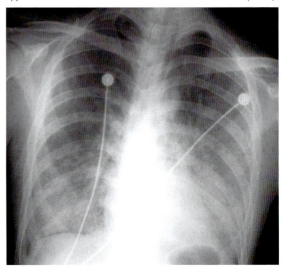

Fig.1d Frontal radiograph of a patient with pulmonary TB with left upper lobe consolidation and cavitation within the lesion (arrow).

Fig.1e An immune-compromised patient with pneumocystis carinii pneumonia (PCP), typically showing bilateral symmetrical perihilar air space opacification which progresses rapidly to involve the entire lung.

Discussion Case 2
Lung collapse

Lung collapse (Fig. 2a)

- The lack of air within collapsed right upper lobe accounts for the increase in radiographic density. The well-demarcated lateral border represents the elevated horizontal fissure.
- The focal bulge at the apex of the collapsed right upper lobe corresponds to the centrally located bronchogenic carcinoma causing the lobar collapse. The combined radiologic appearance on frontal radiograph is known as 'Golden S sign'.
- The hyperinflation and elevated right hemidiaphragm are due to volume loss.

Discussion

- *Other radiologic features of right upper lobe collapse not seen on this chest radiograph include:*
    1. Crowding of ribs in right upper chest wall – due to underlying lung volume loss
    2. Tracheal deviation to the right – due to traction from the collapsed lung
- Lobar collapse in different lobes gives characteristic radiographic appearances on frontal and lateral radiographs (Fig. 2b, c, d).
- In general, lobar collapse represents obstruction to the corresponding lobar bronchus. The underlying etiology may be classified as:
    1. Intraluminal obstruction (e.g. mucus plug / foreign body)
    2. Intramural obstruction (e.g. bronchogenic carcinoma)
    3. Extramural obstruction (e.g. extrinsic compression by enlarged hilar lymph nodes)
- Recognition of lobar collapse is important, especially in elderly patients, as this may be the only radiologic feature of primary lung carcinoma. Further evaluation by sputum cytology, bronchoscopy or CT scan is necessary.

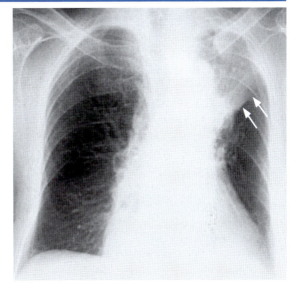

Fig.2b *Left upper lobe collapse. Note the left upper zone opacity (arrows) and signs of volume loss including ipsilateral mediastinal shift.*

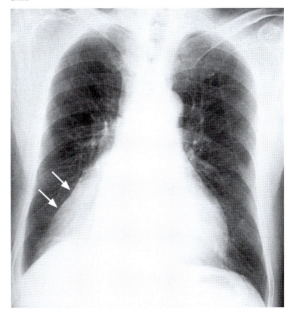

Fig.2c *Right lower lobe collapse – triangular shaped opacity in the medial right lower zone (arrows) with signs of volume loss. Note the right heart border is still seen suggesting it is not a right middle lobe disease.*

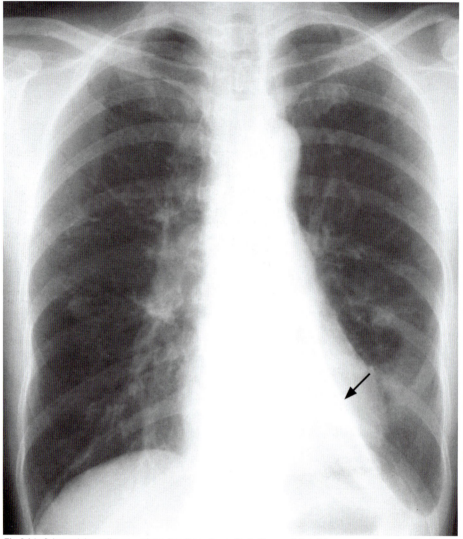

Fig.2d *Left lower lobe collapse - triangular shaped opacity in the medial left lower zone (arrow) with signs of volume loss.*

Note:
(1) Collapse of different lobes produce characteristic radiological appearances.
(2) Search for underlying aetiology causing persistent lobar collapse, especially in elderly patients, is necessary.

Discussion Case 3
Pneumothorax

Pneumothorax (Fig. 3a)
The absence of vascular markings in the periphery of the left hemithorax is due to air in the pleural cavity and not in the lung.

Discussion

- Pneumothorax represents abnormal air accumulation within pleural cavity. This may be due to trauma (accidental or iatrogenic) (Fig. 3b), underlying pulmonary disease (e.g. asthma) or idiopathic in origin
- Erect chest radiograph in full expiration is diagnostic in majority of cases
- If the patient is unable to stand erect, lateral decubitus view may be helpful for diagnosis
- Note *the radiological features of tension pneumothorax* seen in this patient include:
  1. Contralateral mediastinal shift
  2. Depression of ipsilateral hemi-diaphragm
  3. Compressive atelectasis of adjacent normal lung
- All of the above radiological signs indicate the presence of significant increased intra-thoracic pressure in tension pneumothorax which necessitates urgent treatment
- Role of imaging in patients with pneumothorax:
  1. Confirm the clinical diagnosis
  2. Assess extent of pneumothorax
  3. Detect signs of tension pneumothorax
  4. Follow-up examination to monitor resolution of pneumothorax after drainage

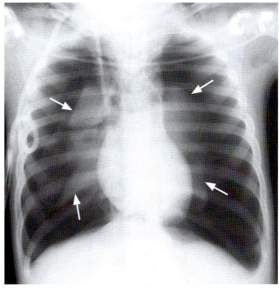

Fig.3b *Bilateral tension pneumothorax due to barotrauma from positive pressure ventilation. Note the flattening of the diaphragm. The presence of bilateral abnormality results in no mediastinal shift. Note the collapsed lungs (arrows) and bilateral hyperlucency.*

Note:

(1) The diagnosis of pneumothorax is confirmed by erect chest radiograph in full expiration.

(2) Signs of tension pneumothorax should be specifically looked for as it is potentially life-threatening and requires urgent treatment.

Discussion Case 4
Pneumomediastinum

Pneumomediastinum (Fig. 4a)
- Which is most likely due to recent oesophageal perforation by fish bone

Discussion:
- Other radiological *findings of pneumomediastinum not seen* in this patient include:
  1. Continuous diaphragm sign – continuous radiolucency connecting both sides of diaphragm (Fig. 4b)
  2. V-sign of Naclerio – air between lower thoracic aorta and diaphragm
- Air may leak into mediastinum via:
  1. Perforation of any air-containing viscus
     - Pharynx/oesophagus (e.g. due to foreign body ingestion, instrumentation etc.)
     - Leak from major or small intrapulmonary airways (e.g. asthma, excessive coughing etc.)
  2. Penetrating thoracic trauma with introduction of air from an external environment
- Water soluble contrast swallow may help to confirm the presence of oesophageal perforation
- CT is more sensitive in detecting small pneumomediastinum (Fig. 4c, d)
- CT thorax detects associated complications such as mediastinitis/mediastinal abscess (Fig. 4d)

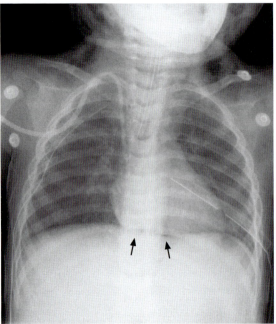

Fig.4b *The 'continuous diaphragm sign (arrows)' of pneumomediastinum.*

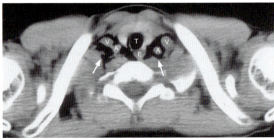

Fig.4c *Axial NECT through the root of the thoracic inlet shows gas (arrows) insinuating between the neck vessels. T=trachea, A=common carotid artery, V=jugular vein, E=oesophagus.*

Pneumomediastinum

Note:
(1) Abnormal air lucency outlining left heart border and aortic knuckle with elevation of mediastinal pleura are suggestive of pneumomediastinum.

(2) Presence of pneumomediastinum warrants careful search for the underlying cause.

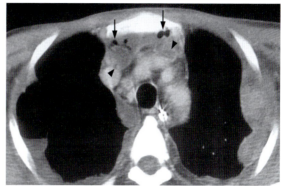

Fig.4d *Contrast enhanced axial CT thorax showing mediastinal abscess formation. Note the presence of air locules (arrows) and rim enhancing abscess cavities (arrowheads) in the mediastinum.*

Discussion Case 5
Primary lung carcinoma

Primary lung carcinoma (Fig. 5a)
- The irregular border is suggestive of an infiltrating lesion.
- The bulging right hilum represents enlarged hilar lymph nodes due to metastatic involvement.
- Thickened paratracheal stripe indicates enlarged right paratracheal lymphadenopathy.

Discussion
- Other possible *radiological features of lung carcinoma not seen in this patient include*:
  1. Bony erosion – due to haematogenous metastases to bone
  2. Pleural effusion – due to lymphatic obstruction by primary tumour or tumour involvement of the pleura
  3. Lobar collapse – due to obstruction by primary tumour or enlarged hilar lymph nodes
  4. Cavitation – indicating tumour necrosis, most common in squamous cell carcinoma
- If a lung mass is identified on chest radiograph, the following features may help to differentiate malignant tumour from benign lesion (such as granuloma):
  1. Margin – spiculated border is more suspicious of malignancy
  2. Intra-lesional calcification – presence of coarse calcification favours benign lesion
  3. Size – large lesion is suspicious of malignancy
  4. Any associated lymphadenopathy (hilar/mediastinal) and bony erosion – suggests metastatic involvement by malignant lung tumour
- Further evaluation aims at confirmation of diagnosis and determination of cell type (sputum cytology/bronchoscopy/imaging-guided fine needle aspiration) and tumour staging (CT thorax including adrenal glands, bone scintigraphy etc)
- The usual diagnostic protocol for suspected Ca lung or suspicious solitary pulmonary nodule on CXR

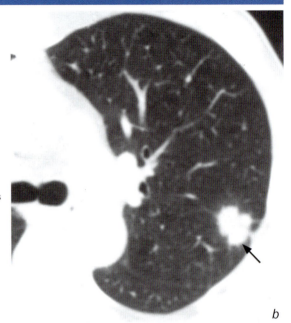

b

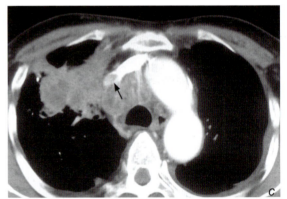

c

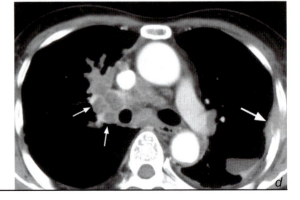

d

Primary lung carcinoma

CXR
⇓
CT
- solitary
- multiple
⇓
bronchoscopy (central lesion)/
imaging-guided FNAC (peripheral
lesion)

- CT is helpful in assessing solitary
  pulmonary nodule seen on CXR
  1. Margins are better defined on CT
     and a spiculated margin (Fig. 5b)
     favours primary lung carcinoma
  2. Cavitation is better seen on CT
  3. Number of lesions are better
     evaluated by CT – multiple lesions
     favour lung metastases rather than
     primary lung carcinoma.
  4. Location – may help in deciding
     the approach for biopsy (i.e.
     bronchoscopy/imaging guided
     FNAC)
  5. Lymphadenopathy – enlarged hilar/
     mediastinal lymph nodes are better
     seen on CT and suggest metastatic
     nodal involvement (Fig. 5c, d).
  6. Liver/adrenal/bone status is better
     seen on CT and any suspicious focal
     lesion may indicate haematogenous
     tumour metastases (Fig. 5e, f).
- Role of imaging in suspected Ca lung
  1. Evaluate the nature (benign/
     malignant) of the pulmonary lesion
  2. Tumour staging (primary tumour,
     nodal status and distant metastases)

Note:
(1) Presence of spiculated
    lung mass on CXR in an
    elderly chronic smoker is
    highly suspicious of
    primary lung carcinoma.
(2) Radiological features
    which help differentiate
    benign and malignant
    mass should be borne in
    mind.

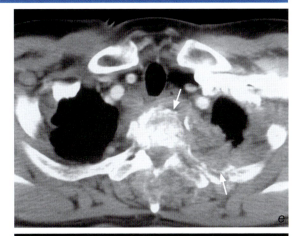

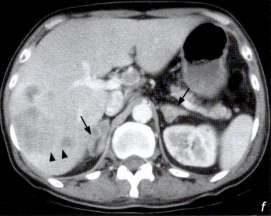

Fig.5b Axial CT of the lung showing a left pulmonary nodule (arrow) with spiculated margins indicating its infiltrative malignant nature.

Fig.5c Contrast enhanced axial CT thorax showing the right lobe tumour together with paratracheal lymphadenopathy. There is tumour which has invaded into the superior vena cava (arrow) i.e. tumour thrombus. Same patient as in Fig.5a.

Fig.5d Contrast enhanced axial CT thorax showing hilar, precarinal and subcarinal metastatic lymphadenopathy (small arrows). Note the left chest wall metastatic deposit near the mid axillary line (large arrow). Same patient as in Fig.5a.

Fig.5e Contrast enhanced axial CT thorax showing metastatic involvement of the upper thoracic vertebra and the adjacent rib (arrows).

Fig.5f Contrast enhanced axial CT of the abdomen showing liver (arrowheads) and bilateral adrenal metastases (arrows).

01 CHEST

Discussion Case 6
Pancoast tumour

Pancoast tumour (Fig. 6a)

Discussion

- Pancoast tumour is a primary lung carcinoma located at lung apices. Because of its close proximity to the adjacent first rib, brachial plexus and sympathetic trunk, these are involved by local tumour infiltration early in the course of the disease producing characteristic clinical signs
- Early case of Pancoast tumour is difficult to detect radiologically, particularly on a CXR as there may be only focal apical pleural thickening instead of apparent mass. Hence detection of subtle bony destruction of adjacent 1st rib is important.
- A lordotic view improves visualization of the apices (Fig. 6b)
- A CT offers better visualization of a suspected lesion in lung apex (Fig. 6c).
- In patients with clinical symptoms and signs of brachial plexus and sympathetic nervous involvement, MRI clearly delineates local tumour infiltration.

Note:
(1) The presence of apical chest pain and ipsilateral Horner's syndrome raise the suspicion of Pancoast tumour.
(2) Apical lung mass with adjacent rib erosion on CXR suggests the diagnosis.

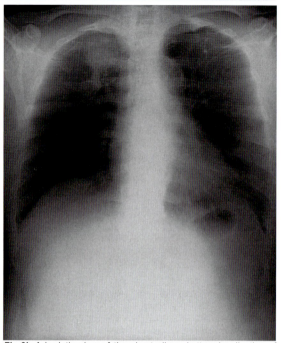

Fig.6b *A lordotic view of the chest allows better visualization of the lung apices as the overlying clavicles are moved out of the way (Courtesy of Dr Esther Hung, Department of Diagnostic Radiology & Organ Imaging, PWH, Hong Kong).*

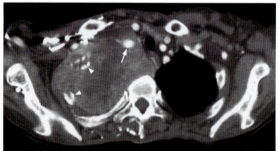

Fig.6c *Same patient as in Fig. 6a. Axial contrast-enhanced CT showing a large mass with has infiltrated and wrapped around the adjacent ribs (arrowheads). The trachea is pushed to left side. The tumour wraps around the right subclavian vein (arrow).*

Discussion Case 7
Pulmonary metastases

Discussion

- Lung is a common site for haematogenous metastases from primary malignant tumours.
- Other *radiological features of pulmonary metastases not seen in this patient* include:
  1. Cavitating lung lesions common in metastases from squamous cell carcinoma (Fig. 7c, d)
  2. Pleural effusion
  3. Hilar/mediastinal lymph node enlargement
  4. Metastatic bony erosion

Two main radiological features to differentiate pulmonary metastases from primary lung carcinoma:

  1. Number of lesions – pulmonary metastases are more likely in the presence of bilateral and multiple lesions
  2. Margin characteristics – spiculated border points to primary lung carcinoma while pulmonary metastases are usually rounded with a smooth well-defined border

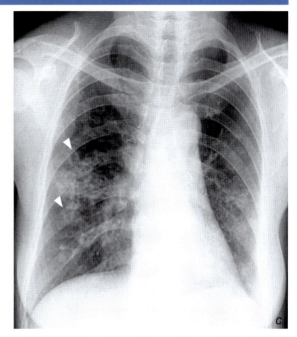

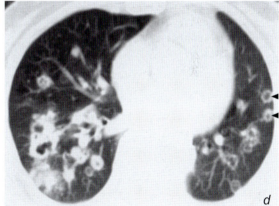

Fig.7c,d *Frontal chest radiograph and axial CT thorax showing squamous cell carcinoma metastases with cavitation (arrowheads).*

Discussion Case 7
Pulmonary metastases

- CT thorax is more sensitive than plain radiograph for early detection of pulmonary metastases. Various appearances of metastases may be seen on CT and these include: 'cannon ball' appearances (Fig. 7a, b), cavitating (Fig. 7c, d), calcifying (from primary osteosarcoma) and miliary (diffuse tiny pulmonary nodules due to haematogenous spread) from papillary carcinoma of the thyroid (Fig. 7e, f)
- The presence of pulmonary metastases usually indicates widespread tumour dissemination.

Note:
(1) Multiple round lung lesions in a patient with known malignancy most likely represents pulmonary metastases.
(2) CT thorax is more sensitive in detection of small pulmonary metastases.

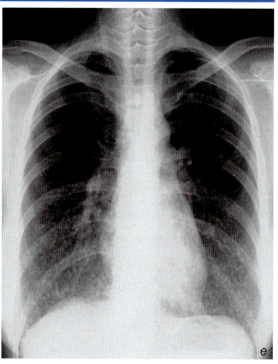

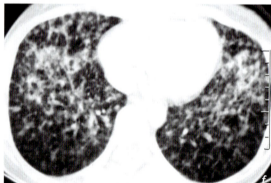

Fig.7e,f Frontal chest radiograph and axial CT thorax showing multiple, small, soft tissue nodules in both lung fields. This patient had a history of papillary carcinoma and the lung nodules represent miliary metastases.

Pleural effusion

Pleural effusion (Fig. 8a)
The complete opacification of the right mid and lower zones is due to fluid in the pleural cavity. Note the meniscus sign, i.e. concavity of the fluid level due to surface tension with the pleura. It is an underlying pneumonia which usually gives rise to para-pneumonic pleural effusion. The pneumonia is often not seen on the CXR as it is obscured by the large amount of pleural effusion

Discussion

- Blunting of costophrenic angle may be due to a small pleural effusion or focal pleural thickening. If it is present on a previous CXR and remains unchanged over a considerable period of time, pleural thickening is more likely.
- Pleural effusion may coexist with pneumothorax (i.e. hydropneumothorax, Fig. 8b) or entrapped within fissures mimicking a tumour.
- If the patient cannot stand, a lateral decubitus CXR is sometimes performed to help in the diagnosis of pleural effusion (as the fluid layers out in the dependent position, Fig. 8c).
- Ultrasound or CT thorax serve as alternative modalities for early detection of small pleural effusion. Ultrasound has the advantage of not involving radiation, and can be used to guide drainage. CT has the advantage of evaluating the underlying lung and mediastinal structures to identify the cause of the effusion.

> ## Note:
> (1) Blunting of costophrenic angle with meniscus sign signifies the presence of pleural effusion.
> (2) Lateral decubitus film, ultrasound or CT thorax helps to detect a small pleural effusion.

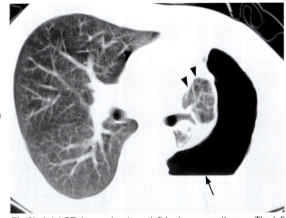

Fig.8b *Axial CT thorax showing a left hydropneumothorax. The left lung is almost completely collapsed (arrowheads). Note the air-fluid level (arrow) and the volume loss of the left hemithorax.*

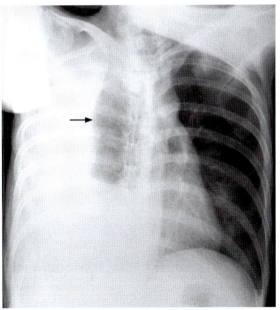

Fig.8c *Lateral decubitus chest radiograph reveals layering of the pleural fluid (arrow) in the dependent portion of the pleural space.*

Discussion Case 9
Empyema

Empyema (Fig. 9a)

CXR shows the presence of a large right pleural effusion with contralateral mediastinal shift. In a septic patient, empyema has to be considered and CT is the best modality to assess the extent of empyema and its mass effect.

On the contrast CT (Fig. 9b) note:

- Fluid collection in the pleural space representing pus accumulation
- Peripheral thick rim enhancement due to hyperaemia within the wall of the empyema
- Note the presence of pleural effusion on the left side. There is no peripheral contrast enhancement within this collection suggesting it is a simple pleural effusion.

Discussion

- Pleural aspiration under clinical or imaging guidance for microscopy and culture allows a definitive diagnosis of empyema and helps to guide appropriate antibiotic treatment.
- For an empyema not responsive to medical treatment drainage may be necessary. In these circumstances, contrast CT plays an important role in mapping the exact extent of pus collection within the pleural cavity.

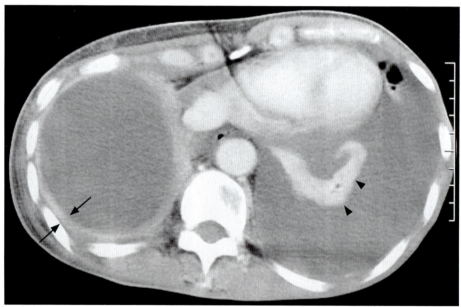

Fig.9b *Contrast enhanced axial CT thorax showing bilateral pleural collections. Note the thick peripheral rim enhancement (arrows) of the empyema on the right and the absence of such a thick rim on the left uncomplicated pleural effusion. Note the collapsed left lung (arrowheads).*

> **Note:**
> (1) The presence of pleural effusion with mass effect in a septic patient should raise the suspicion of empyema.
> (2) Contrast enhanced CT thorax is the imaging modality of choice for assessing the extent of involvement and to provide supporting evidence of active inflammation within pleural spaces.
> (3) Aspiration of pleural fluid clinically or under imaging guidance confirms the diagnosis and helps to institute the appropriate antibiotic treatment.

Lung abscess

Lung abscess (Fig. 10a, b)
The air-fluid level within the lesion is due to accumulation of pus in the dependent part and air in the non-dependent portion. The thick walls are due to inflammatory reaction due to the inciting organism and adjacent air space opacification reflects pneumonic changes in the lung.

Discussion

- In the presence of cavitating lung lesion on CXR, the two main differential diagnoses are lung abscess and cavitating lung tumour (either primary or secondary tumour). The imaging appearances on CXR and CT thorax can be similar and clinical information (e.g. history of known malignancy, clinical evidence of sepsis) are clues towards the final diagnosis.
- Bronchoscopy or imaging-guided aspiration may be necessary to differentiate the two conditions.
- An air-fluid level is sometimes seen in a hiatus hernia reflecting stomach (herniated) contents This classically occurs behind the cardiac silhouette (Fig. 10c, d).

Note:

(1) Thick-walled cavitating lung lesion with air-fluid level, are radiological features of lung abscess. However, cavitating malignancies will also have a similar appearance.

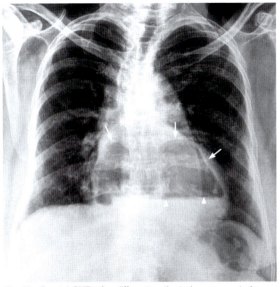

Fig.10c *Frontal CXR of a different patient shows a central mass (arrows) above the diaphragm. An air-fluid level is present within it (arrowheads).*

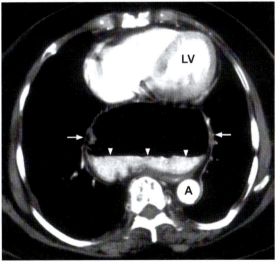

Fig.10d *Axial CECT of the same patient in Fig.10c shows an air-fluid (air-contrast) level (arrowheads) within a herniated stomach (arrows). LV=Left ventricle, A=descending aorta.*

01 CHEST

Post-primary pulmonary tuberculosis

Pulmonary tuberculosis (Fig. 11a)
The cavitation and air-fluid level within
the opacity represents caseous necrosis in
tuberculosis. The involvement of the apex
is a clue towards the diagnosis of TB as
post-primary TB has a predilection for
the lung apex

Discussion

- Other *radiological findings of
  pulmonary TB not seen in this
  patient* include:
  1. Enlarged hilum – representing
     granulomatous inflammation of
     lymph nodes, usually in primary
     TB
  2. Fibrocalcific changes in lung
     apex (Fig.11b) usually
     representing healing of previous
     TB infection
  3. Multi-focal air-space opacities
     representing bronchogenic spread
     of infection (Fig. 11c)
  4. Tiny miliary nodules in both
     lungs (Fig. 11d, e) representing
     miliary TB due to haematogenous
     spread of infection
- Radiological manifestation depends
  on whether the patient had
  previous PTB infection (post-
  primary TB) or not (primary TB)

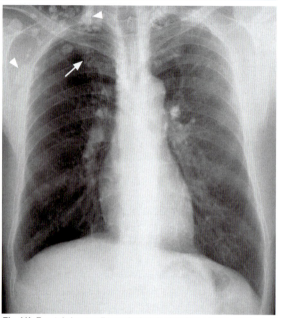

Fig.11b *Frontal chest radiograph showing haziness in the right apical region representing fibrocalcific changes from previous TB (arrow). Note the multiple calcified lymph nodes in both supraclavicular fossae and right axilla (arrowheads).*

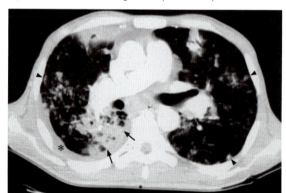

Fig.11c *Axial CT (lung window settings) shows multiple opacities (arrowheads) from bronchogenic spread of TB. This has evolved into consolidation (arrows) in the right lower lobe. A thin pleural effusion is present (asterisk).*

Post-primary pulmonary tuberculosis

Note:

(1) Radiological manifestations are different for each type including primary TB (hilar lymph node involvement), post-primary TB (predilection for lung apex) and miliary TB (small miliary nodules in both lungs).

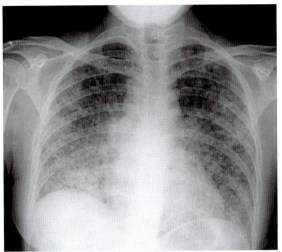

Fig.11d *Frontal chest radiograph showing miliary tuberculosis. Note the innumerable tiny nodules seen throughout both lungs.*

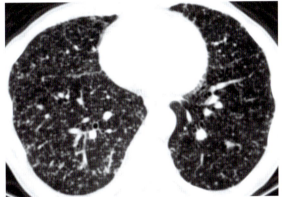

Fig.11e *Axial CT thorax showing miliary tuberculosis as multiple tiny nodules scattered throughout the lung (Courtesy of Dr Patrick Tam, Department of Diagnostic Radiology & Organ Imaging, PWH, Hong Kong).*

Discussion Case 12
Cystic bronchiectasis

Cystic bronchiectasis (Fig. 12a)
The air-fluid levels within the cystic spaces
represent retained secretions within the
dilated bronchioles.

A CT scan (Fig. 12b) was performed as
it better assesses the extent and severity of
the disease. It showed:

- String of cysts appearance
  representing cystic dilatation of
  bronchioles
- Thickening of bronchial wall
  indicating on-going inflammatory
  change
- Air-fluid level representing retained
  bronchial secretions

Discussion

- Majority of bronchiectasis occurs
  peripherally in lower lobes.
  Unusual sites of involvement raise
  the suspicion of certain aetiologies
  of bronchiectasis, e.g. upper zone
  predominance in cystic fibrosis,
  proximal central zone involvement
  in allergic bronchopulmonary
  aspergillosis.
- In the past bronchogram was
  regarded as the gold standard for
  diagnosis by demonstrating
  dilated bronchioles outlined by
  contrast. However, it has been
  replaced by CT as it offers a non-
  invasive method for diagnosis.
- Radiological signs on CT of less
  severe form of bronchiectasis
  include
  1. 'Tram-track' sign (Fig. 12c) due
     to dilated bronchioles with its
     accompanying vessel
  2. 'Signet-ring' sign (Fig. 12d)
     representing dilated bronchiole
     closely related to its adjacent
     vessel
- Role of radiology in bronchiectasis
  includes
  1. Confirm the diagnosis and assess
     the extent of pulmonary
     involvement
  2. Detect complications such as
     pneumonia, lung abscess,
     fibrosis.

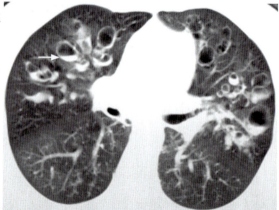

Fig.12b Axial CT thorax showing cystic bronchiectasis. Note the
air-fluid levels (arrows) within the dilated bronchioles

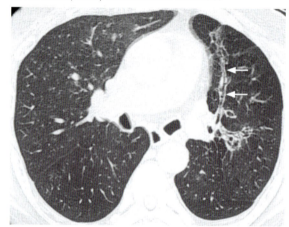

Fig.12c Axial CT thorax showing the 'tram-track' sign (arrows)
of bronchiectasis in the anterior segment of the left upper lobe.

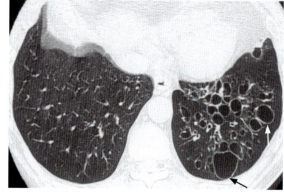

Fig.12d CT thorax showing the 'signet-ring' sign (arrows) of
bronchiectasis in the left lower lobe.

Cystic bronchiectasis

- Patients with previous plombage (Fig. 12e) may demonstrate multiple air-fluid level and should not be mistaken for cystic bronchiectasis.

> **Note:**
> (1) Abnormal dilatation of bronchioles on imaging confirms the diagnosis of bronchiectasis.
> (2) CT thorax is the imaging modality of choice for diagnosis and to demonstrate the extent and severity of the disease.

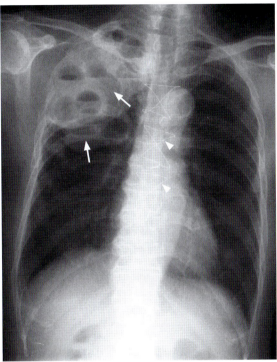

Fig.12e *Plain x-ray showing multiple air-fluid level (arrows) in the right apex. This patient has undergone plombage for treatment of TB and should not be mistaken for cystic bronchiectasis. Note the midline sutures (arrowheads) indicating previous surgery (Image courtesy of Dr Grace Au, Department of Diagnostic Radiology and Organ Imaging, The Chinese University of Hong Kong).*

01 CHEST

Chronic obstructive airways disease

Chronic obstructive airways disease
(Fig. 13a)

Discussion

- Other *radiological features of COAD not seen in this patient* include:
  1. Right heart enlargement which indicates raised pulmonary arterial pressure
  2. Prominent pulmonary vascularity with peripheral pruning due to pulmonary arterial hypertension
  3. Bullae which are seen as round thin-walled lucent lesions devoid of vasculature.

- Hyperinflated lungs are also seen in patients with asthma. The episodic nature and absence of history of chronic smoking may help to differentiate it from COAD
- Role of radiology in patients with chronic obstructive airway disease:
  1. To detect complications, e.g. cor pulmonale, pneumothorax (Fig. 13b)
  2. To detect infective component in case of acute exacerbation

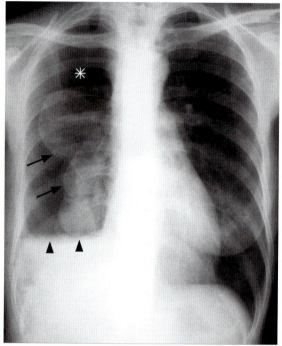

Fig.13b COAD complicated by right hydropneumothorax. Note the collapsed right lung (arrows) and the air-fluid level (arrowheads), and the hyperlucency of pneumothorax (asterisk).

Note:
(1) Chronic obstructive airway disease occurs commonly in chronic heavy smokers with chronic respiratory symptoms.
(2) Hyperinflated lungs is the characteristic radiological feature.

Lymphoma

Lymphoma (Fig. 14a, b)

Discussion

- Other *CT findings of lymphoma not seen in this patient* include:
    1. Soft tissue pulmonary nodule indicating tumour involvement of the lung parenchyma
    2. Pulmonary air-space opacities, another radiological manifestation of tumour infiltration
    3. Pleural effusion

- Common causes for hilar and mediastinal lymph node enlargement include
    1. Lymphoma, especially in young patients
    2. Metastatic disease, patients usually have known history of underlying malignancy (Fig. 14c, d)
    3. Infection such as tuberculosis, usually with lung parenchymal changes in addition to hilar/mediastinal lymphadenopathy
    4. Sarcoidosis, relatively rare in Asians

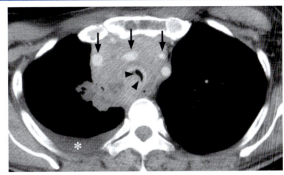

Fig.14c *Axial CECT image through the upper thorax of a patient with mediastinal metastatic disease (squamous cell carcinoma of the skin). The metastatic deposits (most likely in lymph nodes) have widened the mediastinum, splayed the great vessels (arrows) and compressed the lower trachea (arrowheads). The tracheal lumen has been reduced to a slit and liable to obstruction by further compression or even by thick mucus. There is an associated right pleural effusion present (asterisk).*

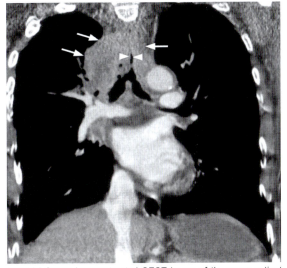

Fig.14d *Coronal reconstructed CECT image of the same patient in Fig. 14c. The mediastinal involvement (arrows) and the tracheal compression (arrowheads) are well demonstrated.*

Discussion Case 14
Lymphoma

- Aside from lymphadenopathy, there are other causes for mediastinal and hilar masses (Fig. 14e, f, g)
- In lymphoma the role of imaging is to assess the extent of disease and in follow-up examinations to evaluate treatment response.

Fig.14e Frontal CXR of a 43- year -old female atient showing an extra 'bulge' (arrow) below the left pulmonary trunk. Note the separate silhouette of the left hilum (arrowheads) meaning that this lesion is not in contact with the left hilum (the 'hilar overlay' sign).

Fig.14f Axial CECT of the same patient in Fig. 14e shows a fluid density lesion (asterisk) wrapped around the root of the pulmonary trunk (P). This is consistent with a pericardial cyst. A=aorta.

Fig.14g Axial T2W MRI of the same patient in Fig.14e shows homogeneous high (fluid) signal within this pericardial cyst (asterisk). p=pulmonary trunk, A=aorta.

Note:
(1) Diagnosis of lymphoma is mainly based on clinical presentation and histology of excised lymph node.
(2) Contrast enhanced CT thorax is the imaging modality of choice to assess extent of intra-thoracic involvement. CT can also help in staging the disease and assessing response to treatment.
(3) Hilar and mediastinal lymphadenopathy are the most common manifestations of intra-thoracic lymphoma.

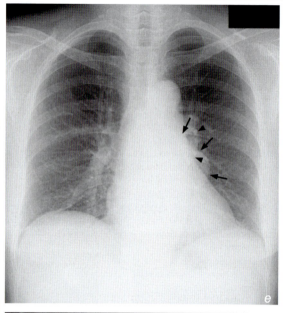

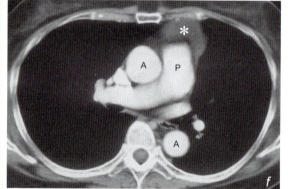

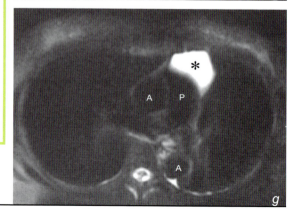

Silicosis

Silicosis (Fig. 15)
The small dense nodular opacities represent inhaled silicone particles with local fibrotic reaction.

Discussion
- Silicosis is an occupational lung disease caused by inhalation of silicone particles
- There is usually a latent period of ~10-20 years before clinical symptoms occur
- Other *radiological findings of silicosis not seen in this patient* include:
  1. Progressive massive fibrosis seen as conglomerate masses in both upper lobes due to coalescence of   nearby inflammatory nodules in advanced stage
  2. Reduction in lung volume due to progressive lung fibrosis
- Apart from diagnosis of silicosis, chest radiograph also helps to detect complications including cor pulmonale, pneumothorax and pulmonary TB
- The differential diagnosis for multiple small pulmonary nodular opacities on CXR include:
  1. Miliary TB – patient is clinically septic and unwell
  2. Miliary metastases – background history of underlying malignancy
  3. Atypical infection (e.g. viral infection)
  4. Extrinsic allergic alveolitis
- Clinical information, particularly relevant occupational history, helps to make the correct diagnosis.

> ## Note:
> (1) Multiple small nodular opacities in both lungs with egg-shell calcification of hilar lymph nodes are characteristic radiological findings of silicosis.

Discussion Case 16
Pulmonary embolism

Pulmonary embolism (Fig. 16a, b)

Discussion

- CXR is usually normal in cases of pulmonary embolism. Radiological signs which may be seen include:
  1. Enlarged pulmonary artery proximal to the obstructed segment - Hampton's hump
  2. Regional oligaemia due to decreased blood supply (Fig. 16c)
  3. Peripheral segmental consolidation due to pulmonary infarction.
- Diagnosis by ventilation-perfusion (V/Q) scan is based on finding of multiple segmental areas of ventilation-perfusion mismatch (i.e. perfusion defects with no corresponding ventilation defects) (Fig. 16d)
- CT pulmonary angiogram is currently the non-invasive imaging modality of choice for diagnosis. Multiple intra-luminal filling defects within pulmonary arteries are diagnostic

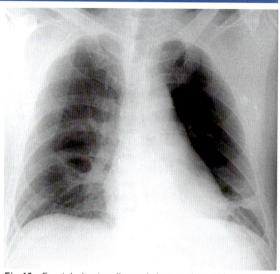

Fig.16c Frontal chest radiograph in a patient with pulmonary embolism showing regional oligaemia at the left upper and mid zones due to emboli restricting the blood supply. Compare it with the vascular markings on the right.

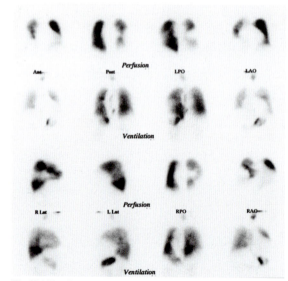

Fig.16d Ventilation-perfusion (V/Q) scan showing multiple perfusion defects without corresponding ventilation defects in a patient suffering from pulmonary embolism.

Pulmonary embolism

- In the past conventional pulmonary angiogram was regarded as the gold standard for diagnosis. However, it is invasive and carries significant morbidity and mortality. CT pulmonary angiogram is able to delineate pulmonary vessels clearly and has largely replaced conventional angiograms in the diagnosis of pulmonary embolism (Fig. 16e)

Note:

(1) In patients with pulmonary embolism a CXR is often unremarkable. It is used as a screening test to rule out other pathology such as a pneumothorax, pneumonia, neoplasm etc. A ventilation / perfusion scintigraphy or CT pulmonary angiogram is used to confirm the diagnosis.

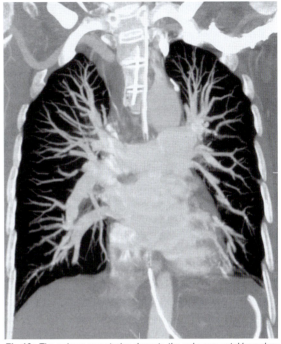

Fig.16e *The pulmonary arteries down to the subsegmental branches can be well demonstrated on CT pulmonary angiogram.*

Discussion Case 17
Re-expansion pulmonary oedema

Discussion

Re-expansion pulmonary oedema:

- May occur when there is rapid re-expansion of a collapsed lung after draining a large pneumothorax or pleural effusion.
- The larger the pneumothorax/hydrothorax, the longer it has been there, and the quicker it has been evacuated, the more likely re-expansion pulmonary oedema will occur.
- Pleural fluid/pneumothorax should therefore not be rapidly drained to avoid re-expansion pulmonary oedema.
- The underlying mechanism is probably alveolar capillary injury initiated by ischaemia.
- It may be asymptomatic and gradually resolve over 5 to 7 days but occasionally may deteriorate to respiratory failure.

Note:

(1) Re-expansion pulmonary oedema may develop after rapid evacuation of a large pneumothorax/pleural effusion.

Discussion Case 18
Trauma

Discussion
- X-rays of the cervical spine, pelvis, chest are routinely performed in patients with polytrauma.
- Other radiological abnormalities possibly seen in patients with thoracic trauma include:
  1. Traumatic aortic injury seen as widened mediastinum due to a haematoma following aortic tear
  2. Skeletal injury, e.g. fractured ribs, scapula, shoulder dislocation
  3. Cardiac injury rarely diagnosed by CXR
- After intubation, it is important to check the position of the ET tube to ensure satisfactory airway protection and lung ventilation. Examples of malposition include insertion into right main bronchus or into the oesophagus (instead of trachea) (Fig. 18b)
- Careful search for injury to other parts of the body (e.g. intra-abdominal visceral injury, intracranial haemorrhage (Fig. 18c)) is important for prompt appropriate treatment

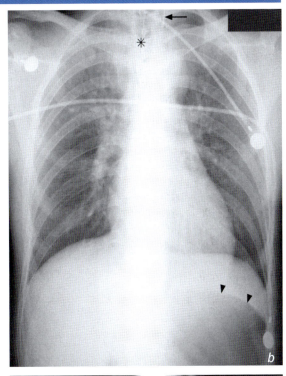

Fig.18b Frontal chest radiograph of a patient soon after intubation. Note that the endotracheal (ET) tube has been inserted into the oesophagus (arrow) and is outside the trachea(*). Attempted ventilation via the malpositioned ET tube has resulted in the large gastric bubble (arrowheads).

Fig.18c Axial CT brain of the same patient showing a depressed fracture (arrowheads), acute right frontal subdural haematoma (small arrow), and right frontal lobe contusion (large arrow).

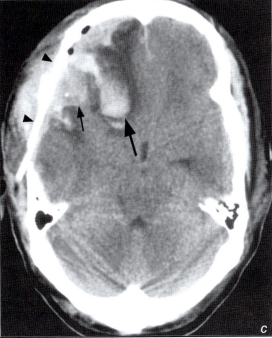

Trauma

- CT is often useful for further evaluation of thoracic trauma if the patient is haemodynamically stable (Fig. 18d, e)

Note:

(1) CXR is useful in initial assessment of intra-thoracic injury in a patient with polytrauma.

(2) Extra-alveolar air (e.g. pneumothorax/ pneumomediastinum/ surgical emphysema), pulmonary contusion and skeletal injury (e.g. rib fracture) are important radiological signs to look for.

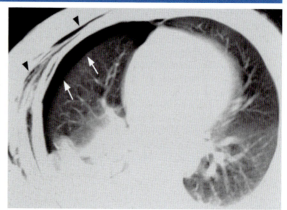

Fig.18d. *Axial CT thorax of the same patient showing the small residual right pneumothorax (arrows) which was difficult to appreciate on radiograph and the surgical emphysema (arrowheads).*

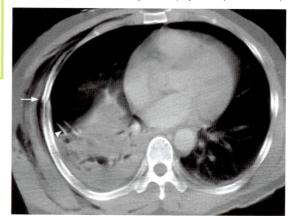

Fig.18e *CT thorax of the same patient showing one of the right rib fracture (arrow) and the right upper zone consolidation. Note the presence of the chest drain (arrowhead).*

Discussion Case 19
Heart failure

Congestive cardiac failure (Fig. 19a) probably secondary to myocardial infarction with the given clinical history.

Discussion

With the development of congestive cardiac failure, left atrial pressure is the first to rise. This causes hydrostatic pressure in the pulmonary capillaries to increase with the formation of interstitial oedema - mainly in the lung bases. This in turn raises the vascular resistance to flow at the lung bases, resulting in shunting of blood to the upper lobe vessels - hence causing upper lobe venous diversion. Upper lobe diversion is diagnosed when, on the erect radiograph, the upper lobe vessels are enlarged to an extent that is equal to or surpasses lower lobe vessels of equal distance from the hilum.

As hydrostatic pressure further increases (to a pulmonary wedge pressure of 18-22 mmHg) the signs of interstitial oedema occur:

- Blurring of the vessel margins
- Peribronchial cuffing
- Perihilar haze
- Kerley A and B lines may be visible when fluid fills and distends the interlobular septa
- Kerley B lines are short horizontal lines which are seen in the periphery of the lung bases
- Kerley A lines which are less frequently seen are lines which radiate from the hilum

As the hydrostatic pressure approaches 25 mmHg, fluid then passes into the alveoli, resulting in pulmonary oedema. This may appear as multiple alveolar densities in the lower half of the lungs. Alternatively, there may be diffuse, poorly defined bilateral airspace densities or 'bat's wings' perihilar densities (Fig. 19b).

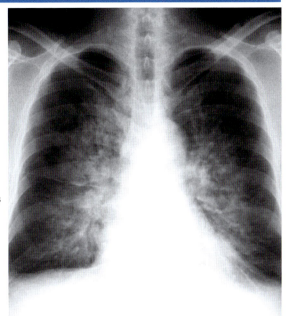

Fig.19b *An example of congestive cardiac failure with perihilar airspace densities in 'bat's wings' distribution representing pulmonary oedema (Image courtesy of Prof. Liu Yuan, Department of Radiology, the First Affiliated Hospital of the Shantou University Medical College).*

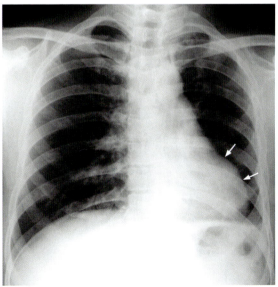

Fig.19c *An example of left ventricular aneurysm shown on chest radiograph, which appears as a focal bulge (arrows) in the left cardiac silhouette (Image courtesy of Radiology Department, KEM Hospital,Mumbai, India).*

Heart failure

The heart size subsequently increases and may be effusion (usually larger on the right).

In the setting of myocardial infarction, it may also be possible to identify the development of left ventricular aneurysms on chest radiographs (Fig. 19c, d).

Note:

(1) Signs of cardiac failure are: cardiomegaly, upper lung venous diversion, pleural effusion.

(2) Progression to pulmonary oedema can be confirmed with : peribronchial cuffing, perihilar haze, Kerley lines, alveolar opacification.

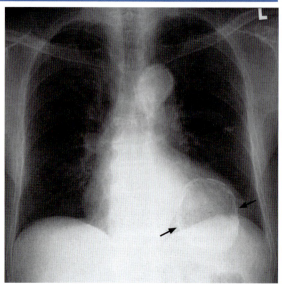

Fig.19d *Frontal radiograph in a patient with previous myocardial infarction. Note the curvilinear calcification (arrows) in a left ventricular aneurysm.*

Mitral stenosis

Mitral stenosis (Fig. 20a) in view of patient's sex, past history of rheumatic heart disease and CXR findings.

Discussion

The most common cause of mitral stenosis is rheumatic heart disease and a history of rheumatic fever may be present in up to 50% of patients with mitral stenosis. A lesion obstructing the left ventricular inflow tract - such as an atrial myxoma or a thrombus - can occasionally cause mitral stenosis.

There is a female predominance - F:M=8:1

Pathophysiology

- Rise in left atrial pressure and subsequent left atrial dilatation. This may lead to atrial fibrillation. Thrombosis of the atrial appendage and thrombus in the left atrium (Fig. 20b) may in turn lead to systemic embolisation (Fig. 20c).
- Rise in pulmonary vascular pressure, medial hypertrophy and intimal sclerosis in pulmonary arterioles leading to pulmonary hypertension

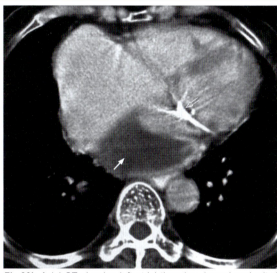

Fig.20b Axial CT showing left atrial thrombus (arrow) and mitral valve leaflet calicification (open arrow). (Image courtesy of Radiology Department, KEM Hospital,Mumbai, India).

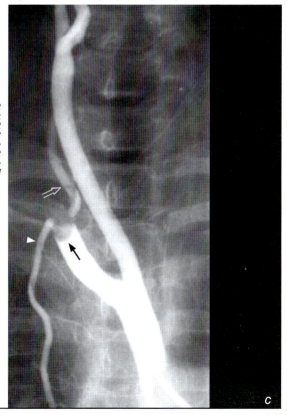

Fig.20c Systemic embolisation to right subclavian artery. Right brachiocephalic trunk angiogram showing a filling defect consistent with an embolus (arrow) in the proximal right subclavian artery around the origin of the right vertebral artery (open arrow) and right internal mammary artery (arrowhead) (Image courtesy of Radiology Department, KEM Hospital,Mumbai, India).

Discussion Case 20
Mitral stenosis

- Right ventricular hypertrophy leading to tricuspid regurgitation, RV dilatation and subsequently right heart failure (Fig. 20d).

Four stages are recognised in mitral stenosis depending on the degree of pulmonary venous hypertension which may be seen on chest radiograph. The findings on CXR range from redistribution of vessels, interstitial and alveolar oedema to haemosiderin deposition and ossification.

The following radiological signs may be seen in mitral stenosis:

Calcification of the mitral valve leaflets (Fig. 20b)
- Prominent pulmonary artery
- Enlarged left atrium (with or without calcification)
- Dilated left atrial appendage
- Right ventricular hypertrophy
- Dilatation of the right ventricle (with associated tricuspid incompetence and pulmonary hypertension) leading to increase in the cardiothoracic ratio
- Displacement of the oesophagus towards the right and posteriorly. This is best seen with the help of a bolus of barium to outline the oesophagus (Fig. 20e, f)

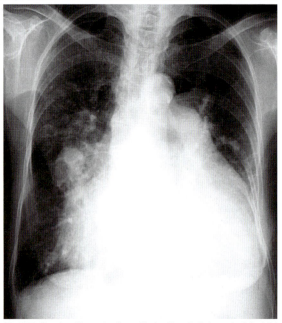

Fig.20d Chest radiograph of a patient with mitral stenosis, left atrial enlargement, pulmonary hypertension, tricuspid regurgitation and right ventricular failure. Note the marked increase in cardiothoracic ratio which is largely due to dilatation of the failing RV.

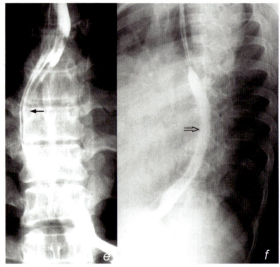

Fig.20e,f Atrial enlargement demonstrated on a barium swallow examination showing deviation of the oesophagus to right (Fig. 20e, arrow) and posteriorly (Fig.20f, open arrow) (Images courtesy of Radiology Department, KEM Hospital,Mumbai, India).

Mitral stenosis

Treatment

Apart from systemic anticoagulation to reduce the risk of thrombus formation in the dilated left atrium, treatment of symptomatic mitral stenosis is primarily surgical - mitral valvotomy or mitral valve replacement (Fig. 20g, h) may be required.

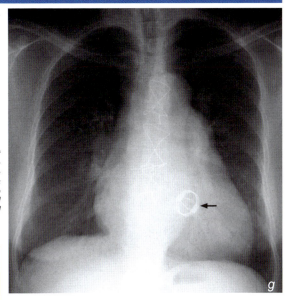

Fig.20g,h Mitral valve replacement. Fig. 20g, h show frontal and lateral chest radiographs of a patient after mitral valve replacement. Note the position of the prosthetic mitral valve (arrows) which is inferior to a line connecting the carina to the anterior costophrenic angle (on a lateral CXR). The aortic valve lies above and anterior to this line.

Note:

(1) Right aterial dilatation (bulging atrial appendage, double atrial contour) in a patient with previous rheumatic heart disease should raise the suspicion of mitral valve disease.

(2) Signs of pulmonary venous hypertension (from mitral stenosis) should be looked for: enlarged pulmonary artery, interstitial/alveolar oedema or calcification/ossification.

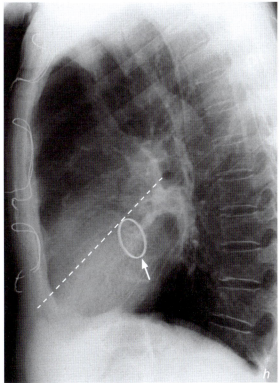

01 CHEST

Tetralogy of Fallot

Tetralogy of Fallot (Fig. 21a)

Discussion:
Tetralogy of Fallot accounts for approximately 8% of all congenital heart disease and is the most common CHD with cyanosis in a child after one year of age. The condition is characterised by:
1. Obstruction to the pulmonary outflow tract usually by pulmonary infundibulum stenosis - occasionally by pulmonary valvular stenosis.
2. Right ventricular hypertrophy resulting from the pulmonary outflow tract obstruction
3. Ventricular septal defect
4. An overriding aorta - the aorta overrides the interventricular septum

Pathophysiology
In fetal life, the pulmonary circulation is filled in a retrograde fashion via the ductus arteriosus and thus RV hypertrophy does not develop. After birth, with closure of the ductus arteriosus, a R to L shunt develops via the VSD, resulting in cyanosis. Pressure overload and RV hypertrophy subsequently develop secondary to the pulmonary infundibulum stenosis.
Tetralogy of Fallot may be associated with other anomalies, the commonest being left pulmonary artery stenosis (40%), bicuspid pulmonary valve (40%) and right sided aortic arch (25%, Fig. 21b).
Treatment is primarily surgical. Palliative operations such as the Blalock-Taussig shunt - which involves end-to-end anastomosis of the subclavian artery to the pulmonary artery opposite the aortic arch - may be performed

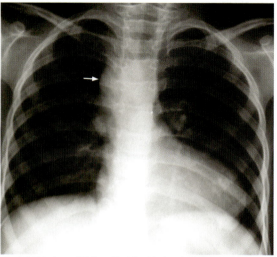

Fig.21b *Tetralogy of Fallot with right sided aortic arch (arrow). Note the boot shaped heart. The pulmonary vessels appear relatively normal (Courtesy of Radiology Department, KEM Hospital, Mumbai, India).*

01 CHEST

> **Note:**
> (1) The presence of a boot shaped heart in a child with cyanosis and heart murmur should raise the suspicion of tetralogy of Fallot.

CENTRAL NERVOUS SYSTEM

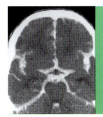

Contributors:

Edmund H.Y. Yuen, Ann D. King, Anil T. Ahuja

Questions

Case 1 - 13	58 - 70

Discussion

Subarachnoid haemorrhage	71 - 75
Extradural haematoma	76 - 77
Subdural haematoma	78 - 80
Obstructive hydrocephalus	81 - 82
Brain abscess	83 - 86
Brain metastases	87 - 90
Depressed fracture	91 - 94
Infarct	95 - 99
Intracerebral haemorrhage	100 - 104
Pituitary macroadenoma	105 - 107
Multiple sclerosis	108 - 112
Meningioma	113 - 114
Astrocytoma	115 - 121

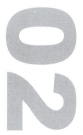

Chapter 02

Case 1

A 55-year-old unconscious man was brought to A&E. He collapsed just after complaining of a sudden onset of severe headache. On admission: GCS 6/15, BP 190/120 mmHg.

An urgent non-contrast CT brain was performed (Fig. 1a, b).

Questions

(1) What does the CT show ?
   - Hyperdense blood in the basal cisterns, Sylvian fissures, ventricles and cortical sulci.

(2) What is the diagnosis ?

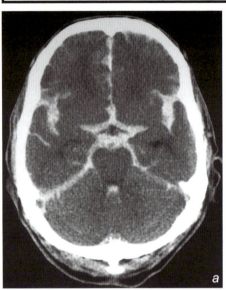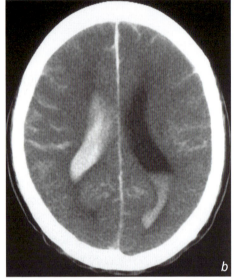

a   *b*

Fig.1a,b *Non-contrast axial CT of the brain shows extensive acute subarachnoid haemorrhage. Note the hyperdense blood in the anterior interhemispheric fissure, bilateral Sylvian fissures, basal cisterns, ventricles and cortical sulci and the intraventricular extension of haemorrhage into the lateral and 4th ventricles. In simplistic terms, the normal CSF spaces are 'black', but in this case all the CSF spaces are 'white' because of the presence of fresh blood.*

Case 2

A young child sustained a head injury and later complained of headache and drowsiness. On admission to A&E the child was unconscious. The vital signs were stable and a skull X-ray did not demonstrate a fracture.
An urgent CT brain was performed (Fig. 2a).

Questions

(1) What does this CT show ?
  - Extra-axial blood in the right temporoparietal area, heterogeneous in density, biconvex in shape with mass effect causing cerebral and ventricular compression and midline shift to the left.

(2) What is the diagnosis ?

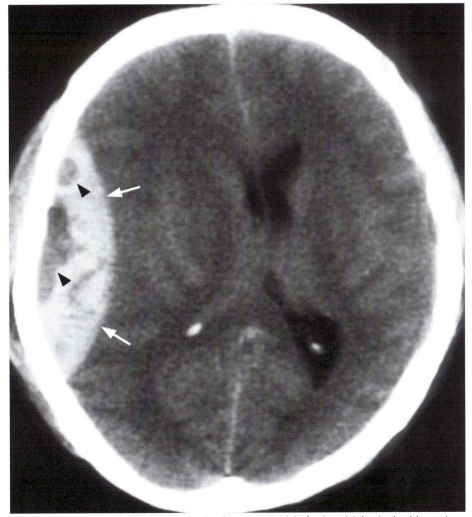

Fig.2a *Non-contrast axial CT of the brain showing an acute right frontoparietal extradural haematoma (arrows) with mass effect on the underlying brain and lateral ventricles, midline shift to the left. The low density areas (arrowheads) within the extradural indicate active bleeding.*

Case 3

A 73-year-old woman presented with chronic headache, occasional vomiting, unsteadiness and frequent falls. In the past few months there had been a progressive deterioration in her mental function and increasing drowsiness. Physical examination showed moderate papilloedema but was otherwise unremarkable. A CT brain was performed (Fig. 3a).

Questions

(1) What is shown on the CT ?
- Crescentic bilateral subdural collections isodense/slightly hyperdense to brain.
- Both the frontal/anterior horns of the lateral ventricles are compressed.
- Mild midline shift to the right.

(2) What is the diagnosis ?

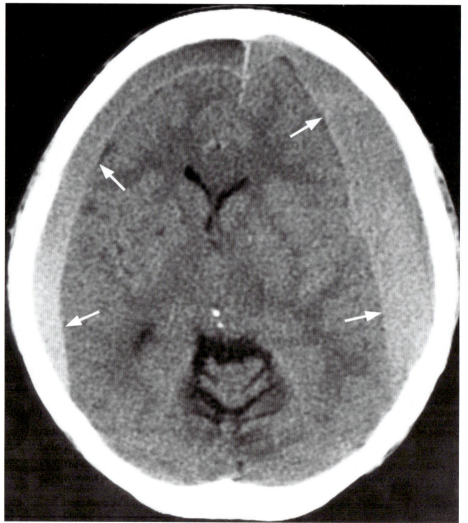

Fig.3a *Non-contrast axial CT of the brain shows bilateral subdural haematomas (arrows) that are acute/subacute.*

Case 4

A 5-year-old boy presented with a one-month history of headache, vomiting and unsteadiness. Physical examination showed ataxia and bilateral papilloedema. A pre- and post-contrast MRI of the brain was performed (Fig. 4a-d).

Questions

(1) What is shown on the MRI ?
   - A large cerebellar vermian mass encroaching onto the 4th ventricle causing proximal ventricular dilatation.
(2) What is the diagnosis ?

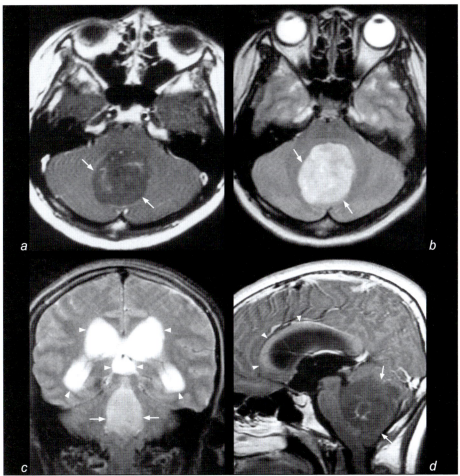

Fig.4a,b *Axial post-gadolinium enhanced T1 (a) and T2 (b) -weighted MR images of the posterior cranial fossa shows a large medulloblastoma (arrows) arising from the cerebellar vermis with mass effect and obliteration of the 4th ventricle.*

Fig.4c *Coronal T2-weighted coronal MR image of the brain shows the medulloblastoma (arrows) causing proximal ventricular dilatation (arrowheads), due to compression/obstruction of 4V.*

Fig.4d *Sagittal post-gadolinium enhanced T1-weighted MR image of the brain shows obstructive hydrocephalus due to extrinsic compression of 4V by the medulloblastoma (arrows). Note the superior bowing of the corpus callosum (arrowheads).*

Case 5

A 23-year-old man was brought to the A&E in a confused and drowsy state. He was a known IV drug addict and complained of headache and high fever for a few days. During his physical examination he suddenly developed generalized tonic-clonic convulsions. He had high fever and laboratory tests revealed a raised white cell count.

An urgent plain and contrast enhanced CT brain was performed (Fig. 5a, b).

Questions

(1) What is shown on the CT ?
- There is a large ring-enhancing lesion in the right frontal lobe.
- Perilesional white matter oedema.
- Mild mass effect on the frontal/anterior horns with slight midline shift to the left.

(2) <u>What is the diagnosis ?</u>

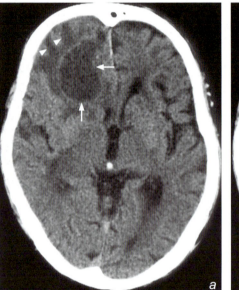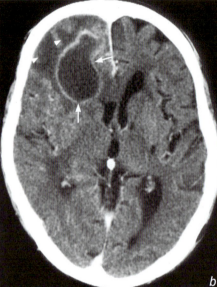

Fig.5a,b *Non-contrast (a) and contrast enhanced (b) axial CT scans show an area of low attenuation in the right frontal lobe with rim enhancement (arrows) and perifocal white matter oedema (arrowheads). Note the mass effect on the ipsilateral frontal/anterior horn. The diagnosis is a brain abscess (in view of clinical signs of symptoms).*

Case 6

A 77-year-old woman had carcinoma of the left breast resected 2 years earlier. Left axillary lymph node dissection was positive for metastases. Following treatment she presented with a sensation of pins and needles and weakness of both arms. Her relatives noticed that she had become increasingly clumsy with progressive memory loss in the last 2 months. A contrast enhanced CT brain was performed (Fig. 6a).

Questions

(1) What is shown on the CT ?
- Multiple, round, enhancing lesions.
- Perilesional oedema.
- Mass effect with compression of the left lateral ventricle and displacement of the midline structures to the right.

(2) What is the most likely diagnosis ?

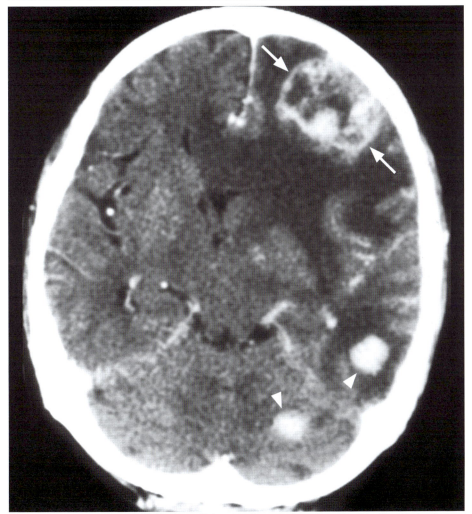

Fig.6a *Axial contrast enhanced CT showing multiple enhancing metastases (arrowheads) with perilesional oedema. Note irregular rim enhancement in the larger left frontal lobe metastasis (arrows).*

Case 7

A 42-year-old man slipped and fell while climbing stairs and sustained a head injury. On arrival at A&E he was fully conscious, complained of headache, GCS 15/15. He had a scalp laceration over the parietal region and skull radiographs and a CT scan were performed (Fig. 7a, b, c).

Questions

(1) What abnormality is shown on this frontal skull radiograph and CT scan ?
- There is a focal area of depression in the left parietal bone.
- Scalp haematoma seen overlying the depressed fracture.
- Associated intracranial injury seen on the CT scan.

(2) What is the diagnosis ?

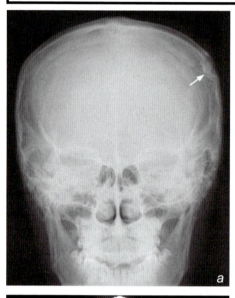

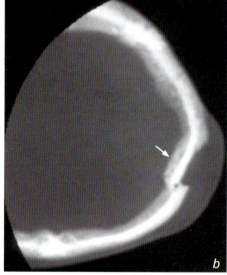

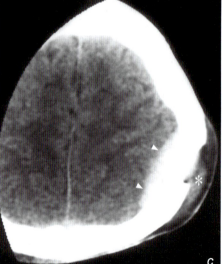

Fig.7a *Frontal skull radiograph shows a cortical break and depression in the left parietal bone (arrow) representing a depressed fracture.*

Fig.7b,c *CT brain on bone window (b) and soft tissue window (c) shows a left high parietal skull fracture with depressed fragment (arrow) with a scalp haematoma (asterisk) overlying the left high parietal skull fracture and the small extradural haematoma (arrowheads) underneath.*

Case 8

A 72-year-old woman with a history of poorly controlled hyperlipidaemia, hypertension and diabetes mellitus suddenly lost consciousness and developed left-sided weakness. Physical examination in A&E showed a BP of 210/120. An urgent CT brain was performed (Fig. 8a).

Questions

(1) What is seen on the CT ?
   - Wedge-shaped low attenuation lesion involving the right frontal and parietal lobe in the right middle cerebral artery (MCA) territory.
   - Hyperdense line running through the low attenuation area along the course of the branches of the right MCA (dense MCA sign).

(2) What is the diagnosis ?

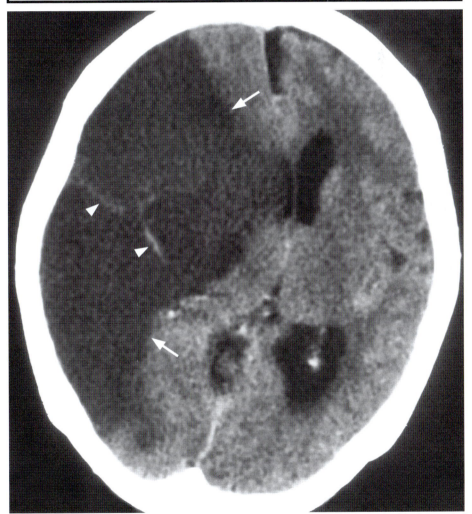

Fig.8a *Non-contrast axial CT scan showing a wedge shaped area of low attenuation (arrows), with effacement of underlying cortical sulci, involving both grey and white matter in the right MCA territory. Also note the mass effect on the ventricles and contralateral shift. The diagnosis is an acute right MCA territory infarct. The arrowheads show a hyperdense thrombus in the branches of the right MCA.*

Case 9

A 75-year-old man with diabetes and uncontrolled hypertension was admitted to the medical ward after suddenly becoming unconscious and developing a hemiparesis. On admission he was hypertensive with a dense left hemiplegia.

An urgent CT brain was performed (Fig. 9a, b).

Questions

(1) What is seen on the CT ?
   - There is an acute intraparenchymal haematoma in the right thalamus and lentiform
     nucleus with intraventricular extension into the lateral ventricles.

(2) What is the diagnosis ?

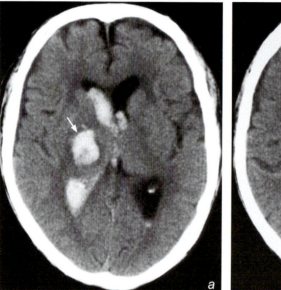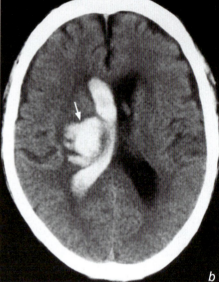

Fig.9a,b *Non-contrast axial CT scan showing a right thalamic and lentiform nucleus haemorrhage (arrow) with extension of blood into the lateral ventricle. The location is typical for a hypertensive haemorrhage.*

Case 10

A 36-year-old woman presented with generalized malaise, oligomenorrhoea and visual disturbance. On physical examination she had bitemporal hemianopia and an MRI was performed (Fig. 10a, b).

Questions

(1) What do you see on the MRI ?
- There is a large pituitary mass with suprasellar extension into the suprasellar cistern.
- Mass effect with compression of the optic chiasm.
- No dilatation of the frontal horns of the lateral ventricles.

(2) What is the diagnosis ?

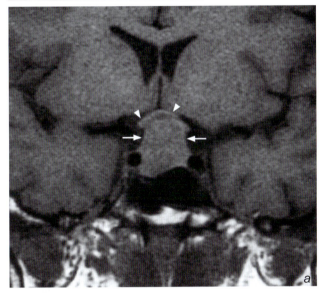

Fig.10a,b *Coronal T1W MR scans before (a) and after (b) gadolinium enhancement showing a well-defined enhancing mass (arrows) arising from the pituitary fossa with suprasellar extension. Note the mass effect and bowing of the optic chiasm (arrowheads). The pituitary floor is depressed. No extension into the cavernous sinus (long arrows).*

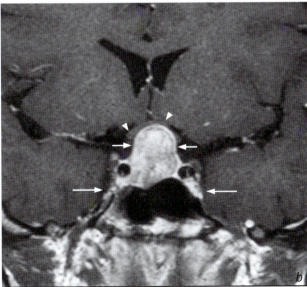

Case 11

A 22-year-old woman with a previous history of optic neuritis two years earlier followed by multiple episodes of relapsing and remitting sensory and motor symptoms involving different parts of the body underwent MRI of the brain (Fig. 11a, b).

Questions
(1) What does the MRI show?
  - Ovoid high signal periventricular lesions perpendicular to the ventricular wall involving the corpus callosum.
(2) What is the most likely diagnosis?

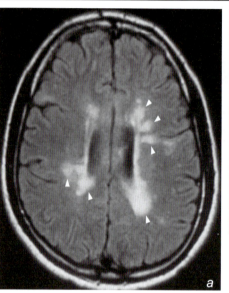
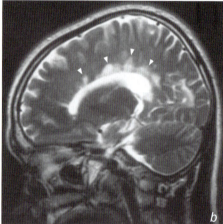

Fig.11a, b *MRI: (a) Axial FLAIR T2-weighted image (the high signal of CSF is suppressed on a FLAIR sequence); (b) sagittal T2-weighted images of the brain shows multiple ovoid periventricular demyelination plaques of high signal (arrowheads) aligned almost perpendicular to the ventricular wall in a patient with multiple sclerosis (MS).*

Case 12

A 68-year-old woman complained of increasing headache and unsteady gait in the past 9 months. Physical examination revealed subtle cerebellar signs but no other neurological deficit. A non-contrast CT (Fig. 12a) and subsequent MRI (Fig. 12b, c) of the brain were performed for further investigation.

Questions

(1) What is seen on the non-contrast CT and contrast enhanced T1W MR image ?
   - On CT there is a well-defined densely calcified right posterior cranial fossa mass.
   - On contrast enhanced MR there is a large well defined enhancing mass which on the coronal image is inseparable from the right tentorium cerebelli and appears extra-axial in origin.
   - No evidence of peritumoural oedema.
   - Slight mass effect on the 4th ventricle.
   - No proximal ventricular dilatation.

(2) What is the diagnosis ?

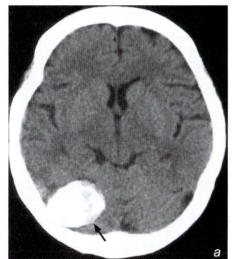
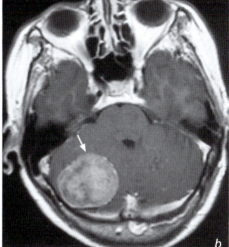

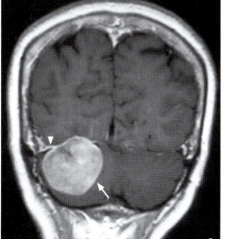

Fig.12a Non-contrast axial CT showing a densely calcified mass (arrow) in the posterior fossa on the right. It does not show peritumoural oedema.

Fig.12b, c Post-gadolinium enhanced T1-weighted axial (b) and coronal (c) MRI images show a homogeneously enhancing tumour (arrow) in the right posterior fossa inseparable from the right tentorium cerebelli with dural enhancement (arrowhead). There is no peritumoural oedema and mild mass effect is seen on the 4V. The diagnosis is a meningioma.

Case 13

A 65-year-old man complained of headache and dizziness for several months and was admitted to A&E department because of loss of consciousness. Physical examination showed bilateral lower limb weakness, papilloedema and bilateral up-going plantar reflex. A pre- and post-contrast CT (Fig. 13a, b) of the brain were performed for investigation.

Questions

(1) What is seen on the CT images (a:pre-contrast, b:post-contrast) ?
  - A large inhomogeneous predominantly isodense supratentorial lesion is present in the left posterior parietal lobe.
  - The lesion shows significant predominantly peripheral contrast enhancement with central non-enhancing area, suggestive of central necrosis.
  - The mass shows considerable vasogenic oedema and mass effect with midline shift to the right, compression of the left lateral ventricle and effacement of the sulci.
  - A small linear calcification in the medial aspect of the lesion is due to calcification of the left choroid plexus within the completely obliterated lateral ventricle.
(2) What is the diagnosis ?

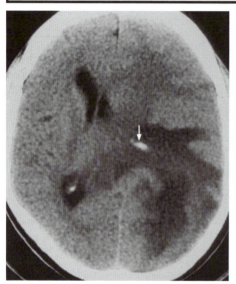 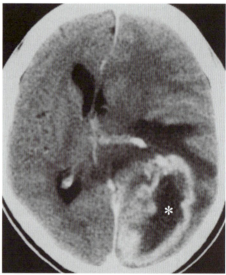

Fig.13a *Non-contrast axial CT showing considerable vasogenic oedema in the left posterior parietal lobe. The mass shows mass effect with midline shift to the right, compression of the left lateral ventricle and effacement of the sulci. A small linear calcification (arrow) in the medial aspect of the lesion is due to calcification of the left choroid plexus within the completely obliterated lateral ventricle.*

Fig.13b *Post-contrast axial CT showing a large inhomogeneous predominantly peripheral contrast enhancing mass with central cavitatory necrosis (asterisk). The vasogenic oedema and the tumour mass are now well delineated.*

Subarachnoid haemorrhage

Subarachnoid haemorrhage

(Fig. 1a, b)

- The most likely cause of SAH is a ruptured aneurysm and further investigations such as a CT angiogram (CTA)/digital subtraction angiogram (DSA) may be required to identify the source of the bleeding.

Discussion:

- Underlying aetiology:
  1. Aneurysm, 90% of the cases (Fig. 1c, d)
  2. Arterio-venous malformation (AVM) (Fig. 1e, f)
  3. Coagulation disorder
  4. Extension from intra-parenchymal haemorrhage
  5. Trauma (Fig. 1g)
  6. Idiopathic

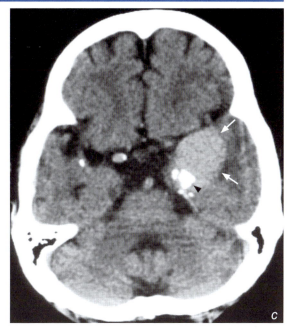

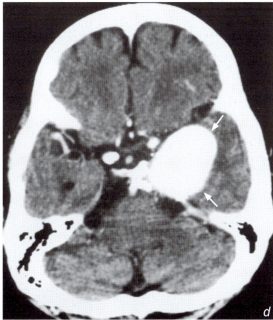

Fig.1c,d *Axial non-contrast (c) and contrast enhanced (d) CT scans show a well defined, slightly hyperdense mass in the left temporal region (arrows) with intense enhancement (similar to adjacent vessels) following the injection of contrast. The appearances are of a giant aneurysm at the skull base. Note the calcification at the edge of the mass (arrowhead), a clue to its vascular nature.*

Discussion Case 1
Subarachnoid haemorrhage

Fig.1e,f *Axial non-contrast CT (e) shows an ill-defined hyperdense area in the right cerebrum (large arrows) with focal areas of calcification (arrowhead). Axial post-contrast CT (f) shows multiple enhancing serpiginous vessels (large arrows) of a large AVM.Note the large draining veins (small arrows)coursing towards the internal cerebral vein.*

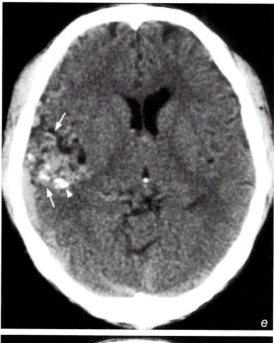

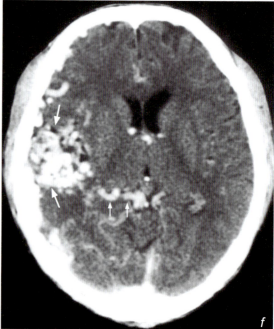

Subarachnoid haemorrhage

Fig.1g *Non-contrast axial CT of the brain showing left acute traumatic subarachnoid haemorrhage (arrows). Note the small air bubble (arrowhead) in the left extra-axial space due to open skull fracture.*

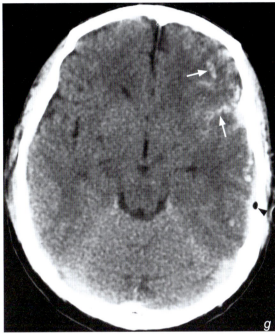

- Complications
  1. Rebleed 50% rate within the first two weeks
  2. Hydrocephalus due to ventricular obstruction or arachnoiditis (Fig. 1h)
  3. Vasospasm, ischaemia, infarction
  4. Leptomeningeal superficial siderosis, cranial nerve (particularly I, II, VIII) palsies
  5. Neurological pulmonary oedema

Fig.1h *Non-contrast axial CT of the brain showing dilatation of the lateral ventricles, 3V and 4V representing hydrocephalus as a late complication of subarachnoid haemorrhage due to arachnoiditis.*

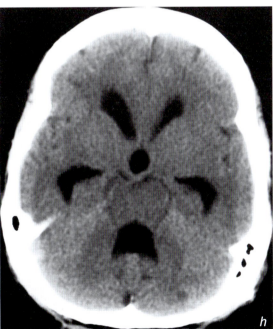

Discussion Case 1
Subarachnoid haemorrhage

- Investigations
- CT is the initial imaging investigation of choice:
  1. Highly sensitive in detecting acute subarachnoid blood within the first 48 hours
  2. The bleeding source may be close to where there is the largest amount of blood (Fig. 1i) and associated intraparenchymal haemorrhage is demonstrated
- Angiogram
- The aim of CTA (Fig. 1j)/DSA is to confirm the diagnosis, locate the aneurysm, identify any other aneurysms (known association of multiple intracranial berry aneurysms with adult polycystic kidney disease)

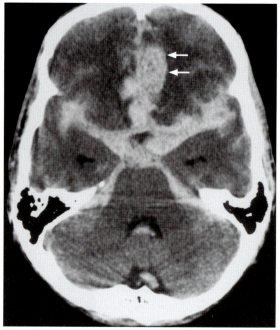

Fig.1i *Non-contrast axial CT of the brain showing blood in the basal cisterns, both Sylvian fissures and the 4V. Note the largest amount of blood is localized in the left parafalcine region anteriorly (arrows), suggesting that a ruptured aneurysm is in its vicinity (ACA, ACoA territory). In this case the SAH was due to a leaking left ACA aneurysm.*

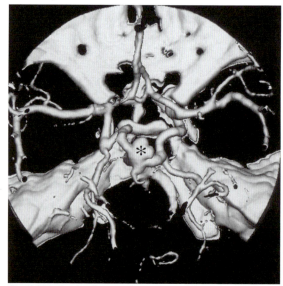

Fig.1j *CTA showing the vascular anatomy of the circle of Willis and a large basilar tip aneurysm (asterisk).*

Discussion Case 1
Subarachnoid haemorrhage

- Interventional radiology
- A diagnostic DSA may be coupled with treatment (endovascular embolization) at the same time (Fig. 1k, l)
- The choice of treatment (surgical clipping or endovascular embolization) depends on the anatomical location, accessibility and configuration of the neck of the aneurysm (aneurysms with 'wide neck' make embolization more difficult since the coils may be dislodged more easily)

Fig.1k,l Pre-embolization (k) DSA shows an anterior communicating artery aneurysm (arrow). Post-embolization (l) DSA shows obliteration of the anterior communicating artery aneurysm by coils (arrowhead).

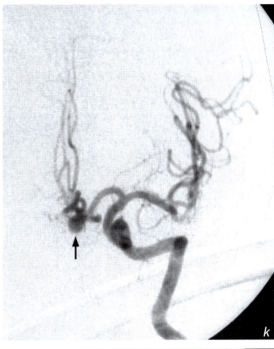

Note:
(1) Spontaneous subarachnoid haemorrhage is usually due to rupture of an aneurysm.
(2) Following the acute event CT sensitively identifies the SAH.
(3) Further imaging (CTA/DSA) is necessary to locate the source of bleeding prior to any treatment.
(4) Treatment options include endovascular embolization or surgical clipping.

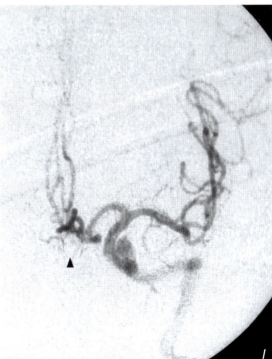

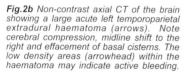

Discussion Case 2
Extradural haematoma

Discussion:

- The bleeding is often from a tear in the right middle meningeal artery and may be associated with a fracture.
- Bleeding sources of extradural haematoma:
- Arterial (90%): tear of the middle meningeal or other meningeal arteries
- Venous (10%): sinus laceration, tear of meningeal vein
- CT features of EDH:
   1. Biconvex/lenticular in shape (Fig. 2b, c)
   2. The haematoma does not cross the coronal and lambdoid sutures
   3. May cross dural reflections falx cerebri and tentorium cerebelli
   4. Most are associated with skull vault fractures (Fig. 2d)
   5. Low density areas within the EDH indicate active bleeding and thus heterogeneity may predict rapid expansion of the haematoma (Fig. 2a, b)
   6. Venous EDHs from low pressure bleed are more variable in shape and may have delayed onset

Fig.2b Non-contrast axial CT of the brain showing a large acute left temporoparietal extradural haematoma (arrows). Note cerebral compression, midline shift to the right and effacement of basal cisterns. The low density areas (arrowhead) within the haematoma may indicate active bleeding.

Fig.2c Non-contrast axial CT of the brain showing an acute right posterior fossa extradural haematoma (arrows) with mass effect on the 4th ventricle. Also note areas of haemorrhagic contusion in the right frontal lobe (arrowheads).

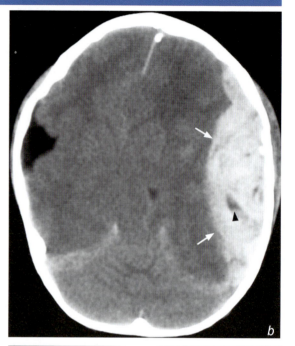

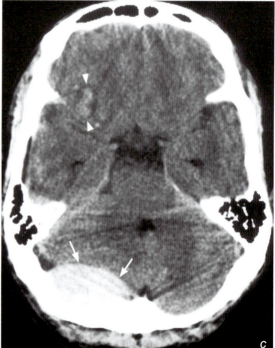

Extradural haematoma

Note:

(1) The presence/absence of skull vault fracture does not predict the presence/absence of intracranial injury.

(2) Skull radiographs have limited value in patients with severe trauma.

(3) In addition to the identification of blood one must also evaluate the heterogeneity within the haematoma, extent of the mass effect, ventricular dilatation if any, the presence of fractures and evidence of any other intracranial injury.

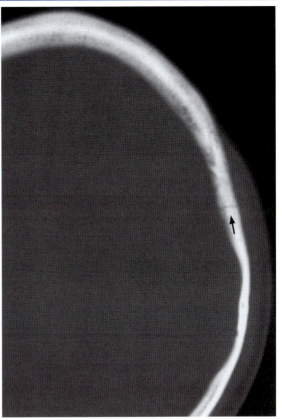

Fig.2d *CT with bone window demonstrates the left temporoparietal skull fracture line (arrow) and the overlying scalp haematoma.*

Discussion Case 3
Subdural haematoma

Subdural haematoma (Fig. 3a)

Discussion:

- Subdural haematomas (SDH) are caused by traumatic tear of bridging veins as they traverse the subdural space to dural venous sinuses, which are more vulnerable in elderly patients with atrophic brain and widened subdural space. Alcoholics and epileptics may develop undetected chronic subdural haematomas as they have repeated falls and the head injuries sustained are trivial and often forgotten (post-ictal state in epileptics).
- Also seen in infants in non-accidental injury (NAI)
- May enlarge gradually over weeks and months with multiple episodes of small haemorrhages
- Symptoms and physical signs are those of an enlarging intracranial space occupying lesion (SOL) and may be confused with an intracranial tumour until CT reveals the diagnosis

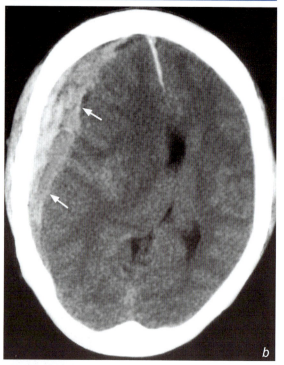

b

Fig.3b,c *Non-contrast axial CT of the brain showing a crescentic, hyperdense acute right subdural haematoma (arrows). Note the compression of the right lateral ventricle and marked midline shift to the left in Fig 3b and the presence of the blood tracking along the anterior interhemispheric fissure (arrow heads) in Fig 3c.*

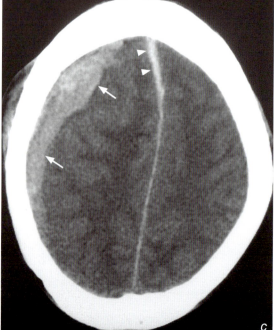

c

Subdural haematoma

- CT features:
  1. Most are supratentorial in location
  2. Crescentic in shape and along the surface of the brain
  3. Unlike extradural haematomas <u>subdural haematomas cross the coronal and lambdoid sutures</u>
  4. Do not cross dural reflections (falx cerebri, tentorium cerebelli)
  5. Acute on chronic haemorrhage results in heterogeneous increase in density and rapid increase in size
- There is no consistent relationship to the presence of skull vault fracture
- Change of haematoma density on CT with time:
  1. Acute SDHs are hyperdense to brain or show mixed heterogeneous density (Fig. 3b, c)
  2. Subacute SDHs (> 1 week) are isodense (Fig. 3a, d) and may be difficult to identify – a clue is when the sulci no longer extend all the way to the skull vault. IV contrast may show enhancing membrane and displaced cortical vessels
  3. Chronic SDHs (> several weeks) are hypodense (Fig. 3e) and may calcify
  4. Fluid level may be seen in subacute or early chronic SDHs in which the denser debris collects in the dependent portion of the haemorrhage (Fig. 3f)

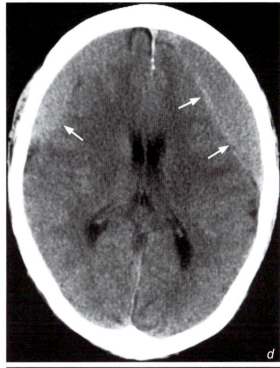

Fig.3d *Non-contrast axial CT of the brain with bilateral isodense subacute frontoparietal subdural haematomas (arrows).*

Fig.3e *Non-contrast axial CT of the brain shows bilateral hypodense (CSF density) chronic frontoparietal subdural haematomas (arrows).*

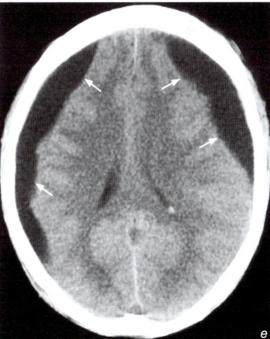

Discussion Case 3

Subdural haematoma

Note:
(1) The density of subdural haematoma changes with time and will become isodense in the subacute stage which may be difficult to identify.

(2) Look for the sulci displaced away from the skull vault.

(3) Note any mass effect or midline shift as these may be the only clues to the presence of an isodense SDH.

(4) Have a high index of suspicion in elderly patients, epileptics and chronic alcoholics.

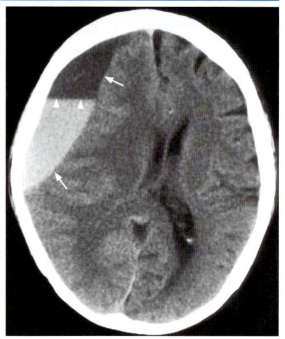

Fig.3f *Non-contrast axial CT of the brain shows a large right frontoparietal subdural haematoma (arrows) with a fluid level (arrowheads). Note the hyperdense acute component at the dependent portion and the hypodense chronic component in the non-dependent portion.*

Discussion Case 4
Obstructive hydrocephalus

Discussion:

- Hydrocephalus is the presence of excessive CSF due to imbalance between CSF formation and resorption resulting in ventricular dilatation and increased intraventricular pressure
- Obstructive hydrocephalus is due to obstruction to the normal CSF flow within the ventricular system and thus absorption:
    1. Extrinsic compression by mass lesion, e.g. tumour (Fig. 4a-e)
    2. Stenosis, e.g. congenital aqueductal stenosis
    3. Malformation, e.g. Dandy-Walker (DW) malformation
- Communicating hydrocephalus (Fig.1h, case 1 CNS) is due to obstruction to normal CSF flow outside the ventricular system or obstruction to CSF absorption usually at arachnoid granulations:
    1. Meningitis
    2. Haemorrhage, e.g. SAH
    3. Carcinomatosis
- Normal pressure hydrocephalus :
    1. Presence of a pressure gradient between the ventricle and brain parenchyma despite normal lumbar CSF pressure
    2. Potential treatable cause of senile dementia
    3. Clinical triad of ataxia, dementia and incontinence

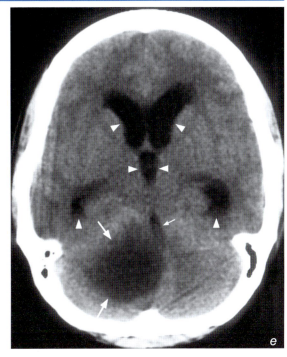

Fig.4e Non-contrast axial CT of the brain showing a low attenuation mass in the right cerebellar hemisphere (arrows) with mass effect on the 4th ventricle (small arrow). Note the ventricular dilatation (arrowheads) of the temporal and frontal horns of the lateral ventricle and the 3rd ventricle (midline).

Fig.4f Axial non-contrast CT of the brain showing generalized atrophy with prominent Sylvian fissures, basal cisterns, ventricles and cerebellar foliae.

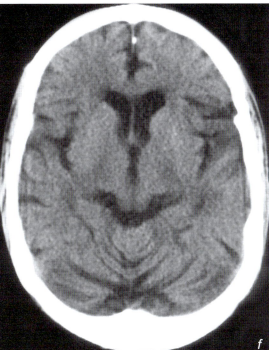

Discussion Case 4
Obstructive hydrocephalus

- Cross-sectional imaging (CT/MRI):
  Hydrocephalus:
  1. Progressive ventricular dilatation
  2. Dilatation of temporal horns and inferior recess of the 3rd ventricle (round rather than a slit like 3V)
  3. Superior bowing of corpus callosum (Fig. 4d)
  4. Transependymal oedema in the form of high T2W, low T1W signal (on MR) and low attenuation (on CT) in the periventricular regions

  Obstructive hydrocephalus:
  - Ventricular dilatation proximal to the obstructive site with normal ventricular size distal to the obstruction

  Communicating hydrocephalus:
  - The 4th ventricle may dilate less than the 3rd and the lateral ventricles

  Hydrocephalus vs atrophy:
  - In hydrocephalus the degree of ventricular dilatation is out of proportion to the degree of sulcal enlargement
  - In hydrocephalus the walls of the 3rd ventricle tend to be biconvex rather than parallel
  - In atrophy, in addition to the ventricular dilatation, the cortical sulci, Sylvian fissures, cerebellar foliae are also prominent (Fig. 4f)
  - Obstruction to CSF flow at the spinal cord level results in syringomyelia (syrinx formation) (Fig. 4g, h).

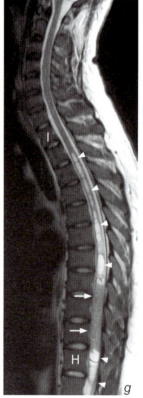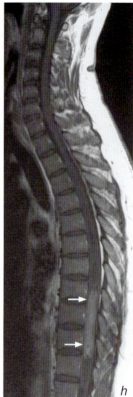

Fig.4g Sagittal T2W MR of a different patient showing a mass (arrows) within the spinal cord with associated syrinx formation (arrowheads) above and below the level of the mass lesion.

Fig.4h Sagittal post-contrast MR of the same patient in Fig.4g. There is contrast enhancement of the mass (arrows) which was later found to be a spinal cord glioma.

Note:
(1) Always look for the cause when you diagnose hydrocephalus.
(2) Dilatation of the temporal horns of the lateral ventricles and rounding of the 3rd ventricle are early clues to identify hydrocephalus.

Discussion Case 5
Brain abscess

Brain abscess (Fig. 5a, b)
The common differential diagnoses for a
solitary ring-enhancing lesion in the brain
include:
- Brain abscess
- Neoplasm: brain metastasis, glioma

However, in view of the high fever, a
history of intravenous drug abuse and
raised white cell count, the most likely
diagnosis in this case is a brain abscess.

Discussion:
- Brain abscess is focal infection of the
  brain parenchyma and may be a result
  of haematogenous dissemination of
  infection. Associated predisposing
  factors include endocarditis, IV drug
  abuse, pulmonary infection, right-to-
  left cardiac shunt or pulmonary AVM
- It may also result from direct
  contagious spread from adjacent
  source of sepsis, e.g. from paranasal
  sinusitis and otomastoiditis or due
  to penetrating trauma with direct
  inoculation.
- Imaging findings on CT:
  1. Initial changes are of cerebritis
     which appears as an ill-defined
     intra-axial lesion of decreased
     attenuation with variable amount
     of oedema and mass effect. There
     is typically no contrast
     enhancement in the early stage
     cerebritis
  2. Contrast enhancement gradually
     develops with eventual formation
     of a ring-enhancing lesion which
     typically shows:
     a. Thin, smooth enhancing rim
     b. Eccentric wall thickness which
        is thicker on the outer grey
        matter side presumably due to
        better blood supply and thinner
        on the inner white matter side
        (Fig. 5c, d) – this gives rise to
        the potential complication of
        abscess rupture into the
        ventricles causing ventriculitis
     c. Formation of adjacent daughter
        abscesses

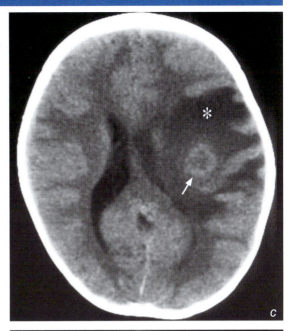

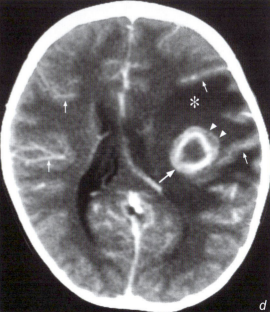

Fig.5c,d *Non-contrast (c) and contrast enhanced (d) axial CT scans
show an area of low attenuation in the left frontoparietal lobe with rim
enhancement (large arrow) and perilesional white matter oedema
(asterisk). Note the thick outer wall of the abscess (arrowheads). In
this case there is prominent enhancement of the meninges (small
arrows) suggesting there may be an element of associated meningitis.
Compare this with no meningeal enhancement in Fig 5b.*

Brain abscess

d. Evaluate if there is any evidence of associated meningitis such as intense meningeal enhancement following injection of contrast and hydrocephalus (Fig. 5c-g).

e. Perilesional oedema and contrast enhancement of brain abscess may be suppressed by steroid therapy.

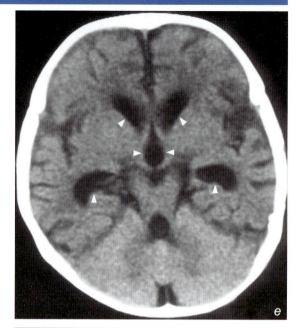

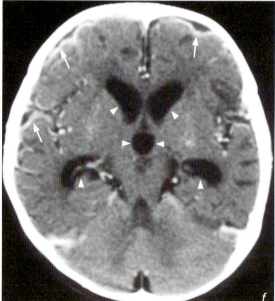

Fig.5e,f *Non-contrast (e) and contrast enhanced (f) axial CT scans show cortical meningeal enhancement (arrows) of meningitis which was causing ventricular dilatation (arrowheads).*

Brain abscess

Fig.5g *Post-gadolinium enhanced axial T1W MR showing meningeal enhancement (arrows) and ventricular dilatation (arrowheads) due to meningitis.*

Fig.5h *Post-gadolinium enhanced coronal T1W MR showing irregular rim enhancing lesion (arrows) in the left temporal lobe. This patient had no fever, raised WCC or any other evidence of infection. Biopsy revealed a glioma. Note its similar rim enhancement to an abscess.*

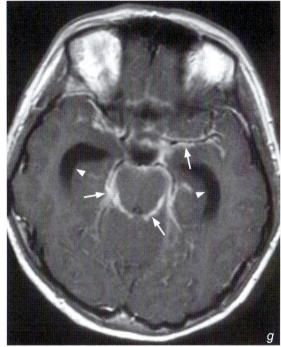

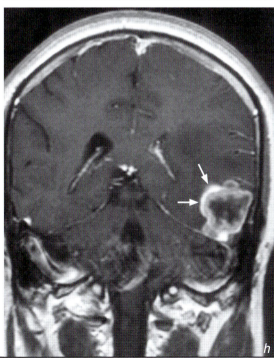

Brain abscess

Note:

(1) On CT a brain abscess appears similar to other lesions such as gliomas (Fig. 5h) and metastases (Fig. 5i). The diagnosis is made in relation to the clinical history and MR spectroscopy may help.

(2) The rim enhancement in abscesses may be absent in patients on steroid therapy.

(3) Look for associated meningitis and hydrocephalus.

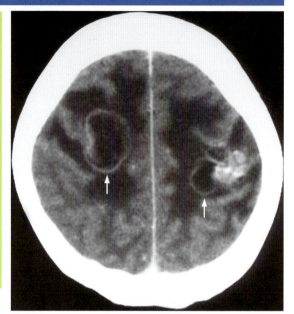

Fig.5i *Post-contrast enhanced axial CT of the brain showing multiple rim enhancing lesions (arrows) with perilesional oedema in a patient with carcinoma of the breast. In view of the patient's history the lesions represent metastases.*

Brain metastases

Brain metastases (Fig. 6a)
- In view of the patient's previous history of a carcinoma breast the most likely diagnosis is ***multiple brain metastases***

Discussion:
The most common primary tumours giving rise to metastatic brain deposits include:
Bronchogenic carcinoma
Breast carcinoma
Colorectal carcinoma
Renal cell carcinoma
Melanoma
Choriocarcinoma
Leukaemia/lymphoma
Neuroblastoma (in children)
- Brain metastases are the result of haematogenous spread, are more likely to be multiple than solitary, and are of varying sizes
- The corticomedullary junction is the typical location and most are deposited in the cerebral hemispheres, followed by the cerebellum and brainstem
- Usually associated with perilesional oedema that may be disproportionately large compared to size of the metastases. In a patient with a known cancer the presence of white matter oedema on a non-contrast CT must be viewed with suspicion for metastatic disease (even if no obvious masses/nodules are seen). A post-contrast CT/MRI will improve the identification of small metastases associated with the white matter oedema (Fig. 6b, c). However, in patients on steroid therapy the perilesional oedema may be missing.

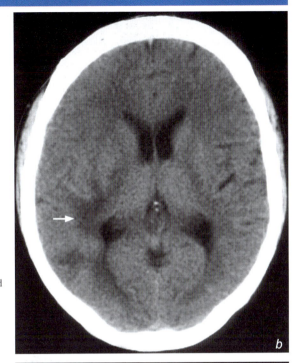

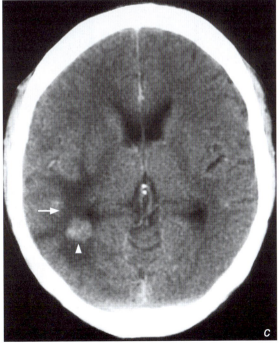

Fig.6b,c *Axial non-contrast (b) and contrast enhanced (c) CT scans show the presence of white matter oedema in the right posterior parietal lobe (arrow). Following contrast the metastasis is clearly seen (arrowhead). In a patient with a known primary the presence of white matter oedema on a non-contrast CT is highly suspicious for metastasis and a contrast enhanced CT or MR is indicated.*

02 CENTRAL NERVOUS SYSTEM

Brain metastases

However, in patients on steroid therapy the perilesional oedema may be missing.

- Imaging findings on CT/MRI:

   1. Metastases appear as round intra-axial lesions of decreased attenuation on plain CT (except for haemorrhagic [Fig. 6d] or calcified brain metastases [Fig. 6e]) and high T2W signal on MRI

   2. Some primary tumours produce haemorrhagic metastases in the brain, and these include:

      1. Melanoma
      2. Choriocarcinoma
      3. Oat cell carcinoma of lung
      4. Renal cell carcinoma
      5. Thyroid carcinoma

Fig.6d Non-contrast axial CT scan shows the presence of haemorrhagic metastases (arrowhead) and white matter oedema (asterisk).

Fig.6e Non-contrast axial CT scan shows multiple densely calcified metastases (arrowheads). This case is unusual because there is an absence of peritumoural white matter edema.

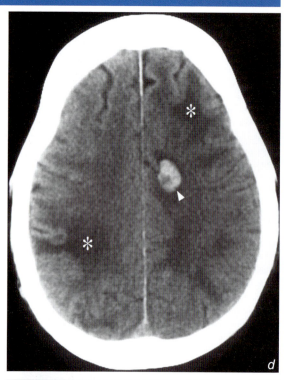

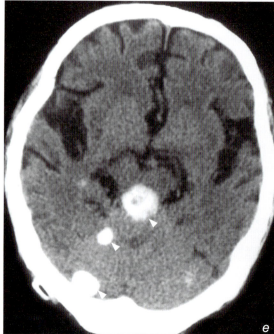

Brain metastases

3. Metastases may also be identified in the dura, leptomeninges (Fig. 6f, g) and skull.
4. Gadolinium-enhanced MRI is very sensitive for the detection of brain metastases which usually show high T2W signal and enhance avidly

Fig.6f,g *Non-contrast (f) and contrast enhanced (g) axial CT scans in a patient with a known cancer, showing enhancement following the cortical sulci (arrows) on the left in a patient with leptomeningeal metastases.*

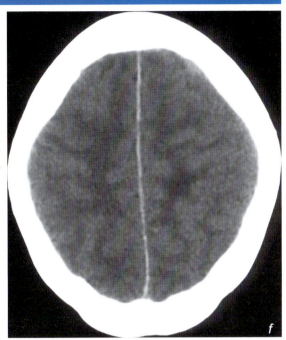

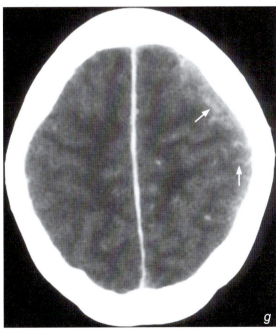

5. Small tuberculomas (Fig. 6h, i) will mimic metastases on imaging and therefore the patient's clinical history and associated laboratory tests must be taken into account before suggesting the diagnosis.

Note:

In a patient with a known primary tumour
(1) Multiple intra-axial brain lesions are highly suspicious of brain metastases but beware because even a solitary enhancing lesion may be a metastatic deposit.
(2) The presence of white matter oedema on a non-contrast CT may be the only clue of brain metastases and a contrast CT/MR should be performed. The oedema may be out of proportion to the size of the metastases.

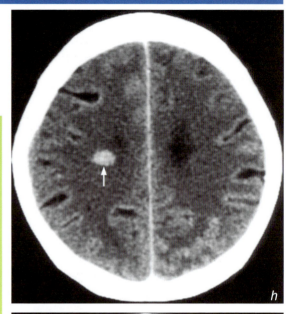

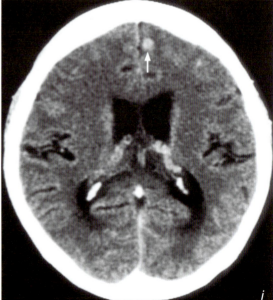

Fig.6h,i Contrast enhanced axial CT scans of a patient with a previous history of pulmonary TB showing small enhancing cerebral tuberculomas (arrows).

Depressed fracture

Discussion:

- Fractures of the skull, similar to fractures elsewhere in the skeleton, may be simple or comminuted; in the latter event the bone fragments are often depressed towards the brain parenchyma.
- Compound fracture is one in which there is real or potential communication between the intracranial cavity and the external environment with an increased risk of infection.
- A fracture passing through the paranasal sinuses or mastoid air cells is essentially considered a compound fracture.
- Although intracranial injury is better evaluated by a CT scan it may miss a fracture when the fracture line is oriented parallel to the axial plane of imaging.
- Simple skull vault fractures usually appear as linear, well-defined, fine lines of lucency (Fig. 7d), and should be distinguished from vascular markings and sutures, which are present at known anatomical locations and have a branching pattern (vessels) or interdigitations (sutures).
- Skull fractures may be associated with widening of sutures/diastasis (Fig. 7e, f).

Fig.7d Frontal skull radiograph showing a non-branching lucent line (arrowheads) running through the skull vault representing a fracture line. Compare it with the interdigitations seen in a suture (arrow).

Fig.7e,f Skull radiograph and axial CT (bone window), showing sutural diastasis/ widening of the left lambdoid suture (arrows) in a patient with skull trauma.

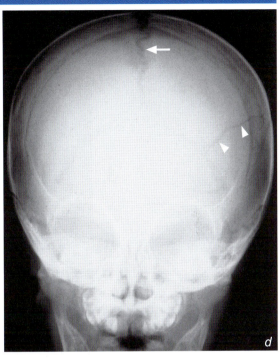

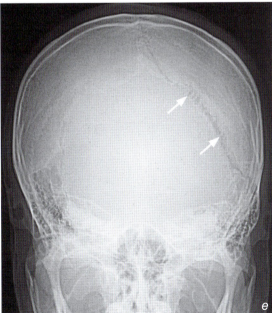

Discussion Case 7
Depressed fracture

- A depressed fragment of skull bone on plain radiograph will have increased density because of overlap with adjacent bone (Fig. 7g). This may be confirmed by tangential views; however, a CT scan is indicated to evaluate the presence of any underlying brain contusion

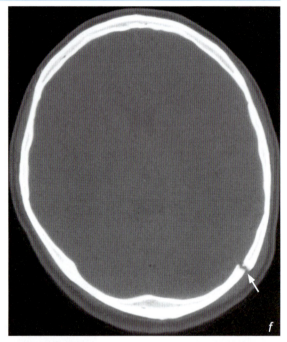

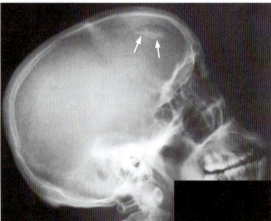

Fig.7g *Lateral skull radiograph of a patient with skull trauma shows a focal linear area of increased density in the frontal region (arrows), the only radiographic clue for a depressed fracture in this patient.*

Depressed fracture

- The only clue to the presence of skull base fractures on plain radiographs or CT may be opacification or air-fluid level of the sphenoid sinus (Fig. 7h) or mastoid air cells (Fig. 7i), due to bleeding or CSF leakage. CT demonstrates the presence of associated intracranial injuries (Fig. 7j).
- Fracture of the petrous temporal bone, especially when longitudinal, may be associated with traumatic disruption of the ossicular chain causing traumatic conductive hearing loss. A multiplanar HRCT (1-3 mm slice thickness) will assess better the temporal bone fracture.
- The presence of intracranial air is suggestive of a fracture running through air containing structures such as sinuses and mastoid air cells (Fig. 7k).

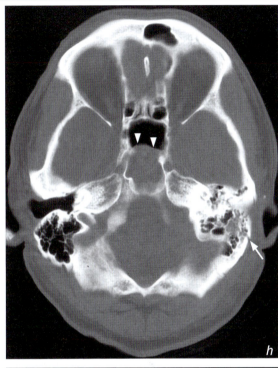

Fig.7h *Axial CT scan (bone window) showing fluid in the sphenoid sinus (arrowheads) indicating the presence of a skull base fracture in a patient with skull trauma. A careful examination reveals a fracture through the left mastoid (arrow).*

Fig.7i. *Axial CT scan (bone window) shows haziness in the left mastoid compared to the normal aeration in the right mastoid. Note the presence of a fracture line through the mastoid and fluid in the mastoid air cells indicating post-traumatic haemorrhage or CSF leak.*

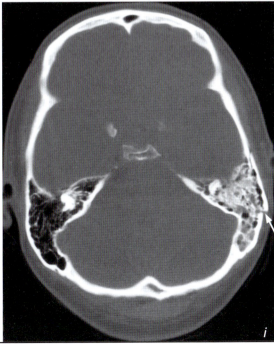

Depressed fracture

Fig.7j *Same patient as in Fig. 7i. Note the extensive haemorrhage in the frontal lobes with significant mass effect. Low attenuation area (asterisk) is also seen in the frontal and parts of temporal lobe indicating significant trauma due to shearing/diffuse axonal injury.*

Fig.7k *Axial CT scan (bone window) showing the presence of free intracranial air (arrowheads) suggesting a fracture through air containing structures such as sinuses, and mastoid air cells.*

Note:

(1) The presence of a skull fracture alone cannot predict the presence/ extent of intracranial injury.

(2) Depressed/compound fractures are often associated with cerebral contusion and patients are at an increased risk of acquiring infection.

(3) In acute trauma CT is the investigation of choice for evaluating intracranial injury and complications/sequelae associated with head injury.

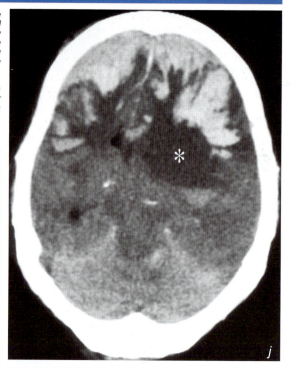

j

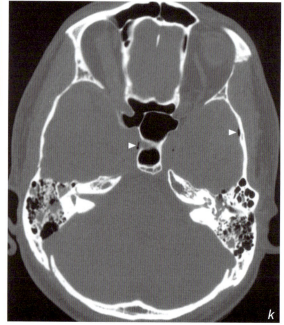

k

Infarct

Discussion:

- Cerebral infarction is the irreversible loss of brain tissues due to ischaemia or haemorrhage
- Role of imaging:
    1. To confirm the clinical diagnosis
    2. To identify any intracranial haemorrhage
    3. To detect other lesions which may clinically mimic an infarct, e.g. tumour, vascular malformation, subdural haematoma
    4. To detect early complications such as subfalcine/transtentorial herniation and haemorrhagic transformation
- CT is the initial imaging of choice for acute stroke. However, it may not demonstrate a cerebral infarct during the first 12 hours. At this time its role is to rule out the presence of intracranial haemorrhage as this defines the treatment options. An infarct may be treated by anticoagulants/ thrombolytics whereas these are contraindicated in the presence of an intracranial haemorrhage.
- Early signs of cerebral infarction on CT:
    1. Loss of grey-white matter interface
    2. Sulcal effacement
    3. Hyperdense clot within thrombosed artery (dense MCA sign [Fig. 8a, b])
- Luxury perfusion (seen on contrast CT): represents hyperaemia in an ischaemic area; the increased perfusion is due to compensatory vasodilatation due to parenchymal lactic acidosis
- Subacute infarcts on CT:
    1. Grey-white matter oedema
    2. Gyral enhancement on contrast CT
    3. Haemorrhagic component seen in up to 40%
- Chronic infarcts on CT (Fig. 8c):
    1. Parenchymal tissue loss
    2. Cystic encephalomalacia

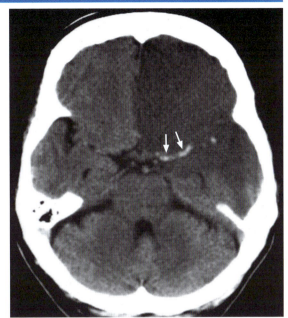

Fig.8b *Non-contrast axial CT showing a dense MCA (arrows) in a patient with a left MCA infarct. Note the low attenuation of the acute infarct in left frontal and temporal lobes (Courtesy of Dr Judy Lam, Department of Diagnostic Radiology & Organ Imaging, PWH, Hong Kong).*

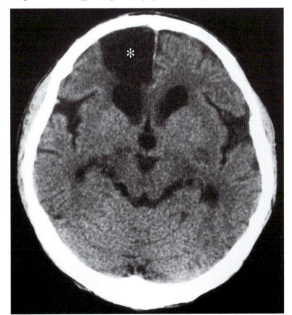

Fig.8c *Non-contrast axial CT showing an area (asterisk) of low attenuation (CSF density) in the right frontal lobe in the ACA territory. The right frontal horn is dilated compared to the left. The appearances are of an old right ACA infarct.*

02

CENTRAL NERVOUS SYSTEM

Infarct

In the presence of occlusion of the main ICA a large area of infarct/oedema will be seen involving multiple vascular territories in the cerebral hemisphere with mass effect and contralateral shift of midline structures (Fig. 8d). Structures supplied by the posterior circulation through the vertebral arteries are unaffected as these vessels remain patent.

Ischaemic areas limited to the posterior circulation (Fig. 8e) should raise the suspicion of vertebral artery dissection which may be due to minor trauma, twisting/hyperextension of the neck.

Fig.8d *Non-contrast axial CT showing diffuse low attenuation in the right cerebral hemisphere involving grey and white matter affecting multiple vascular territories. The right lateral ventricle is obliterated and there is contralateral shift of the midline. The appearances are of an acute right ICA infarct. In these patients parts of the brain supplied through the posterior circulation are spared.*

Fig.8e *Non-contrast axial CT scan showing basilar territory infarct involving both occipital lobes (arrows).*

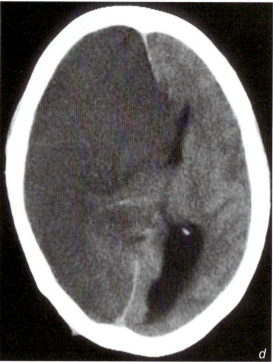

d

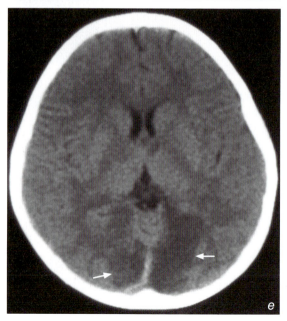

e

Infarct

In the event of an acute episode of hypotension (e.g. during surgery) the vessels involving the basal ganglia are most susceptible and areas of ischaemia may be seen in the thalami, caudate nuclei, globus pallidus and lentiform nucleus (Fig. 8f, g)

Fig.8f,g *Non-contrast axial CT scan showing infarcts in both the caudate nuclei (arrowheads), lentiform nuclei (arrows) and thalami (asterisk) in a patient with an acute prolonged hypotensive episode.*

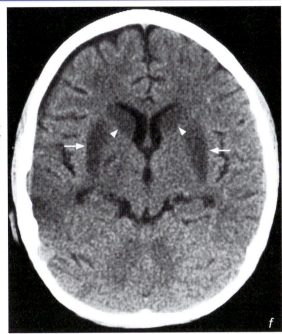

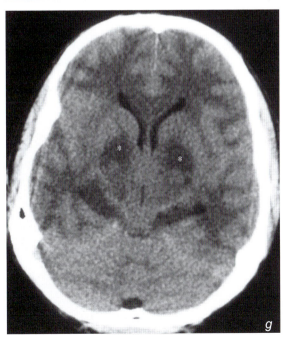

02 CENTRAL NERVOUS SYSTEM

Infarct

In CT scans of elderly patients one may find areas of ischaemia or small lacunar infarcts, often with no associated clinical signs or symptoms (Fig. 8h).

- MR Diffusion Weighted Imaging (DWI):
  Is very sensitive in identifying areas of brain ischaemia early in stroke (first six hours [Fig. 8i]). It identifies the cytotoxic oedema and along with perfusion imaging defines the extent of the vascular insult.

Fig.8h *Non-contrast axial CT scan showing a small low attenuation area (arrow) in the left internal capsular territory, consistent with a lacunar infarct.*

Fig.8i *Axial Diffusion Weighted Image (DWI) showing a high signal (fluid restriction) in the left MCA territory consistent with an infarct (Courtesy of Dr Wynnie Lam, Department of Diagnostic Radiology and Organ Imaging, The Chinese University of Hong Kong).*

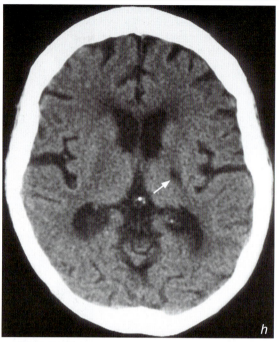

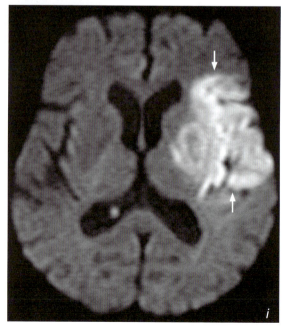

Discussion Case 8
Infarct

Patients with an intracerebral infarct on anticoagulants may develop haemorrhage and show deterioration in their clinical status. A CT scan will demonstrate the haemorrhagic transformation of the infarct (Fig. 8j)

Note:

(1) Role of imaging:
  1. To confirm clinical diagnosis
  2. To rule out any intracranial haemorrhage
  3. To detect other lesions which may clinically mimic infarct, e.g. tumour, vascular malformation, subdural haematoma
  4. To detect early complications such as herniation and haemorrhagic transformation

(2) Intracranial haemorrhage is a contraindication to anticoagulation/ thrombolytic therapy.

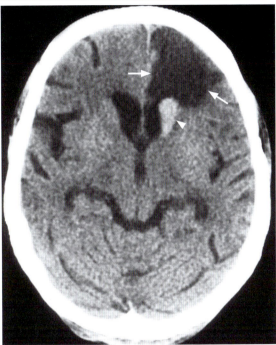

Fig.8j *Non-contrast axial CT scan in a patient with a known left ACA infarct (arrows) on anticoagulant therapy with recent clinical deterioration showing the presence of a haemorrhage in the left caudate nucleus (arrowhead).*

Discussion Case 9
Intracerebral haemorrhage

Intracerebral haemorrhage
(Fig. 9a, b)
Note that both infarcts and haemorrhage cause stroke and their clinical presentation may be very similar. A CT scan is indicated to differentiate the two as the treatment options are very different. Anticoagulation/thrombolytic treatment is contraindicated in patients with intracranial haemorrhage.

Discussion:
- Common causes of intraparenchymal haemorrhage:
    1. Hypertensive haemorrhage:
        a. Typical location: basal ganglia (Fig. 9a, b), brainstem (Fig. 9c), cerebellum (Fig. 9d)
        b. Variable secondary intraventricular and subarachnoid extension
        c. May cause hydrocephalus or brain herniation due to its mass effect
        d. Often not associated with much surrounding oedema.
    2. Ruptured/leaking aneurysm
    3. Bleeding from an ateriovenous malformation (AVM)
    4. Trauma
    5. Intra-tumoural (Fig. 9e) or peritumoural haemorrhage. Haemorrhagic tumours:
        a. Glioblastoma multiforme (GBM)
        b. Anaplastic astrocytoma
        c. Oligodendroglioma
        d. Ependymoma
        e. Primitive neuroectodermal tumours (PNETs)
        f. Pituitary adenoma
        g. Metastases
        Contrast CT may show enhancement of the non-haemorrhagic component in tumour haemorrhage. The presence of persistent white matter oedema around the haemorrhage may suggest that the haemorrhage is probably within an underlying

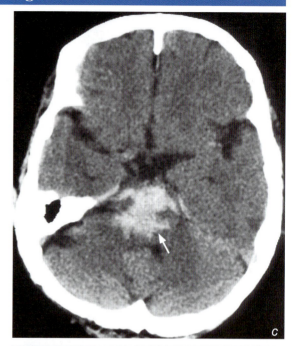

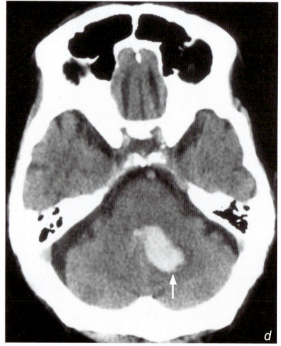

Fig.9c,d *Non-contrast axial CT showing haemorrhage (arrow) in the pons and cerebellum.*

Discussion Case 9
Intracerebral haemorrhage

tumour and further imaging with contrast enhanced CT or MRI is necessary.

6. Haemorrhagic infarct
7. Coagulation disorder

- Venous haemorrhage:

This may be due to thrombosis of the intracranial venous sinuses/ veins which results in increased back-pressure and therefore haemorrhage and/or cerebral oedema.

Common causes of venous sinus thrombosis include

1. Idiopathic
2. Adjacent septic focus,
   e.g. mastoiditis
3. Trauma
4. Tumour compressing or
   invading into adjacent sinus
5. Hypercoagulability,
   e.g. oral contraceptives,
   pregnancy, antiphospholipid
   syndrome

- The superior sagittal sinus is most commonly involved. Others include transverse, sigmoid and straight sinuses.
- Non-contrast axial CT scan shows unilateral or bilateral parenchymal haemorrhage which is typically close to a venous sinus (Fig. 9f).

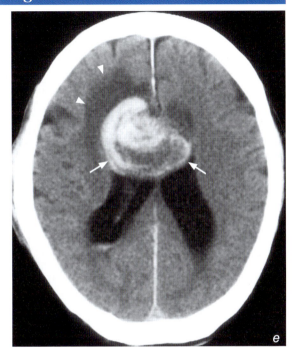

Fig.9e Non-contrast axial CT showing a heterogeneous collection of blood in the region of the corpus callosum (arrows), extending across the midline with associated white matter oedema (arrowheads). Note the mass effect on the lateral ventricles. The appearances are suggestive of haemorrhage into a tumour of the corpus callosum and a contrast enhanced CT/MRI is indicated for further evaluation.

Fig.9f Non-contrast axial CT brain of a different patient shows acute haematomata (arrows) in both fronto-parietal regions with peri-focal oedema. There is also general effacement of all cerebral sulci suggesting more extensive cerebral oedema. Note that the haematomata lie close to the superior sagittal sinus (arrowheads).

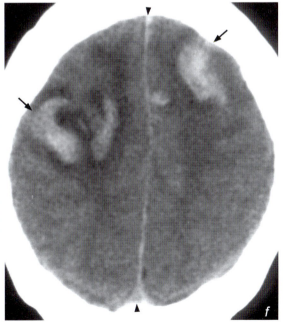

02 CENTRAL NERVOUS SYSTEM

101

Intracerebral haemorrhage

- CT scan may show a thrombus (Fig. 9g) or a contrast filling defect in the adjacent sinus (termed the 'delta sign' for the superior sagittal sinus) with/without outward bowing of sinus wall.

- The venous phase of a cerebral angiogram (Fig. 9h) is currently the gold standard for diagnosing venous sinus thrombosis but it is an invasive procedure. Multi-detector CT venography shows promising potential (Fig. 9i).

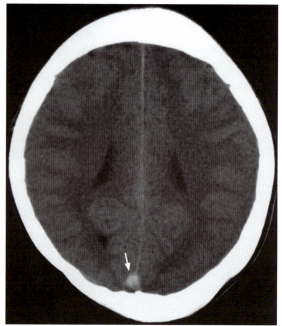

Fig. 9g *Non-contrast axial CT shows a hyperdense triangular thrombus (arrow) in the posterior aspect of the superior sagittal sinus (Courtesy of Dr Judy Lam, Department of Diagnostic Radiology & Organ Imaging, PWH, Hong Kong).*

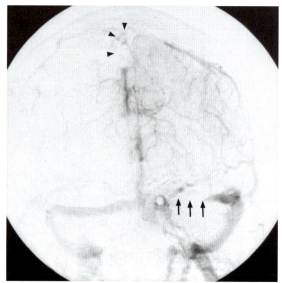

Fig.9h *Cerebral venogram frontal view showing multiple filling defects along the superior sagittal sinus (arrowheads) and left transverse sinus (arrows) in keeping with venous sinus thrombosis.*

Intracerebral haemorrhage

- MR venogram offers a radiation-free alternative. The technique relies on a loss of   flow-related signal within the venous sinus for diagnosis (Fig. 9i) or the presence of a filling defect (Fig. 9k, l).

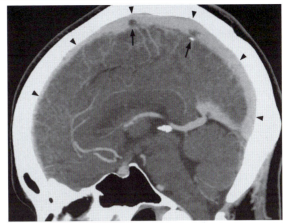

Fig.9i *Multi-detector CT venography clearly delineates the superior sagittal sinus (arrowheads) with filling defect within (arrows).*

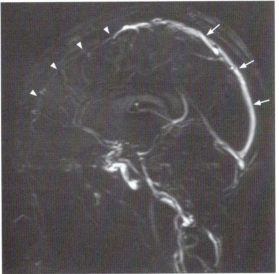

Fig.9j *MR venogram of a different patient with thrombosis involving the anterior aspect of the superior sagittal sinus. This MRI sequence relies on the normal flow of venous blood in the veins and sinuses to produce signal (arrows). In this patient, there is a lack of flow (therefore no signal, arrowheads) in the anterior aspect of the superior sagittal sinus indicating thrombosis.*

Intracerebral haemorrhage

Note:

(1) Chronic uncontrolled hypertension is the most common cause of intracerebral haemorrhage.

(2) Patients with intracerebral infarcts and intracerebral haemorrhage may have a similar presentation and clinical signs. A CT scan is necessary to differentiate the two prior to starting any treatment.

(3) Atypical location/ appearance of the haemorrhage may prompt further investigation to exclude other causes.

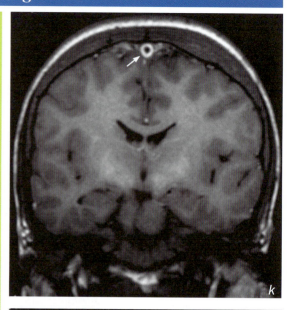

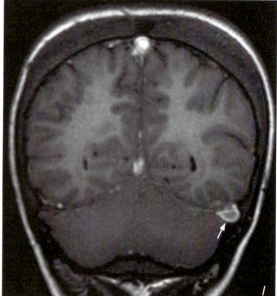

Fig. 9k, l *Contrast enhanced coronal T1W MR images show a filling defect (arrow) within the superior sagittal sinus (Fig. 9k) and left transverse sinus (Fig. 9l) (Courtesy of Dr Judy Lam, Department of Diagnostic Radiology & Organ Imaging, PWH, Hong Kong).*

Discussion Case 10
Pituitary macroadenoma

Pituitary macroadenoma (Fig. 10a, b) with suprasellar extension and compression of optic chiasm.

- Patients with a visual field defect due to a large pituitary tumour require surgical decompression. The chance of recovery of vision depends on the time lapse since the visual field defect began. The chance of a full recovery is remote in patients who have been symptomatic for a longer time (4 months).

Discussion:
- Pituitary adenomas
  - The most common sellar/juxtasellar mass
  - Microadenoma (<10 mm): often endocrinologically functional
  - Macroadenoma (>10 mm): often endocrinologically nonfunctional
- Patients may present with:
  - Endocrine symptoms
  - Mass effect: bitemporal hemianopia due to compression of optic chiasm
  - Pituitary gland compression resulting in hypopituitarism
  - Pituitary apoplexy: sudden haemorrhage into a pituitary adenoma causing headache and visual disturbance
  - CT is unable to identify small pituitary microadenomas.
  - Large pituitary tumours can be seen on CT scans (Fig.10c); however, MRI is the investigation of choice for pituitary lesions.
  - MR is far superior to CT in defining the extent of tumour, its adjacent relationships, associated complications and post-treatment follow up/evaluation.

MRI appearances of a pituitary macroadenoma:
- · Intermediate T1W and T2W signal
- · Heterogeneous signal if there is a haemorrhagic or cystic component (Fig. 10d)

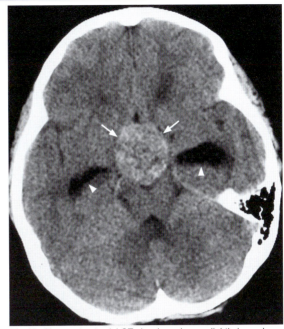

Fig.10c *Non-contrast axial CT showing a large, slightly hyperdense mass (arrows) in the region of the pituitary fossa. Note the dilatation of the temporal/inferior horns (arrowheads) of the lateral ventricles suggesting obstructive hydrocephalus due to the mass. A MRI is the investigation of choice for further evaluation.*

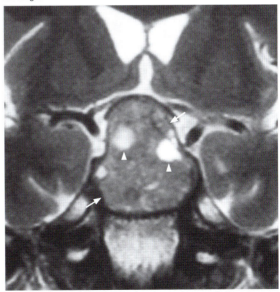

Fig.10d *Coronal T2W MR showing a large pituitary tumour (arrows) with suprasellar extension, compression of optic chiasm with heterogeneous signal intensity. The focal area of high signal (arrowheads) represents cystic/necrotic change.*

105

Pituitary macroadenoma

- Enhances following injection of gadolinium (Fig. 10e), except for cystic (Fig. 10f), necrotic or haemorrhagic components
- There may be superior extension into suprasellar cistern, compression of optic chiasma (causing visual field defects) and floor of 3rd ventricle (causing proximal hydrocephalus)
- May invade the cavernous sinus and encase intracavernous portion of internal carotid artery

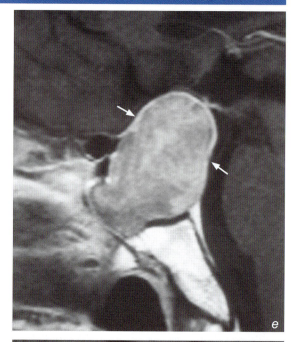

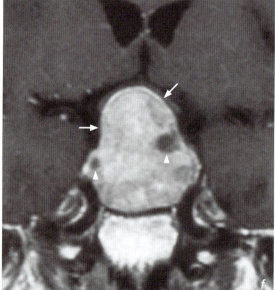

Fig. 10e,f *Post-gadolinium enhanced T1W sagittal and coronal scans showing uniform enhancement of the large pituitary macroadenoma (arrows) with focal non-enhancing areas (arrowheads) within, suggestive of cystic/necrotic change. Same patient as in Fig.10d.*

Pituitary macroadenoma

MRI appearances of pituitary microadenoma:

- Hypointense or isointense on non-contrast T1W images
- May cause mild asymmetry or deviation of the infundibular stalk
- Following injection of gadolinium there is absent (Fig. 10g) or delayed enhancement of the microadenoma compared to the rest of the pituitary gland.

Incidental finding of small cysts or non-functioning microadenomas is common and usually of no clinical significance

Empty sella syndrome

- Following involution of a pituitary neoplasm or an enlarged pituitary gland (Sheehan's syndrome in pregnancy), the sella turcica communicates with the subarachnoid space (thus subjected to normal CSF pulsation). The pituitary gland may be pushed inferiorly giving the sella an empty appearance (Fig. 10h).

Note:
(1) MRI is the investigation of choice for pituitary lesions.
(2) Microadenomas (<10 mm) are often endocrinologically functional.
(3) Macroadenomas (>10 mm) are often endocrinologically non-functional and present with signs and symptoms caused by an enlarging mass.

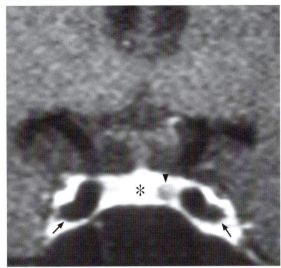

Fig.10g *Coronal T1W dynamic MR scans following gadolinium injection show a small, well-defined non-enhancing lesion (arrowhead) in the pituitary gland on the left. Note the intense enhancement of the normal pituitary gland (asterisk). Arrows indicate the tip of the ICA on both sides.*

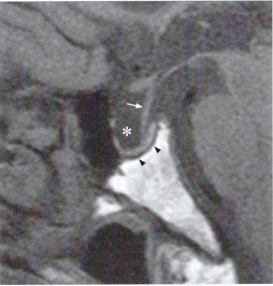

Fig.10h *Sagittal T1W MRI shows most of the sella contains CSF (asterisk). The pituitary gland is pushed postero-inferiorly (arrowheads). The infundibulum (arrow) is displaced posteriorly and extends to the floor of the sella (the 'infundibulum sign').*

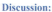
Discussion Case 11
Multiple sclerosis

Multiple sclerosis (Fig. 11a, b)
In view of the patient's history (optic neuritis and multiple episodes of remitting and relapsing sensory and motor symptoms) and high signal periventricular lesions on MR, the most likely diagnosis is multiple sclerosis.

The lesions in the corpus callosum represent areas of demyelination and similar lesions/plaques may also be found in the optic nerves (Fig. 11c) and the spinal cord (Fig.11d).

Discussion:
Multiple sclerosis:
- Autoimmune demyelinating disease with a typical history of multiple focal neurological deficits with a remitting and relapsing course
- Symptoms depend on anatomical location of lesions but visual loss, gait and sensory disturbances are common

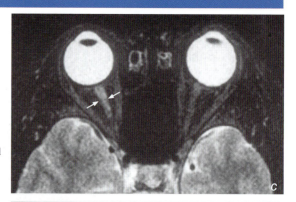

Fig.11c Axial T2W fat suppressed MR scan of the orbit shows a high signal demyelination plaque (arrows) in the right optic nerve in a patient with multiple sclerosis.

Fig.11d Sagittal T2W MR of the spine showing a high signal demyelinating plaque (arrows) in the cervical cord (C2-5) in a patient with multiple sclerosis (Courtesy of Dr Wynnie Lam, Department of Diagnostic Radiology and Organ Imaging, The Chinese University of Hong Kong).

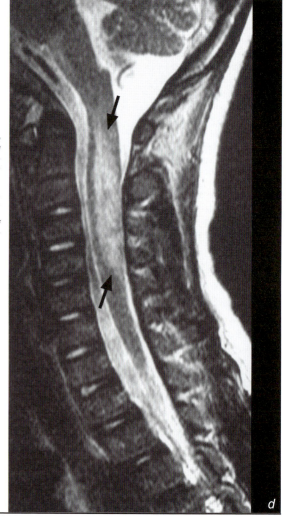

Multiple sclerosis

MRI is the imaging investigation of choice for multiple sclerosis:

1. Plaques are usually multiple and may be found anywhere in the CNS
2. On T1W scans inactive plaques show low signal intensity and do not enhance following the injection of gadolinium. The enhancement in active plaques is variable and may be homogeneous, heterogeneous or ring-like (Fig. 11e, f)

Fig.11e,f *Axial T1W MR scans before (e) and after (f) gadolinium showing a small, low signal intensity lesion (arrowhead) in the medulla oblongata which enhances (arrowhead, f) following the injection of gadolinium in a patient with multiple sclerosis. The enhancement suggests it is an active plaque.*

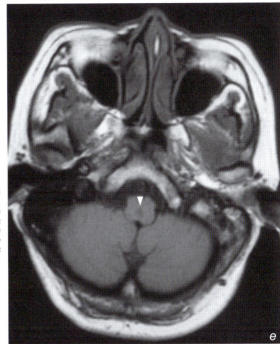

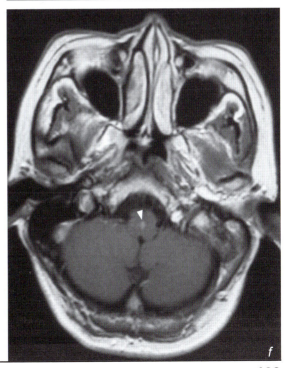

Multiple sclerosis

3. Plaques show high signal on FLAIR (Fig. 11g) and T2W images (Fig. 11h) and typically appear as oblong, elliptical lesions at the callososeptal interface and subependymal periventricular white matter extending into the deep white matter (Dawson's fingers).

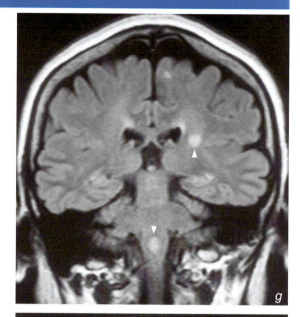

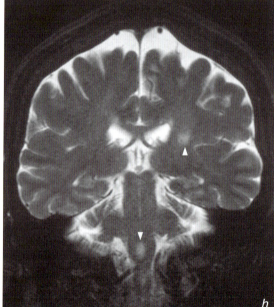

Fig.11g,h Coronal FLAIR (g) and T2W (h) scans showing the high signal plaques (arrowheads) in a patient with multiple sclerosis.

Multiple sclerosis

Ischaemic/inflammatory change and other causes of demyelination also appear as focal or multiple areas of high signal on FLAIR and (Fig. 11i) T2W scans (Fig. 11j, k), in the periventricular region. The diagnosis of multiple sclerosis therefore depends on a combination of clinical, laboratory and imaging findings.

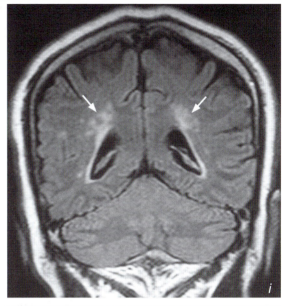

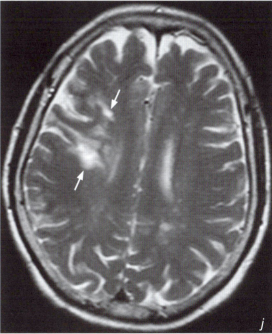

Fig.11i,j *Coronal FLAIR (i) and axial T2W (j) MR scans showing high signal lesions in the periventricular areas (arrows). In this patient they represent areas of ischaemia and may mimic the lesions seen in multiple sclerosis. It is therefore important to correlate the clinical picture with the imaging in order to diagnose multiple sclerosis.*

Discussion Case 11
Multiple sclerosis

Note:
(1) Although MR can demonstrate plaques in multiple sclerosis the diagnosis depends on a combination of clinical, laboratory and imaging findings.
(2) MR is also used for monitoring treatment response.

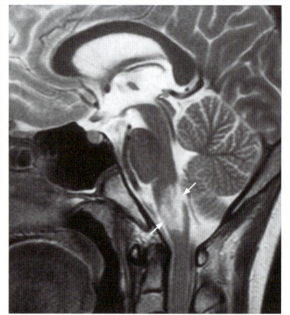

Fig.11k *Sagittal T2W MRI of a patient with brainstem encephalitis showing a high signal lesion (arrows) in the brainstem.*

Meningioma

Meningioma (Fig. 12a, b and c)

- In view of its extra-axial location, dense calcification, close relationship to the tentorium cerebelli and enhancement of the adjacent dura, the diagnosis is a meningioma.

Discussion:

- Meningioma is the most common extra-axial intracranial tumour with a predilection for elderly females
- Location: majority are supratentorial–cerebral convexity, parasagittal, sphenoid ridge; infratentorial–cerebellar convexity, tentorium cerebelli, cerebellopontine angle
- CT appearances: well-defined, may be calcified hyperdense mass with wide attachment to adjacent dura and intense homogeneous enhancement; hyperostosis of adjacent skull may be seen
- MRI appearances: hypointense/isointense on T1-weighted images and isointense/hyperintense on T2-weighted images with intense contrast enhancement
- 'dural tail' sign: curvilinear enhancement tapering off from the tumour margin along dural surface (Fig. 12d)
- Meningiomas are almost always supplied by the external carotid artery and may be complicated by local invasion into the venous sinuses (Fig. 12e)

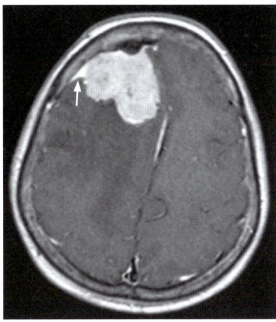

Fig.12d Post-contrast T1-weighted axial MR scan showing a large meningioma with a dural tail (arrow)

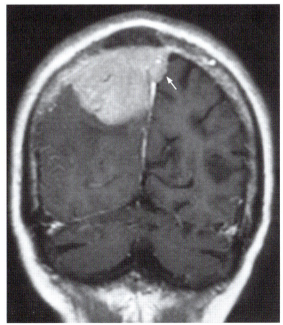

Fig.12e. Post-contrast T1-weighted coronal MR scan showing a large meningioma with invasion into the sagittal sinus (arrow)

Meningioma

- Simple meningiomas do not demonstrate significant peritumoural oedema in contrast to other aggressive lesions.
- Meningiomas show intense homogeneous enhancement unlike some of the other tumours such as glioma (Fig. 12f) and lymphoma.

Note:

(1) Meningioma is the most common extra-axial intracranial tumour.
(2) Has a predilection for elderly females.
(3) Calcification, intense contrast enhancement and dural tail sign are characteristic.

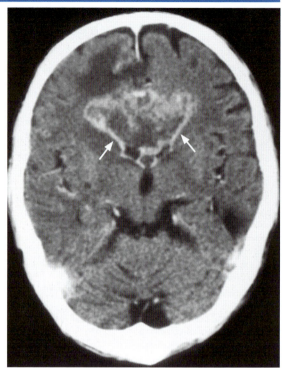

Fig.12f *Post-contrast axial CT showing an ill-defined heterogeneously enhancing glioma in the corpus callosum (arrows). Note the peritumoural oedema.*

Discussion Case 13
Astrocytoma

Discussion:

- Brain tumours can be classified by location (supratentorial and infratentorial) or histology (glioma, lymphoma etc.). Primary tumours in adults are most commonly supratentorial. The most common form of the supratentorial primary tumour is astrocytoma. Glioblastoma multiforme is the most malignant form of all gliomas.
- Spread by direct extension along the white matter tracts, subependymal, CSF or haematogenous
- Imaging findings on CT (Fig. 13c-d):
  1. Inhomogeneous low-density mass with irregular shape and poor-defined margins
  2. Associated central necrosis and peritumoural vasogenic oedema
  3. Considerable mass effect with compression on the ventricles and brain parenchyma
  4. Rarely calcifies

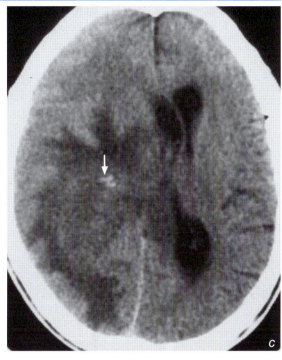

Fig.13c *Non-contrast axial CT showing an isodense mass lesion with ill-defined margins present in the right parietal lobe associated with significant vasogenic oedema. The mass shows considerable mass effect with midline shift to the left, compression on the left lateral ventricle and effacement of the sulci. Spots of calcification are present within the mass lesion (arrow).*

Fig.13d *Post-contrast axial CT showing the mass lesion has predominantly peripheral contrast enhancement. The medial wall of the tumour shows ill-defined margins.*

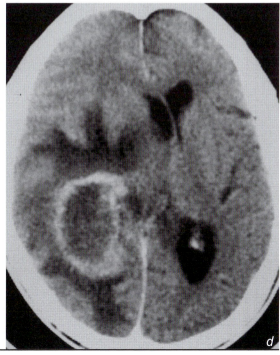

Discussion Case 13
Astrocytoma

- Imaging findings on MR (Fig. 13e-g)
  1. Mass lesion with significant mass effect and vasogenic oedema, same as CT findings.
  2. The tumour can contain haemosiderin and haemorrhage deposits.

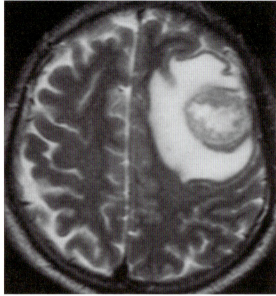

Fig.13e *Axial T2W MRI image showing a roundish heterogeneous lesion in the left frontal lobe with significant surrounding vasogenic oedema and effacement of the adjacent sulci.*

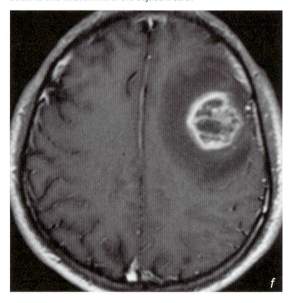

Astrocytoma

- Brain tumours are usually located in the cerebral hemispheres, but can also be present in the corpus callosum (Fig. 13h, i), brainstem (Fig. 13j, k), posterior cranial fossa (Fig. l-o) and even extra-axial in location.

Fig.13f, g Axial (f) and coronal (g) with gadolinium T1W MRI images showing the mass lesion with irregular wall and heterogeneous contrast enhancement. Surrounding vasogenic oedema with no contrast enhancement is present around the lesion. Associated mass effect with midline shift and compression on the frontal horn of left lateral ventricle (arrow).

Fig.13h Non-contrast axial CT showing a heterogeneous mass lesion with ill-defined margins present in the frontal lobe, splaying out and compressing on the frontal horns of the bilateral and lateral ventricles. Features are suggestive of callosal origin, showing a butterfly appearance. There is associated mild peritumoural vasogenic oedema.

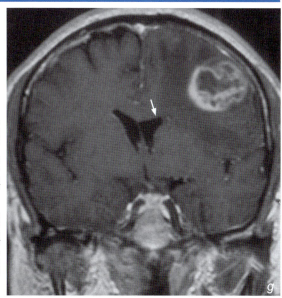

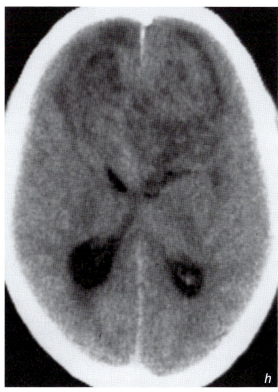

Discussion Case 13
Astrocytoma

Fig.13i *Post-contrast axial CT showing the mass lesion has heterogeneous contrast enhancement. The mass shows irregular and poorly defined margin.*

Fig.13j *Coronal FLAIR T2W MRI image shows a glioma with high signal intensity present in the midbrain (arrow).*

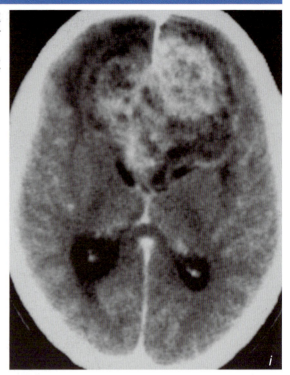

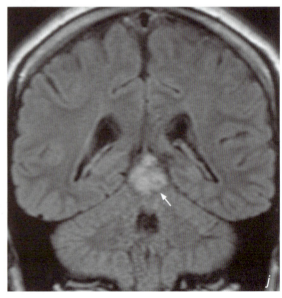

Astrocytoma

Fig.13k *Sagittal T1W with gadolinium MRI image shows the glioma has moderate contrast enhancement present in the tectal plate of the midbrain (arrows). Associated mass effect with compression on the aqueduct causes mild dilatation of the lateral ventricle.*

Fig.13l *Non-contrast axial CT showing a well-defined midline vermian hyperdense mass in the posterior cranial fossa. The tumour encroaches on the fourth ventricle (arrow) with hydrocephalus as evident by dilated temporal horns (open arrows). A tiny hyperdense nodule (arrowhead) is present in the third ventricle which is suspicious of subependymal metastasis.*

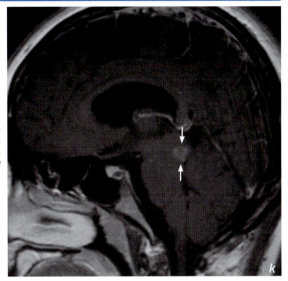
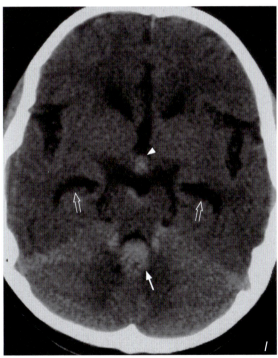

Astrocytoma

Fig.13m *Post-contrast axial CT showing the mass lesion has intense homogeneous contrast enhancement. The tiny hyperdense nodule also shows mild contrast enhancement. Another tiny nodule on the left which is not evident on the non-contrast axial CT image is now enhanced and compatible with the subependymal metastasis (arrow). Biopsy proven medulloblastoma with subependymal spread.*

Fig.13n *Axial T1W with gadolinium image of the same patient in Fig. 16m also shows intense contrast enhancement of the medulloblastoma in the vermis. Significant linear enhancement of the quadrigeminal cisterns (arrows) suggestive of direct invasion by medulloblastoma.*

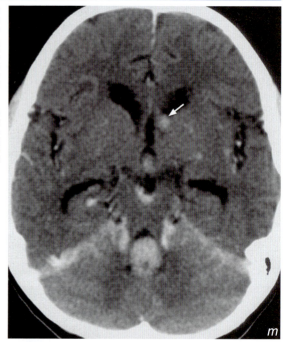

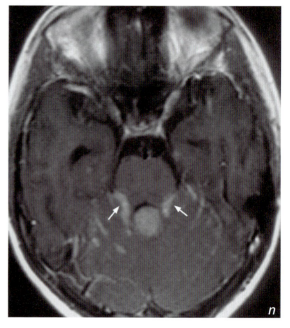

Astrocytoma

Fig.13o *Coronal T1W with gadolinium image showing the invasion of the roof of the fourth ventricle (arrows) on top of the tumour mass in the vermis. Tumour deposit is also present in the right lateral ventricle (open arrow).*

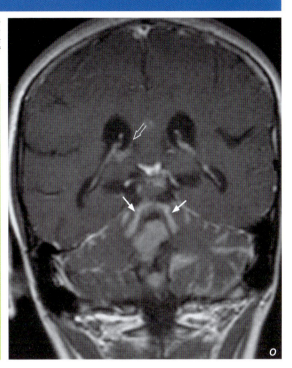

Note:
(1) Primary brain tumours in adults are most commonly supra-tentorial.
(2) The neoplasm may induce considerable surrounding oedema which in turn results in significant mass effect and symptoms.
(3) Imaging is crucial for determining the size, location and mass effect of these lesions.

VASCULAR

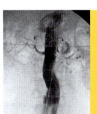

Contributors:

**Simon S.M. Ho, Gregory E. Antonio,
Simon C.H. Yu, Stella S.Y. Ho**

Questions

Case 1 - 11   124 - 134

Discussion

Ruptured intracranial aneurysm   135 - 138
Carotid artery stenosis   139 - 140
Abdominal aortic aneurysm   141 - 143
Iliac artery stenosis   144 - 145
Occlusion of superficial femoral artery   146 - 148
Dissecting abdominal aortic aneurysm   149 - 152
Gastrointestinal bleeding   153 - 155
Renal artery stenosis   156 - 159
Ruptured hepatocellular carcinoma   160 - 161
Deep vein thrombosis   162 - 164
Superior vena cava obstruction/syndrome   165 - 167

Chapter 03

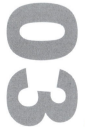

Case 1

A 35-year-old man presents to the Accident & Emergency Department with acute onset headache and vomiting. Clinical examination reveals reduction in level of consciousness with a GCS of 12/15. A CT brain was performed as an initial investigation (Fig. 1a, b).

Questions
(1) What abnormalities are seen on this non-contrast CT scan ?
  - A small amount of hyperdense (indicating its relatively recent nature) blood is seen in the basal cistern surrounding the left side of the pons and in the left Sylvian fissure.
  - The temporal horns are prominent for patient's age and the development of early hydrocephalus has to be considered.
(2) What is the most likely diagnosis ?

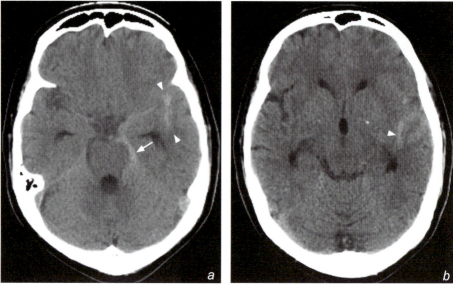

Fig.1a, b *Hyperdense acute subarachnoid haemorrhage is seen in the basal cistern around the left side of the pons (arrow) and in the left Sylvian fissure (arrowheads). This suggests that the site of bleeding is likely to be on the left side. Note the early dilatation of the third ventricle and the temporal/inferior horns of the lateral ventricle.*

Case 2

A 70-year-old man presents with recurrent episodes of transient ischaemic attacks and a confirmed episode of retinal infarct on the left despite the use of aspirin. A Duplex Doppler was performed on his left internal carotid artery (Fig. 2a).

Questions

(1) <u>What abnormality has been demonstrated and what is the diagnosis ?</u>

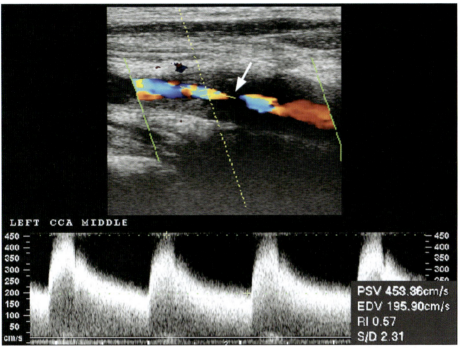

LEFT CCA MIDDLE

PSV 453.36cm/s
EDV 195.90cm/s
RI 0.57
S/D 2.31

Fig.2a *A longitudinal Duplex colour Doppler sonogram showing a stenosis (arrow) in the left common carotid artery.*

Case 3

A 70-year-old man, a smoker with a history of myocardial infarction, presents with a pulsatile mass in the abdomen. An ultrasound (Fig. 3a, b) followed by a contrast CT (Fig. 3c, d) of the abdomen were performed.

Questions

(1) <u>What are the abnormalities shown on ultrasound and CT ?</u>

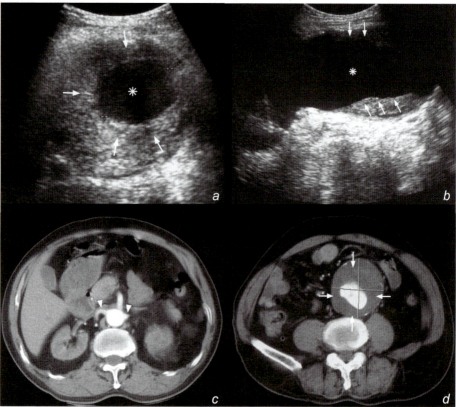

Fig.3a, b *Transverse (a) and longitudinal (b) ultrasound images of an abdominal aorta with mural thrombus (arrows). Note the true aortic lumen (asterisk)*

Fig.3c, d *Two axial images of a contrast enhanced CT scan of an infrarenal abdominal aorta with mural thrombus (arrows). Note the lack of involvement at the level of the renal arteries (arrowheads)*

Case 4

A 48-year-old man who has been smoking 30 cigarettes a day for over 25 years presents with a 3 year history of increasing bilateral buttock claudication worse on the right side with a claudication distance of 100 – 200 m. An arteriogram of the lower limbs was performed (Fig. 4a).

Questions

(1) What abnormalities are present on this investigation ?
- Bilateral proximal common iliac arteries stenoses, likely to be caused by atheromatous plaques.
- The right external iliac artery also appears more narrowed than the left.
(2) What risk factors for this condition should you extract from your history taking and what do you expect to find when you examine this patient's femoral pulses ?

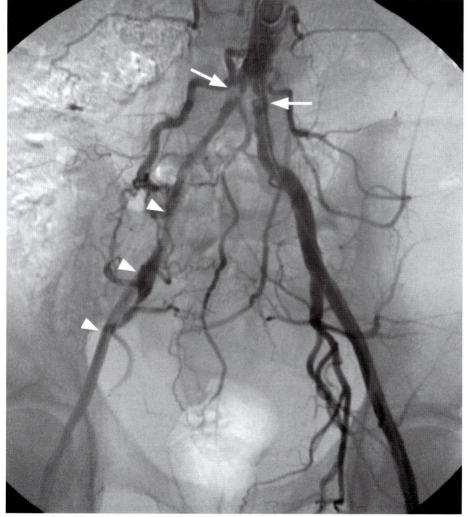

Fig.4a Digital subtraction angiogram (DSA) of the iliac arteries showing bilateral proximal common iliac stenoses (arrows) and a relatively narrowed right external iliac artery (arrowheads).

Case 5

A 65-year-old man with diabetes, hyperlipidaemia and ischaemic heart disease presents with a two year history of right calf claudication. A gadolinium contrast enhanced MR angiogram of the lower limb arteries was performed (Fig. 5a).

Questions

(1) What is the main abnormality demonstrated on this investigation ?

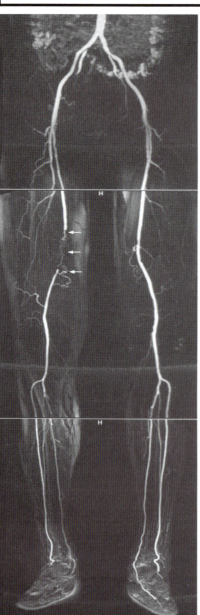

Fig.5a A multistation gadolinium enhanced magnetic resonance angiogram of the lower limb arteries showing a right superficial femoral artery occlusion (arrows).

Case 6

A 70-year-old man with a known history of hypertension presents to the Accident and Emergency Department with acute onset epigastric/upper abdominal pain radiating to the back. An urgent ultrasound examination of the abdomen was performed (Fig. 6a).

Questions

(1) <u>What is the abnormality shown on this examination ?</u>

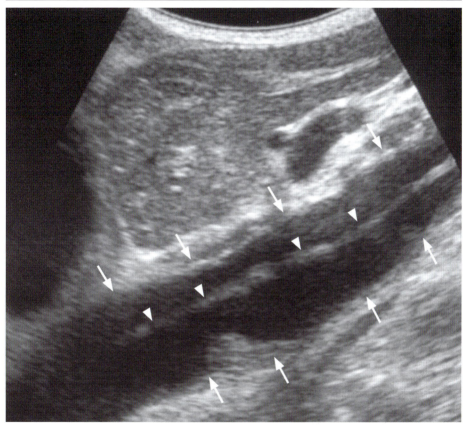

Fig.6a *Longitudinal sonogram of the abdominal aorta with a dissection flap (arrowheads) seen within the abdominal aorta (arrows).*

Case 7

An 86-year-old man presents with gastrointestinal bleeding and chronic anaemia. Upper GI endoscopy and colonoscopy done previously and on this admission failed to identify the source of bleeding. Patient continued to pass tarry stools. A Technetium (Tc-99m) labelled red cell (RBC) scan was performed (Fig. 7a, b).

Questions

(1) What abnormalities are shown on Figure 7a and b ?

Fig. 7a, b Tc-99m labelled red cell scan.

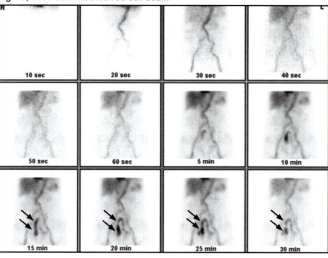

Fig.7a Dynamic images taken at 5 min show abnormal tracer accumulation (arrows) in a loop of bowel, most probably distal small bowel.

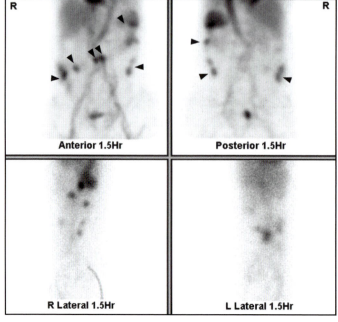

Fig.7b Delayed images taken at 1.5 hr show transit of the isotope into the large bowel (arrowheads).

Case 8

A 55-year-old man presents with a history of hypertension that is becoming more difficult to control despite the use of three antihypertensive drugs over the last two years. Clinical examination reveals a vascular bruit in the region of the right kidney. Renal function is normal. An MRI and MR angiogram of the renal arteries was performed (Fig. 8a, b).

Questions
(1) <u>What abnormalities are seen on these coronal MRI images (Fig. 8a, b) ?</u>

Fig.8a, b MRI and MRA of the kidneys.

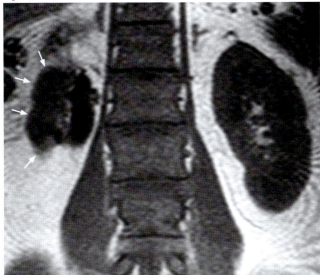

Fig.8a Coronal T1 weighted MRI through the kidneys showing marked reduction in size of the right kidney (arrows) as a result of renal artery stenosis.

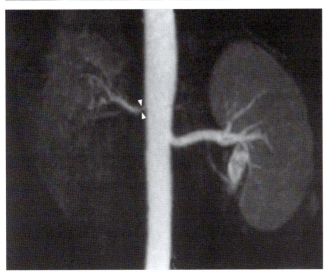

Fig.8b MRA of the renal arteries confirming the presence of a >75% stenosis at the ostium of the right renal artery (arrowheads).

Case 9

A 35-year-old Chinese man, a chronic hepatitis B carrier with a known liver tumour, presents with sudden onset of right upper quadrant pain. Clinical examination reveals sweatiness, pallor, tachycardia with pulse of 120/min, BP 90/60 and guarding over the abdomen. An arterial phase contrast enhanced CT of the abdomen was performed (Fig. 9a, b).

Questions

(1) What abnormalities are seen on this CT ?

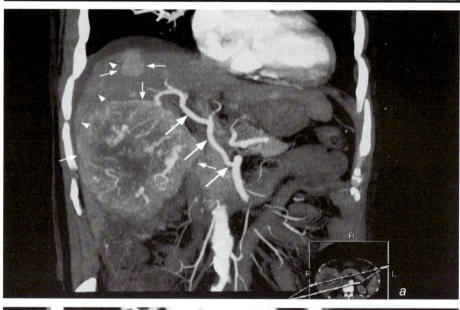

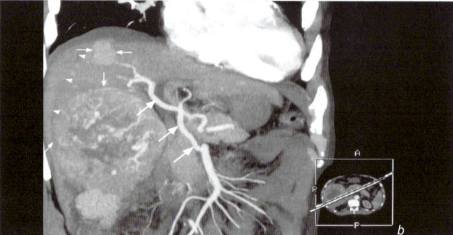

Fig.9a,b *Multifocal HCC with spontaneous rupture. These two coronal oblique multiplanar reformat images show at least one large and one small arterially enhancing hepatocellular carcinomas in the right lobe of the liver (small arrows). Central necrosis is seen in the larger of the two tumours. There is a rim of hyperdense subcapsular haematoma (arrowheads) seen overlying the right lobe of the liver indicative of spontaneous rupture. A replaced right hepatic artery is also shown (large arrows).*

Case 10

A 35-year-old lady with a history of a known pelvic gynaecological malignancy on chemotherapy treatment presents with acute swelling of the left thigh and left calf. A Duplex Doppler of the left lower limb veins has been performed (Fig.10a – Doppler of left common femoral vein, Fig. 10b – Doppler of the left popliteal vein).

Questions

(1) <u>What abnormalities are present on these two images ?</u>

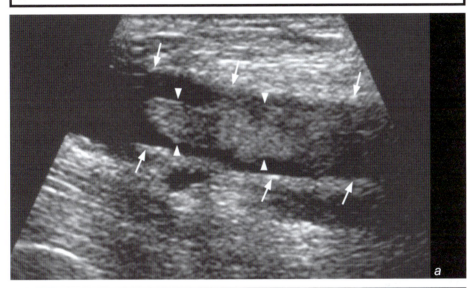

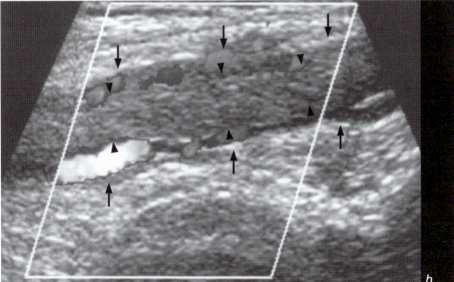

Fig.10a, b *Duplex Doppler ultrasound of deep vein thrombosis. Fig. 10a and b are longitudinal scans of the left common femoral vein (arrows) and left popliteal vein (arrows) respectively. Echogenic thrombus (arrowheads) is seen in both scans.*

Case 11

A 53-year-old heavy smoker for over 30 years presents with dyspnoea, facial and bilateral upper limb swelling, head fullness and light-headedness. Clinical examination reveals venous distension in the chest wall and neck, facial and upper limb oedema. A CT scan of the thorax was performed (Fig. 11a, b, c).

Questions

(1) <u>What abnormalities are present on these images ?</u>

Fig. 11a, b, c CT of the thorax

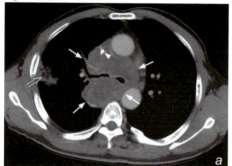

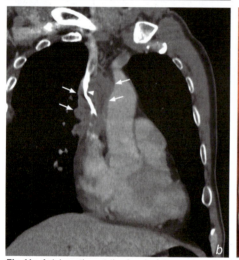
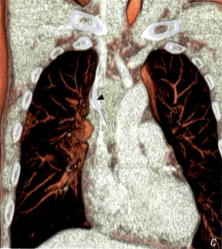

*Fig.11a Axial section at the level of the carina showing a large 10 cm tumour (arrows) encasing the SVC (arrowhead) - narrowing its diameter to 4-5 mm - and encasement of the carina. The tumour abuts the ascending and descending aorta. A wedge shaped area of consolidation is seen peripherally in the right lung (open arrow). **Fig.11b** Coronal oblique multiplanar reformat image showing encasement of the SVC (arrowhead) by the large tumour (arrows). **Fig.11c** Volume rendered reconstruction depicting encasement of the SVC (arrowhead) by the tumour.*

Discussion Case 1
Ruptured intracranial aneurysm

Ruptured intracranial aneurysm (Fig. 1a, b)
- The most likely diagnosis is subarachnoid haemorrhage due to rupture of an intracerebral aneurysm.
- A CT angiography will be useful for assessment of the Circle of Willis. A cerebral angiogram may also be required especially when embolisation of the cerebral aneurysm is to be performed.

Discussion:
- Subarachnoid haemorrhage may be spontaneous or post-traumatic in origin. The most common cause for acute spontaneous subarachnoid haemorrhage in a relatively young patient is rupture of an intracerebral aneurysm.
- Other causes include AV malformation, hypertensive haemorrhage, haemorrhagic tumour, embolic haemorrhagic infarction and bleeding tendencies (including iatrogenic causes such as anticoagulants).
- Acute blood appears relatively high in attenuation on an unenhanced CT brain. The presence of blood should be looked for in all the CSF containing spaces – the basal cistern, suprasellar cistern, quadrigeminal cistern, Sylvian fissures, cerebral sulci and within the ventricles. A normal CT does not entirely exclude a diagnosis of subarachnoid haemorrhage.
- Complications of acute subarachnoid haemorrhage include vasospasm which may lead to infarction, hydrocephalus due to obstruction to CSF flow (in the cerebral aqueduct or outlet of the fourth ventricle) or reduced reabsorption of CSF and mass effect related to the amount of blood present.

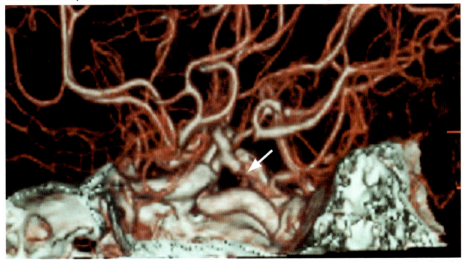

Fig.1c *CT angiography (CTA) of the Circle of Willis of the same patient showing a small aneurysm arising from the meningohypophyseal trunk of the left internal carotid artery(arrow).*

Ruptured intracranial aneurysm

Role of imaging in patients with acute subarachnoid haemorrhage

- Confirm the presence and assess the amount and extent of subarachnoid blood.
- Assess for presence of hydrocephalus or significant mass effect.
- A CT angiogram may demonstrate the exact location of the aneurysm causing the bleeding (Fig. 1c) and act as a guide for neurosurgical (clipping) or endovascular (coiling) intervention. Digital subtraction angiography is still considered the 'gold standard' for the diagnosis of intracerebral aneurysms (Fig. 1d) and is particularly useful when embolisation of the aneurysm is to be performed. The most commonly used embolic agent for intracerebral aneurysms are detachable coils (Fig. 1e). A cerebral angiogram, however, carries a 1% risk of producing a stroke in the patient (from distal emboli, dissection or induction of vasospasm).

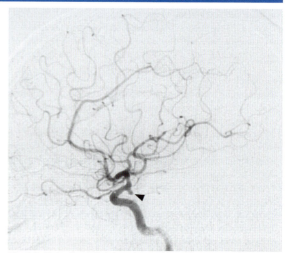

Fig.1d *Selective left internal carotid angiogram confirming the presence of the aneurysm (arrowhead) shown on CTA.*

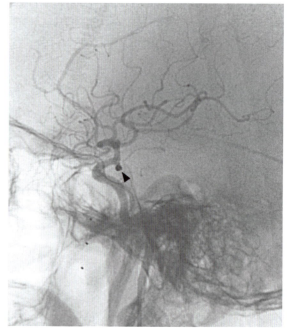

Fig.1e *Post-embolisation image showing complete occlusion of the main bulk of the aneurysm by detachable coils (arrowhead) with preservation of flow through the left internal carotid artery.*

Ruptured intracranial aneurysm

Fig.1f, g *Pre- and post-contrast enhanced scan of another patient with subarachnoid haemorrhage showing subarachnoid blood around the Circle of Willis (arrows) with enhancement of an aneurysm in the region of the right middle cerebral artery (arrowhead). Note the early dilatation of both temporal/inferior horns of the lateral ventricles.*

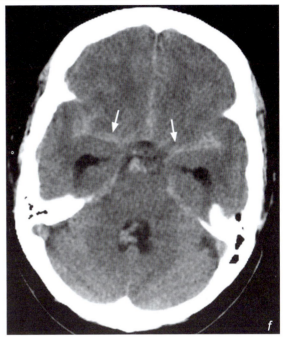

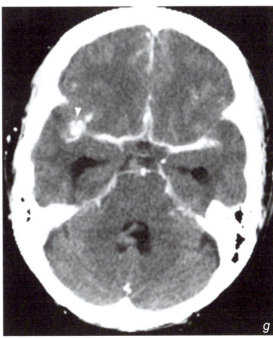

03 VASCULAR

Discussion Case 1
Ruptured intracranial aneurysm

Note:

(1) While CT brain scan is useful for detection of subarachnoid haemorrhage, a normal study does not entirely exclude the diagnosis.

(2) A CT angiogram of the Circle of Willis may be useful for identifying intracerebral aneurysms.

(3) Digital subtraction cerebral angiography remains the gold standard for diagnosis of intracerebral aneurysms, and embolisation by detachable coils has become a widely used treatment option.

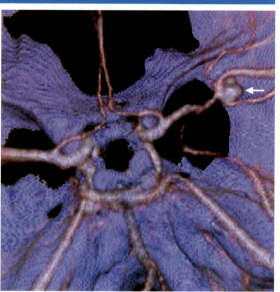

Fig.1h CTA of the patient in Fig. 1f and g showing a 2 cm aneurysm (arrow) centred over the first division of the right middle cerebral artery. Note that the right middle cerebral artery is seen on the left side of the image as this gives the neurosurgeon's perspective observing from cranial to caudally.

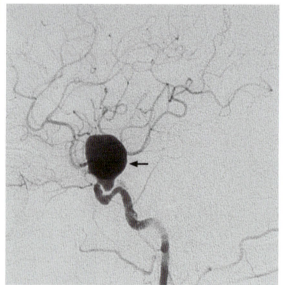

Fig.1i An example of a larger aneurysm (arrow) arising from the distal internal carotid artery.

Discussion Case 2
Carotid artery stenosis

Carotid artery stenosis (Fig. 2a)
- There is a short segment narrowing in the left internal carotid artery suggesting ICA stenosis.
- Treatment is normally recommended if there is a >70% stenosis in the internal carotid artery or the common carotid artery. The two options currently available are carotid endarterectomy and carotid artery stenting.

Discussion:
- High grade internal carotid and common carotid stenoses are associated with increased risk for transient ischaemic attacks and stroke from carotid occlusion or emboli from the site of stenosis.
- The European Carotid Surgery Trial (ECST) and the North American Symptomatic Endarterectomy Trial (NASCET) have shown significant reduction of ipsilateral stroke in treated patients with high grade stenosis and have recommended >80% and >=70% diameter stenosis as their threshold for surgery respectively.
- Carotid artery stenting is an alternative to surgical treatment for treatment of symptomatic carotid stenosis. With the refinement of stenting techniques, increasing experience of the operators and the routine use of cerebral protection devices, the results from carotid stenting are similar to those of surgery. Carotid stenting is associated with a high technical success rate of up to 99% and 30 days stroke or death rate has been reported between 3 and 7%.

Fig. 2b shows a selective angiogram of the left common carotid artery demonstrating a complex atheromatous stenotic segment at the origin of the left internal carotid artery (arrows) - the narrowest portion has a >90% diameter stenosis.

Fig. 2c shows the post-stenting angiogram after a self expanding metallic stent (arrows) has been placed from the common carotid artery across the stenotic segment into the proximal left internal carotid artery with good results.

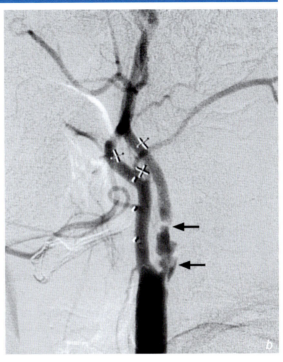

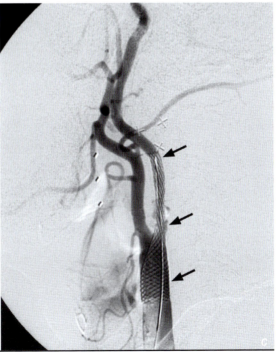

Carotid artery stenosis

Role of imaging in carotid artery stenosis

- The role of Duplex Doppler ultrasound in the imaging of extracranial common carotid and internal carotid stenotic disease is well established.
- MRA and CTA will play an increasingly crucial role in the non-invasive assessment of carotid artery stenosis, especially when the intracranial portions of the internal carotid arteries are not accessible by ultrasound.
- Diagnostic digital subtraction angiography carries a < 1% chance of causing a stroke (from embolic complications or dissection) and is usually reserved for difficult cases after all non-invasive options have been exhausted or done as part of an interventional procedure.

Note:

(1) High grade stenoses in the common carotid artery and the internal carotid artery are associated with increased risk of transient ischaemic attacks and stroke.

(2) Most institutions would recommend surgical or endovascular intervention when stenoses within the common carotid artery or internal carotid artery are >= 70% in symptomatic patients.

(3) Duplex Doppler ultrasound, MRA and CTA are all possible non-invasive methods for assessing the common and internal carotid arteries. The latter two imaging modalities have the capability to image the intracranial portions of the internal carotid arteries.

(4) Carotid artery stenting is now becoming an alternative to surgery.

Abdominal aortic aneurysm

Abdominal aortic aneurysm (Fig. 3a-d)
- There is aneurysmal dilatation of the abdominal aorta on both the ultrasound and CT images.
- In the absence of anaesthetics or other contraindications, elective surgery may be considered in this patient as the diameter of the aneurysm exceeds 5.5 cm.

Discussion:
- Focal dilatation of the abdominal aorta of greater than 3 cm is considered aneurysmal. Atherosclerosis is the most common cause accounting for around four-fifths of cases. Other causes include trauma, inflammation/vasculitis and infection.
- Most centres consider 5.5 cm as the cut-off limit for recommending elective surgical or endovascular intervention. The surgical mortality for non-ruptured aneurysm is around 2-4% while the mortality for ruptured aneurysm is around 50%
- Ruptured abdominal aortic aneurysm can be diagnosed on the demonstration of obscuration or anterior displacement of the aneurysm by an irregular, high density mass or collection, which extends into one or both perirenal spaces and, less commonly, pararenal spaces. The psoas muscles may also be obscured (Fig. 3e). Although intravenous contrast is not required for the diagnosis of ruptured aortic aneurysm, contrast enhancement may document active arterial extravasation (Fig. 3f).
- In recent years, endovascular repair has evolved as a plausible alternative to surgical repair in selected patients (Fig. 3g-j)
- Apart from being less traumatic, endovascular repair may be used in patients with poor cardiovascular reserve in whom cross clamping of the aorta from surgical repair may be potentially hazardous.

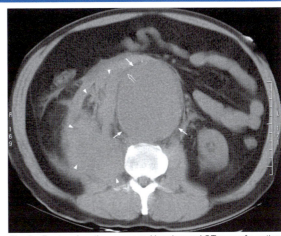

Fig. 3e *Ruptured aortic aneurysm. Unenhanced CT scan of a patient with a 9.5 X 8.0 cm (AP X TS) aortic aneurysm (arrows) which has ruptured. Note the disruption to the wall of the aorta at the 10 o'clock position (open arrow) and the large amount of irregular soft tissue strands representing acute haemorrhage (arrowheads) extending from the right side of the aorta into the right perirenal space and around the right psoas. This patient required urgent surgery straight after the CT scan.*

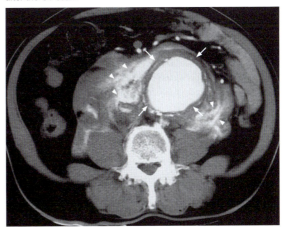

Fig. 3f *Ruptured aortic aneurysm. Contrast enhanced CT scan of a patient with a large aortic aneurysm (arrows) which has ruptured and demonstrates active leakage of the hyperdense contrast (arrowheads) around the aortic aneurysm at the time of scanning. This patient was transferred to the operating theatre for urgent surgery straight after the CT scan.*

141

Abdominal aortic aneurysm

- Follow up CT scanning is mandatory following endovascular repair to rule out endoleaks.

Role of imaging in patients with abdominal aortic aneurysm

- Confirm the diagnosis
- Define the proximal (relationship with renal arteries) and distal (iliac arteries involvement) extent of the aneurysm to determine the site for cross clamping at surgery (supra- or infra-renal in position), the type of surgical graft required, the possibility of endovascular repair.
- In the acute setting, imaging helps to rule out rupture or impending rupture in haemodynamically stable patients. Haemodynamically unstable patients with suspected aortic aneurysm rupture often go straight to the operating theatre and precious minutes are not spent waiting for imaging.
- While ultrasound is good for screening and monitoring of size increase of abdominal aortic aneurysms, CT is the modality of choice for pre-operative and pre-interventional assessment. CT is also the investigation of choice in the haemodynamically stable patients presenting acutely with suspected rupture or leakage of abdominal aortic aneurysm.

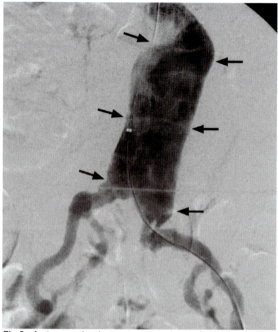

Fig.3g *Aortogram showing an aneurysmal aorta (arrows).*

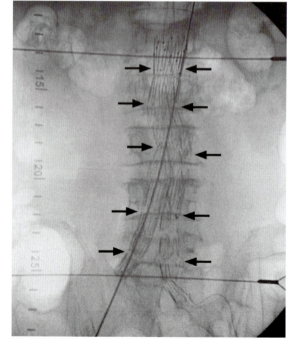

Fig.3h *Full deployment of an endovascular aortic stent graft (arrows) below the origin of the renal arteries.*

Abdominal aortic aneurysm

Fig. 3i *Angiographic image post deployment of the endovascular aortic stent graft showing exclusion of the aneurysm by the stent graft.*

Fig. 3j *A 3D reconstruction of the abdominal aorta from a CT angiogram of the aorta following endovascular repair.*

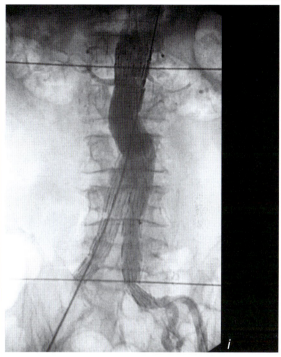

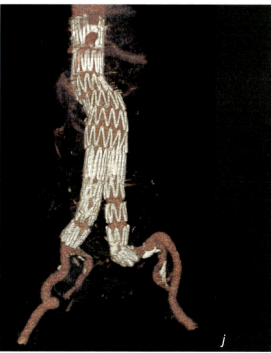

Note:

(1) The abdominal aorta is considered aneurysmal over 3 cm in maximal diameter and elective surgery should be considered in patients with aneurysms over 5.5 cm in diameter.

(2) Ultrasound is useful for confirming the diagnosis and follow up of the size of abdominal aortic aneurysms while CT is the investigation of choice for pre-operative/ pre-endovascular repair assessment. CT is also the investigation of choice for suspected rupture/ aneurysm leakage in the acute setting in the haemodynamically stable patient.

(3) Haemodynamically unstable patients with suspected ruptured aortic aneurysm often go straight to operating theatre rather than waiting for imaging.

Discussion Case 4
Iliac artery stenosis

Iliac artery stenosis (Fig. 4a)
- The patient's femoral pulses are likely to be weak bilaterally, and the patient may have risk factors such as smoking, diabetes, hyperlipidaemia, hypertension and a family history of arterial disease.
- The common iliac arteries and the right external iliac artery are amenable to angioplasty and stenting   (Fig. 4b and c).

Discussion:
- Endovascular treatment for stenotic disease in the iliac segment is highly successful, and the technical success rate from angioplasty and stenting in the iliac segment is around 95-99%.
- For iliac occlusions of less than 5 cm, technical success with endovascular treatment drops to 83%.
- For occlusions greater than 5 cm in length, surgical bypass will be the treatment of choice.
- The 3 and 5 year patency for iliac stenoses angioplasty and stenting are 66% and 74%, and 61% and 72% respectively. The 3 year patency for iliac occlusion angioplasty and stenting are 60% and 64% respectively.
- Endovascular treatment can be repeated should patient again become symptomatic and does not preclude surgical bypass options.
- The possible complications from angioplasty and stenting include:
  1. Major complications (4%):
     a. Distal embolisation
     b. Vessel rupture
     c. Acute occlusion at the site of angioplasty/stenting
  2. Damage to the femoral artery at the arterial puncture site (0.3%)
  3. Groin haematoma from the puncture site (2-3%)
  4. Urgent surgery (1-3%).

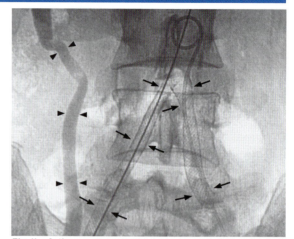

Fig.4b *Self expanding metallic stents (arrows) deployed in both common iliac arteries and in the right external iliac artery . Arrowheads identify the right ureter following excretion of angiographic contrast.*

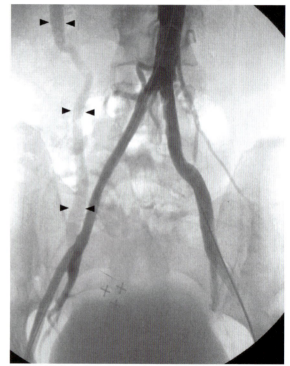

Fig.4c *Digital subtraction angiogram following stenting of both common iliac arteries and the right external iliac artery showing good technical results. Arrowheads identify the right ureter following the excretion of angiographic contrast.*

Iliac artery stenosis

Note:
(1) Endovascular treatment of peripheral vascular disease involving the iliac segment with angioplasty and stenting is highly successful, repeatable and does not preclude surgical bypass options.
(2) Groin haematoma at the puncture site is the most common complication for most angiographic procedures (2-3%).
(3) The overall major complication rate for angioplasty/stenting is around 4% with a need for urgent surgery of around 1-3%.

03 VASCULAR

Occlusion of superficial femoral artery

Occlusion of superficial femoral artery
(Fig. 5a)

- There is an occlusion in the distal right superficial femoral artery just above the region of the adductor canal.
- The patient is likely to have weak / absent popliteal, dorsalis pedis and posterior tibial pulses on the right and normal peripheral pulses on the left.
- The treatment options include exercise therapy, endovascular intervention and surgical bypass.

Discussion:

- Conventional imaging of peripheral vascular disease relied heavily on digital subtraction angiography (DSA) which has the disadvantage of being invasive.
- Duplex Doppler ultrasound (Fig. 5b and c) subsequently emerged to be the widely used non-invasive imaging modality of the peripheral vascular tree. Unfortunately, ultrasound has the disadvantage of being operator dependent, time consuming and imaging of the iliac segments is often suboptimal due to patient's habitus or bowel gas.
- Magnetic resonance angiography (MRA) is becoming the non-invasive investigation of choice for peripheral vascular disease. The entire arterial tree from the iliac arteries to the foot arteries can be assessed on this single examination. Many studies have shown excellent correlation of MRA (Fig. 5d) with DSA (Fig. 5e), and in many centres, DSA is reserved for patients who require endovascular intervention.
- With the increasing use of multidetector CT, CT angiography is also likely to have a role in the assessment of peripheral vascular disease, particularly in patients in whom MRA is either contraindicated or unavailable.
- The majority (75%) of patients with claudication have stable symptoms. Only a minority of patients with limb claudication would progress to

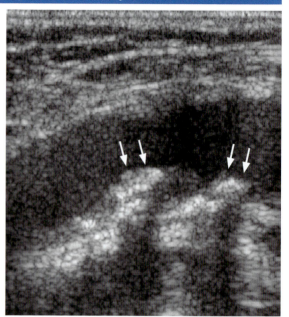

Fig.5b *Grey-scale sonogram of the right external iliac artery with calcified atheromatous plaques (arrows) casting acoustic shadows in the posterior wall of the artery.*

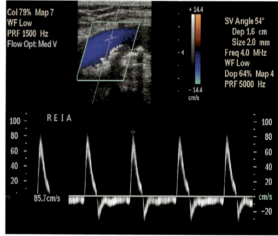

Fig.5c *Colour Doppler flow and spectral Doppler tracing of flow through the right external iliac artery.*

Occlusion of superficial femoral artery

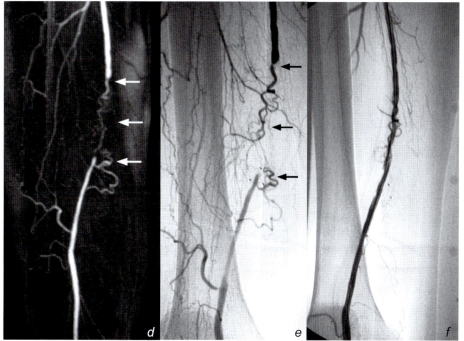

d e f

03 VASCULAR

Fig. 5d, e, f Figure 5d and e shows the correlation between the MRA image and the DSA image of the right superficial femoral artery occlusion (arrows). Fig. 5f shows the DSA image of the right superficial femoral artery post angioplasty with restoration of flow following a successful procedure

critical limb ischaemia – rest pain, ulcers, gangrene and tissue loss, and between 2 and 8% would progress to limb loss.
- In the absence of tissue loss, the decision to perform endovascular intervention or surgical bypass depends on the severity of symptoms and limitation of daily activities. In general, short stenoses and short occlusions (<10 cm not involving the popliteal artery) are amenable to treatment with angioplasty while longer occlusions and diffuse femoropopliteal disease are better treated with surgical bypass.
- The technical success rate for angioplasty of stenotic lesions is around 90-95% while that for occlusions <10 cm is in the region of 60-80%. The long term secondary patency rate of angioplasty for stenoses and occlusions at 5 years are 68% and 35% respectively, with an overall patency rate of around 40% at 5 years. Although this does not compare with the 5 year patency of femoropopliteal bypasses - femoropopliteal vein graft 80%, above-knee femoropopliteal PTFE graft 75% and below knee femoropopliteal PTFE graft 65% - angioplasty is less invasive and does not usually preclude surgical bypass options.
- The use of stents in the femoropopliteal segment is still a controversial issue. While some studies have shown increased immediate technical success and improved long term patency compared with angioplasty, others have shown no significant difference in long term patency.

Role of imaging in patients with peripheral vascular disease
The main goals of imaging in peripheral vascular disease are as follows:
1) Assess severity of disease
  a) Distribution of vessel involvement
  b) Stenoses vs occlusions
  c) Distal run-off

Occlusion of superficial femoral artery

2) Assess suitability for intervention
  a) Endovascular intervention
  b) Surgery
3) Improve procedure planning
  a) Antegrade vs retrograde puncture
  b) Angioplasty vs stenting
  c) Transluminal vs subintimal approach
4) Improve informed consent
  a) Stenosis vs occlusions
  b) Chance of success
  c) Distal run-off assessment which relates to the chance of major complications from distal emboli

Note:

(1) Non-invasive methods including Duplex Doppler ultrasound and particularly MRA are increasingly replacing diagnostic DSA as the investigation of choice for the assessment of peripheral vascular disease. CT angiography also has a role to play in patients in whom MRA is either contraindicated or not available.

(2) Angioplasty is the main endovascular intervention option for stenotic and occlusive disease (<10 cm) in the femoropopliteal segment. Although long term patency is not as good as surgical bypass, angioplasty has the advantage of being less invasive, repeatable and does not usually preclude surgical bypass options.

Dissecting abdominal aortic aneurysm

Dissecting abdominal aortic aneurysm
(Fig. 6a)
- The image shows a flap within the abdominal aorta, suggesting a dissecting aortic aneurysm.
- A CT scan of the aorta from the level of the aortic arch down to the level of the aortic bifurcation is indicated for further evaluation.

Discussion:
- Aortic dissection is caused by spontaneous separation of the intima from the adventitia by blood gaining access into the media of the aortic wall and separating it in two. This can be the result of degeneration of the media, increase in haemodynamic forces accentuated by hypertension and stress in the aortic wall as a result of persistent aortic motion secondary to cardiac motion.
- The dissection may extend proximally or distally. Proximal extension may compromise the arch vessels and the coronary arteries. Further proximal dissection can compromise the aortic root and also cause haemopericardium.
- Distal extension may compromise the visceral vessels, renal arteries and even the lower limb arteries.
- Aortic dissection rarely occurs in aortic aneurysms <5 cm in diameter with a peak incidence in patients around 60 years old.
- Predisposing factors include:
Hypertension
Trauma
Aortic valve disease
  - aortic stenosis, bicuspid aortic valve, prosthetic heart valves
Syndromes
  - Marfan, Turner, Ehlers-Danlos

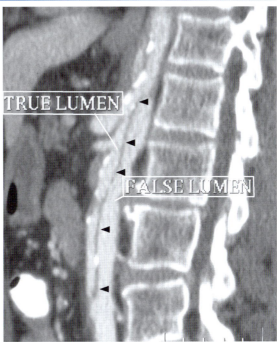

Fig.6b *Sagittal reconstruction from a 16 slice multidetector CT scanner showing dissection of the abdominal aorta. Note the intimal flap (arrowheads) which contains displaced internal calcification separating the true and false lumen.*

03 VASCULAR

Discussion Case 6
Dissecting abdominal aortic aneurysm

- The imaging modality of choice for dissection is CT as it has high sensitivity (87-94%) and specificity (92-100%) for aortic dissection and is readily available in most institutions (Fig. 6b-i).
- The Stanford classification is the most commonly used classification for aortic dissection because of its simplicity. Stanford Type A proximal dissections affect the aorta proximal to the left subclavian artery and usually require urgent surgical management. Stanford Type B distal dissections affect the aorta distal to the left subclavian artery and can usually be managed conservatively.
- Transoesophageal echocardiogram and MRI (Fig. 6j) have similar sensitivities and specificities to CT and may be used instead of CT or in conjunction with CT in some centres. Aortography is seldom performed for the diagnosis of dissection these days. It may be useful for showing the exact site of entry of a dissection if endovascular stenting were to be considered.

Role of imaging in aortic dissection
- Confirm the diagnosis
- Delineate the extent of the dissection, particularly the relationship of the dissection with the left subclavian artery for the Stanford classification.

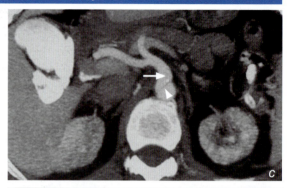

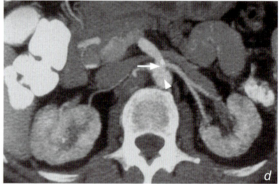

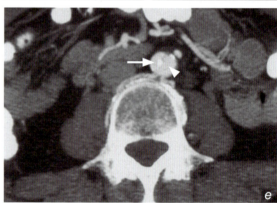

Fig.6c, d, e Axial CT of the same patient (Fig. 6b) at the level of the coeliac axis, renal arteries and infrarenal aorta respectively. The true lumen (arrows) still supplies the coeliac axis and the renal arteries, but its diameter is considerably compromised by the false lumen (arrowheads). The reduction in renal blood flow led to deterioration in renal function in the patient.

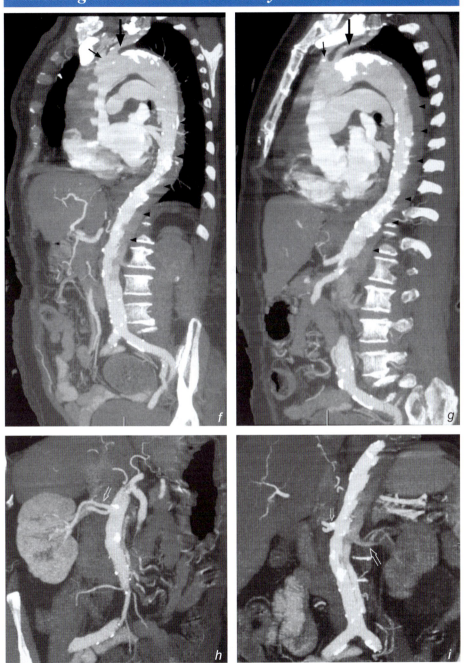

Fig.6f, g, h, i - *Figure 6f, g shows an extensive dissection of the aorta extending proximally from the aortic arch down to the infrarenal aorta. The left subclavian artery (large arrow) and the left common carotid artery (small arrow) appear patent. The false lumen (arrowheads) is thrombosed and note the intimal calcification displacement. Figure 6h, i shows the right renal artery to be supplied by the true lumen (small open arrow) while the left renal artery (large open arrow) is occluded within the thrombosed false lumen.*

Dissecting abdominal aortic aneurysm

Note:

(1) CT is the main imaging modality for aortic dissection. Ultrasound may have a limited role in imaging within the abdomen.

(2) The distinction between Stanford Type A and Type B dissection is key to management.

(3) Dissection may extend proximally or distally. Occlusion of vessels involved may occur and cause complications relating to the corresponding vessel.

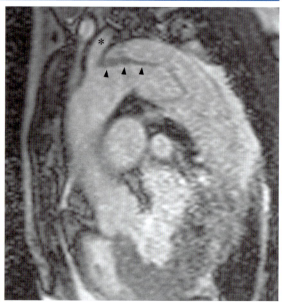

Fig.6j Sagittal oblique MRI showing a Stanford Type B dissection with the intimal flap (arrowheads) involving the thoracic aorta just distal to the left subclavian artery (asterisk).

Gastrointestinal bleeding

Gastrointestinal bleeding (Fig. 7a, b)
- In Figure 7a, an abnormal focal area of tracer accumulation appeared at 5 minutes after injection of the isotope in the lower abdomen, likely to be in the distal small bowel. Transition of the isotope to the large bowel is seen on the 1.5 hr delay scan (Fig. 7b).

Discussion:
- Upper GI endoscopy and colonoscopy are the most important tools for the investigation of gastrointestinal bleeding and can detect up to 95% of causes of chronic GI bleeding. The remaining 5% of causes fall into the category of bleeding from obscure origin (negative upper and lower GI endoscopy), and the small bowel is usually the culprit.
- The amount of bleeding is often small and these patients tend to present with chronic iron deficiency anaemia, although occasionally the bleeding may be more severe. These patients are best investigated when they are actively bleeding with a Tc-99m labelled scan or with visceral angiography.
- In vivo labelling Tc-99m red cell scan is the most widely used. Labelled red cell scan can detect bleeding rates as low as 0.1 ml/min and is a good investigation when there is intermittent bleeding. However, labelled red cell scan can only localise the site of bleeding and does not usually shed any light on the aetiology of the bleeding lesion.
- Visceral angiography on the other hand is less sensitive (can detect bleeding rates of at least 0.5-1 ml/min) and invasive requiring femoral artery puncture. Angiography can localise the site of bleeding in 50-72% in patients with massive GI bleeding, but the yield drops to 25-50% in patients without active bleeding.

Fig. 7c, d Visceral angiogram with embolisation.

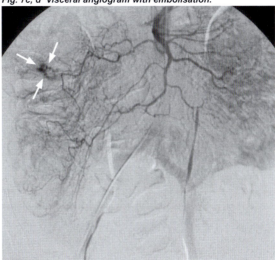

Fig.7c Selective angiogram of the superior mesenteric artery with a focus of abnormal contrast extravasation (indicative of active bleeding) in the ascending colon (arrows).

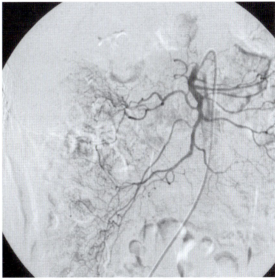

Fig.7d Post-embolisation image with cessation of contrast extravasation.

03 VASCULAR

Discussion Case 7
Gastrointestinal bleeding

Angiography can be used to diagnose the nature of the bleeding lesions (e.g. angiodysplasia, tumours) and, in suitable cases, embolisation to stop bleeding can be attempted at the same time.

- The main causes for bleeding from obscure origin are listed below. The majority occur in small intestine distal to duodenal bulb and proximal to ileocaecal valve:
  • Angiodysplasia 70-80%
  • Tumours   5-10%
Others:
  • Crohn's disease
  • Meckel's diverticulum
  • Zollinger-Ellison syndrome
  • Infections
  • Drugs
  • Vasculitis
  • Radiation enteritis
  • Jejunal diverticulosis
  • Pancreatic pseudocysts

- Meckel's diverticulum when presenting with GI bleeding, usually contains gastric mucosa and is caused by persistence of the omphalomesenteric duct (also known as the vitelline duct) which usually obliterates by week 5 of gestation. The well known rule of 2 applies:
Occurs in 2% of the population
Around 2 inches (5 cm) in length
Located within 2 feet (0.6 m) of the ileal caecal valve
Patients present usually before the age of two

- A dedicated nuclear medicine examination called the Meckel's scan can be performed for the detection of Meckel's diverticulum with an i.v. injection of Tc-99m pertechnetate (which is excreted by mucoid cells of gastric mucosa). The Meckel's diverticulum on a positive study would appear as a focus of increased tracer accumulation, usually around the right iliac fossa with the activity mirroring that of gastric mucosa (Figure 7e and f). Alternatively,

Fig. 7e, f Meckel's scan.

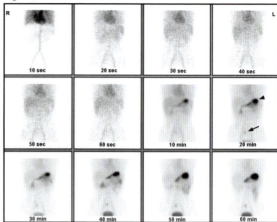

Fig.7e Dynamic images with an abnormal focus of tracer accumulation seen in the right iliac fossa (arrow) at 20 minutes mirroring the timing of tracer accumulation in the stomach (arrowhead).

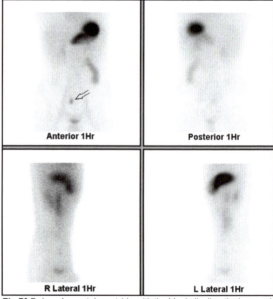

Fig.7f Delayed scan taken at 1 hr with the Meckel's diverticulum again shown in the right iliac fossa (open arrow).

Gastrointestinal bleeding

a Meckel's diverticulum can be diagnosed at angiography by demonstration of the vitello-intestinal artery (Fig. 7g and h).

Role of imaging in gastrointestinal bleeding

- Upper GI endoscopy and colonoscopy remain the first line investigations for gastrointestinal bleeding
- Imaging has a crucial role particularly in the investigation of small bowel pathology and in identifying and possibly embolising the source of bleeding in the acute situation.

Note:

(1) In the bleeding patient, labelled red cell scan is the most sensitive test for localising the site of bleeding (can detect bleeding at rates as low as 0.1 ml/min).

(2) Angiography, although less sensitive (can detect bleeding rates at 0.5-1.0 ml/min), may shed light on the cause of bleeding and may facilitate embolisation at the site of bleeding.

Fig. 7g, h Angiographic appearance of Meckel's diverticulum.

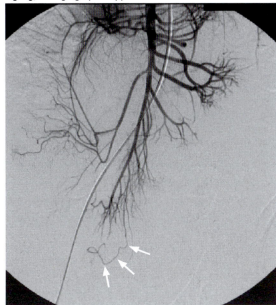

Fig.7g *Selective angiogram of the superior mesenteric artery demonstrating the persistence of a vitello-intestinal artery which is diagnostic of a Meckel's diverticulum (arrows) (Courtesy of Dr. James Jackson, Hammersmith Hospital, London, U.K.).*

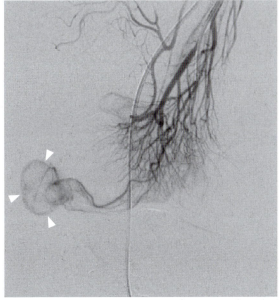

Fig.7h *Super-selective angiogram of the vitello-intestinal artery demonstrating the Meckel's diverticulum (arrowheads) (Courtesy of Dr. James Jackson, Hammersmith Hospital, London, U.K.).*

Renal artery stenosis

Renal artery stenosis (Fig. 8a, b)
- The right kidney is significantly smaller than the left.
- There is ostial stenosis of the right renal artery.

Discussion:

- Renal artery stenosis is the most common cause of secondary hypertension and is the cause of hypertension in up to 6% of hypertensives. Renal artery stenosis should be suspected if a patient has:
  - Hypertension refractory to multiple drugs treatment (3 or more)
  - Abnormal renal function while receiving ACE inhibitors
  - Age of onset of hypertension <30 or >50
  - Hypertension previously well controlled becoming difficult to control
  - Imaging study, e.g. ultrasound suggesting significant difference in size of the kidneys
  - A vascular bruit over the abdomen in the region of the renal arteries
  - Other vascular disease, e.g. coronary arterial, cerebral vascular and peripheral vascular disease
  - Sudden onset of pulmonary oedema

Fig.8c, d Duplex Doppler ultrasound of the renal artery of a transplant kidney.

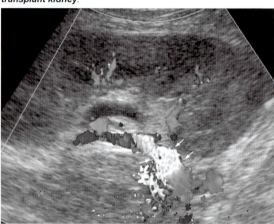

Fig.8c Colour Doppler examination of the graft renal artery showing turbulent flow (arrows).

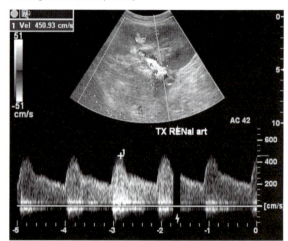

Fig.8d Spectral Doppler assessment of the graft renal artery revealing abnormally high peak systolic velocity of 450 cm/s (>200 cm/s is taken as abnormal) diagnostic of stenosis of the graft renal artery.

Renal artery stenosis

- The conventional imaging modality of choice used to be Duplex Doppler ultrasound (Fig. 8c, d) - commonly used parameters for diagnosing renal artery stenosis include main renal artery velocity of >200 cm/s, acceleration time of > 70 ms, and intrarenal tardus parvus waveform.
- Ultrasound, however, is operator dependent, affected by patient's body habitus and bowel gas, and is a time consuming investigation.
- The above problems with ultrasound can be overcome by both magnetic resonance angiography (MRA) and computed tomography angiography (CTA). MRA and CTA have both been shown to have good correlation with digital subtraction angiography findings, and have both been adopted by different institutions as the non-invasive screening modality of choice for renal artery stenosis depending on local expertise and availability.
- MRA has the advantage of not using ionising radiation, uses gadolinium rather than iodinated contrast (potentially nephrotoxic and has a slightly higher incidence of anaphylactic reactions) and is less affected by calcification in vessels.
- CTA (Fig. 8e, f), on the other hand, is faster and more available in most institutions.
- Both techniques allow 3D visualisation and simultaneous assessment of the kidneys.
- DSA is usually reserved for patients in whom the diagnosis remains in doubt after the non-invasive tests or for patients who are to receive endovascular intervention (Fig. 8g, h).
- The ultimate purpose for imaging of the renal arteries is to identify treatable disease for endovascular intervention or surgical revascularisation.

Fig.8e, f CT angiography of the renal arteries.

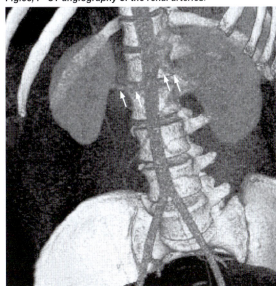

Fig.8e *Volume rendered image of the renal arteries (arrows) from a normal subject.*

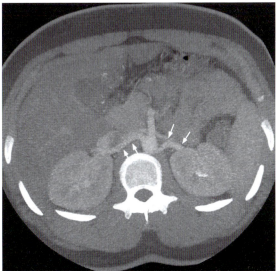

Fig.8f *Multiplanar reconstructed image on the normal renal arteries (arrows) from the same subject.*

Renal artery stenosis

- There are two main types of renal artery stenosis: (i) atheromatous disease and (ii) fibromuscular dysplasia. Atheromatous disease tends to affect older patients and the ostium (origin) of the renal arteries. With the advent of metallic stents, technical success of endovascular intervention for renal artery stenosis has increased substantially (90%), although re-stenosis remains problematic (rate of 15-20%/year).
- Fibromuscular dysplasia, on the other hand, tends to occur in younger patients (children and young adults, 30-40) and mainly affects the mid portion of renal arteries.
- Stenting can also be performed on renal arteries from transplant kidneys that are prone to develop stenoses around their anastomotic sites (Fig. 8i, j).

Role of imaging in renal artery stenosis
- Confirm the diagnosis of renal artery stenosis.
- Allow simultaneous assessment of renal size, cortical thickness, function (by contrast excretion) and presence of other significant renal lesions (e.g. tumours)
- Allow patient selection for endovascular intervention or surgery.
- Performed as part of endovascular intervention.

Fig.8g, h Stenting of a native right renal artery.

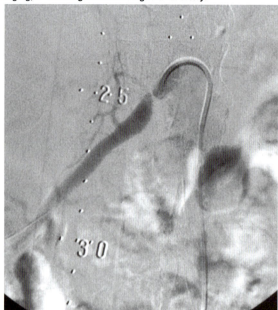

Fig.8g Tight >90% stenosis (next to the 25 cm marker) at the ostium of the right renal artery.

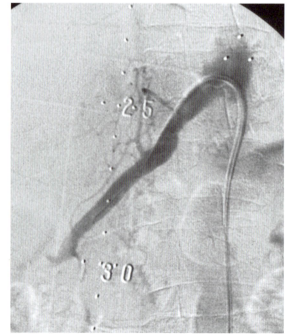

Fig.8h Post-stenting image – note the marked improvement.

Renal artery stenosis

Note:

(1) Although the majority of hypertensive patients have primary hypertension (90-95%), renal arterial stenosis is the most common cause of secondary hypertension.

(2) Non-invasive techniques for imaging the renal arteries, in particular MRA and CTA are increasingly replacing DSA for the assessment of renal arteries.

(3) DSA tends to be reserved for patients in whom diagnostic doubts remain after MRA or CTA, or be performed as part of renal artery endovascular stenting.

Fig.8i, j Stenting of two renal arteries from a transplant kidney.

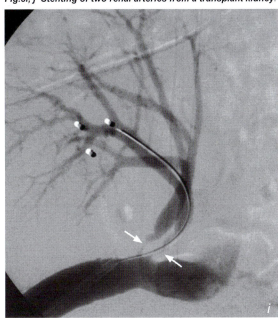

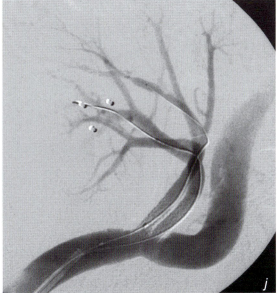

Fig.8i Hypertensive renal transplant patient with a serum creatinine of 850 µmol/l and >90% stenoses of both the renal arteries of his graft (arrows). He was due to be transferred onto the dialysis list. Two renal artery stents were inserted with good technical results (*Fig. 8j*) and the patient's creatinine dropped to 180 µmol/l over the course of 10 days and was discharged home.

Ruptured hepatocellular carcinoma

Ruptured hepatocellular carcinoma
(Fig. 9a, b)

- At least one large and one small arterially enhancing lesions are seen in the right lobe of the liver. The larger of the two lesions shows central low attenuation change likely to represent central necrosis. A rim of hyperdense material is seen in the subcapsular region overlying the right lobe of the liver likely to represent a subcapsular haematoma. Further lower attenuation free fluid is also seen around the upper abdomen. The appearances are likely to represent multifocal hepatocellular carcinoma with rupture of the larger of the two lesions and subcapsular haematoma.
- Incidentally, a replaced right hepatic artery – the right hepatic artery arising from the superior mesenteric artery (occurs in 25% of the population) – is seen.

Discussion:

- Hepatocellular carcinoma (HCC) is the most frequent primary visceral malignancy worldwide, and accounts for 80-90% of primary liver malignancies.
- Its incidence is higher (5.5-20%) in geographical regions where hepatitis B and hepatitis C are prevalent - Southeast Asia, Japan, sub-Saharan Africa, Greece, and Italy.
- HCC is highly associated with cirrhosis, and between 60 and 90% of HCCs arise from cirrhotic livers.
- HCC is a vascular tumour and usually derives its blood supply from the hepatic artery, and thus HCC classically shows early arterial phase enhancement on CT.
- The majority of HCCs are multifocal (65%), while the rest are predominantly solitary (30%) with a small proportion being infiltrative (5%).
- Invasion of the portal vein is a common finding (57%) and calcification may be seen in a tenth of HCCs.

Fig.9c, d Embolisation of HCC.

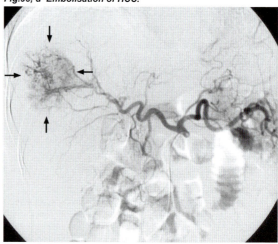

Fig.9c *Selective angiogram of the coeliac axis with demonstration of a hypervascular tumour (arrows) in the right lobe of the tumour.*

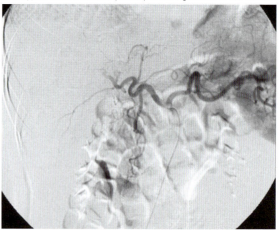

Fig.9d *Post-embolisation image demonstrating obliteration of the vascular blush from the tumour after superselective cannulation of the right hepatic artery with a microcatheter and embolisation with polyvinyl alcohol particles.*

Ruptured hepatocellular carcinoma

- Extrahepatic spread is also common via nodal spread and haematogenous spread (typically to lungs or adrenals).
- As HCCs are vascular tumours, and up to 8% may present with spontaneous rupture, embolisation of the hepatic artery may be performed for treatment of HCC rupture

Role of imaging in spontaneous hepatocellular carcinoma rupture
- In the patient who is stable haemodynamically, CT has an important role in establishing the diagnosis of a ruptured HCC and for evaluating the extent of intraperitoneal bleeding. While ultrasound may play a role in diagnosis and follow up of HCC, its role is limited in the acute situation of rupture.
- Angiography can be diagnostic and therapeutic, and embolisation has become an established treatment option for ruptured HCC (Fig. 9c, d).

<u>**Note:**</u>
(1) The most common aetiological factors for HCC are cirrhosis, chronic HBV and HCV infections.
(2) HCC is a vascular tumour and usually receives its blood supply from the hepatic artery.
(3) In spontaneous rupture, CT is the imaging modality of choice. Angiography can be diagnostic and therapeutic as embolisation has become an established treatment option for ruptured HCC.

Discussion Case 10
Deep vein thrombosis

Deep vein thrombosis (Fig. 10a, b)
- Echogenic thrombi are seen on both of these images diagnostic of deep vein thrombosis in the left common femoral vein and the left popliteal vein.
- The left deep vein thrombosis is likely to be caused by compression of the iliac veins from the known pelvic malignancy. A contrast enhanced CT venogram (Fig. 10c, d) or a magnetic resonance venogram (MRV) (Fig. 10e) may be useful for further assessment of the iliac veins and IVC if they are not adequately seen on ultrasound.

Fig.10c, d CT venogram (same patient as in Fig. 10a, b)

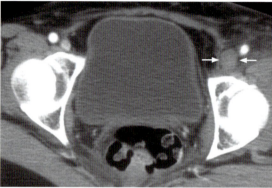

Fig.10c *Axial section at the level of the femoral veins showing non-opacification and expansion of the left common femoral vein (arrows) consistent with deep vein thrombosis.*

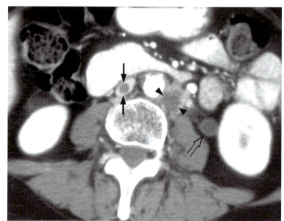

Fig.10d *Extension of the thrombus into the IVC with a filling defect seen centrally within the IVC (arrows). Note also that there is a necrotic lymph node (arrowheads) with a low attenuation centre seen to the left of the aorta and the left ureter is dilated (open arrow) likely from compression by the same pelvic mass which caused the deep vein thrombosis.*

Deep vein thrombosis

Discussion:

- Deep vein thrombosis above the knee joint is a common medical emergency. Unless promptly treated, it may cause pulmonary embolism and become life threatening to the patient.

- The more central the location of the thrombus, the higher the risk of pulmonary embolism (PE). The assessment of the iliac veins and IVC may be obscured by bowel gas and hampered by patient's body habitus.

- A CT venogram can be performed, with acquisition of the images performed 3-4 minutes after injection of an i.v. contrast bolus.

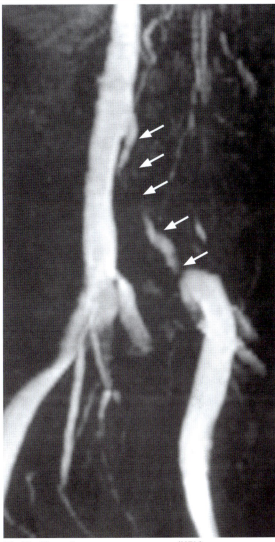

Fig.10e Magnetic resonance venogram (MRV)
MRV of the left lower limb of another patient presenting with swelling of the lower limb. Notice the long segment stenosis in the left common iliac vein (arrows). This examination utilised a technique called 'time of flight' where the property of flowing blood was used to create contrast between the vein and the surrounding structures that are stationary. No i.v. contrast agent was necessary.

Deep vein thrombosis

Role of imaging in deep vein thrombosis

- Establish the diagnosis of deep vein thrombosis.
- Determine the upper extent of the thrombus.
- An IVC filter can be deployed below the renal veins to reduce the risk of pulmonary embolism (Fig. 10f, g). IVC filters act predominantly by fragmenting large clots into smaller ones rather than trapping them. The main complication of IVC filter deployment is thrombosis of the IVC with extension to the renal veins.
- Imaging for pulmonary embolism.

Fig. 10f,g IVC filter deployment
Fig. 10f   IVC cavogram done with a pigtail catheter inserted via the right internal jugular approach. This is done to determine the position of the renal veins.

Fig.10g   Deployment of a retrievable IVC filter (arrows) below the left renal vein.

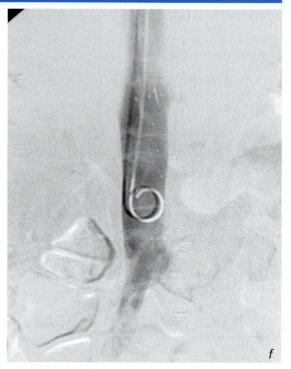

f

Note:

(1) Duplex Doppler ultrasound is the first choice modality for the investigation of deep vein thrombosis.

(2) CT is useful for assessing the pelvic veins and IVC for thrombus extension. It may also be possible to assess the pelvis for masses at the same time.

(3) The deployment of an IVC filter can reduce the risk of pulmonary embolism and is particularly useful in patients in whom anticoagulation is contraindicated or when the risk of pulmonary embolus is high.

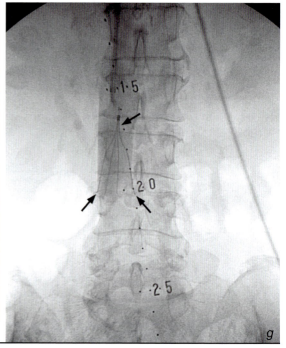

g

Discussion Case 11
Superior vena cava obstruction/syndrome

*Superior vena cava obstruction/
syndrome* (Fig.11a-c)
- Fig.11a shows a large soft tissue mass
  encasing the superior vena cava and
  narrowing its lumen. The mass abuts
  the ascending and descending aorta
  and also encases the carina. An area
  of consolidation is seen peripherally
  in the right hemithorax.
- On the coronal oblique multiplanar
  reconstruction in Fig. 11b and the
  volume rendered reconstruction in
  Fig. 11c, the encasement of the SVC
  by the mass can be better appreciated.
  The features are consistent with SVC
  obstruction (SVCO) or SVC syndrome
  caused by a malignant tumour -
  bronchogenic carcinoma is the most
  likely.

Discussion:
- Malignancies are the most common
  cause of superior vena cava syndrome,
  accounting for 80-90% of cases -
  bronchogenic carcinoma (>50%) and
  lymphoma are the most common
  tumours.
- Benign causes include central venous
  catheters and pacing wires (accounting
  for around a quarter of all benign
  causes), central venous stenosis in
  renal haemodialysis patients,
  granulomatous mediastinitis/infection,
  substernal goitre, ascending aortic
  aneurysm and constrictive pericarditis.

Fig. 11d, e, f, g, h SVC stenting
*Fig.11d A haemodialysis patient with
superior vena caval obstruction due to
multiple central venous catheter insertion.
A left internal jugular catheter is seen in situ
with the tip in the left brachiocephalic vein.
The right internal jugular vein was punctured
and a venogram was performed confirming
complete SVCO (arrows).*

*Fig.11e Venogram performed after a
hydrophilic guidewire (arrows) was passed
through the site of obstruction in the SVC
and manipulated past the right atrium into
the IVC.*

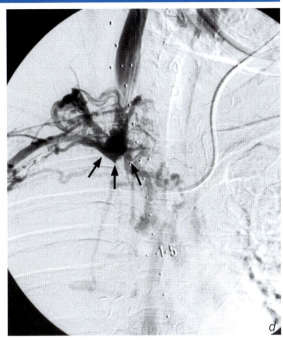

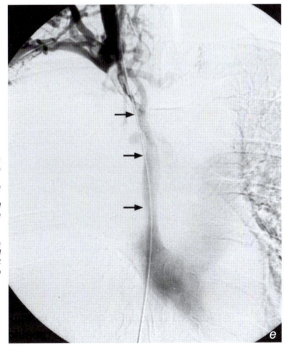

Superior vena cava obstruction/syndrome

- The treatment for malignant SVCO tends to be palliative as by this stage the tumour would usually be inoperable. Apart from lymphoma which may have dramatic response to chemotherapy, radiotherapy and SVC stenting are the two main treatment options for other malignant tumours.
- SVC stenting provides near immediate relief from symptoms.
- SVC stenting can also be used in selective cases on benign SVCO.
- One of the most common uses is in venous stenosis in haemodialysis patients caused by intimal hyperplasia (Fig. 11d-h).

Role of imaging in superior vena cava obstruction/syndrome

- Establish the diagnosis and differentiate between benign and malignant causes
- Assess the severity of the obstruction
  - narrowing vs complete obstruction
- Assess for suitability for SVC stenting
- Assess and follow up of treatment response

Fig.11f Deployment of the self expanding SVC stent (arrows) across the site of SVCO. The stent was expanded to its intended size (16 mm diameter) with an angioplasty balloon (Fig. 11g).

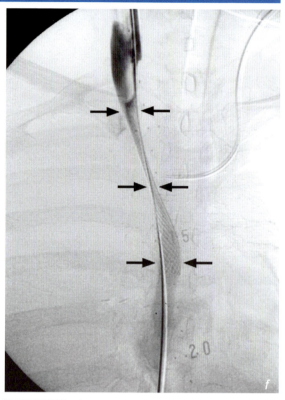

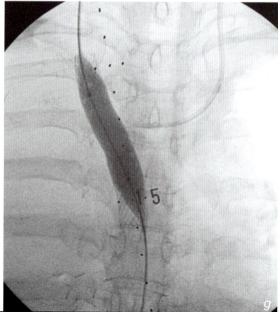

Superior vena cava obstruction/syndrome

Note:

(1) Malignant tumours are the most common cause of superior vena cava obstruction/syndrome.

(2) CT of the thorax is the investigation of choice.

(3) SVC stenting is an important treatment option for SVC obstruction/syndrome, especially as relief from symptoms is more immediate than after radiotherapy or chemotherapy.

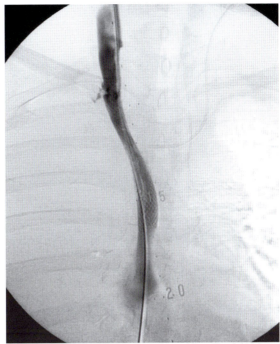

Fig.11h *Post-stenting venogram performed from the right internal jugular vein showing free flow of contrast through the SVC into the right atrium.*

03 VASCULAR

MUSCULOSKELETAL

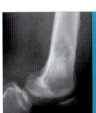

Contributors:

Gregory E. Antonio, James F. Griffith, Simon S.M. Ho, Anil T. Ahuja

Questions

Case 1 - 16   170 - 185

Discussion

Hyperparathyroidism	186 - 188
Multiple myeloma	189 - 192
Septic arthritis	193 - 195
Rheumatoid arthritis	196 - 197
Degenerative joint disease	198 - 199
Ankylosing spondylitis	200 - 201
Avascular necrosis of the femoral head	202 - 203
Gouty arthritis	204 - 205
Osteosarcoma	206 - 209
Ewing's sarcoma	210 - 211
Multiple bone metastases	212 - 214
Haemophilic arthropathy	215
Vertebral discitis/osteomyelitis	216 - 217
Chronic suppurative osteomyelitis	218 - 219
Pathological spinal fracture	220 - 221
Degenerative disc disease	222 - 225

Chapter 04

Case 1

A 40-year-old man, with good past health, complained of lethargy, polydipsia and polyuria for 3 months. Physical examination was unremarkable aside from muscle hypotonia and bone tenderness. Laboratory investigations revealed hypercalcaemia and hypophosphataemia. Alkaline phosphatase and parathyroid hormone levels were elevated. Hyperparathyroidism was suspected and radiographs of the hands and the skull were performed (Fig. 1a to c).

Questions

(1) What abnormalities do you see on these radiographs ?

    Frontal view of hand: Generalized osteopenia

                                Cortical bone tunneling

                                Subperiosteal bone resorption

    Lateral skull view: Mottled calvarium (salt and pepper skull)

                                Blurred inner and outer tables

                                Well-defined lucent lesion in the parietal bone

(2) <u>What is the diagnosis ?</u>

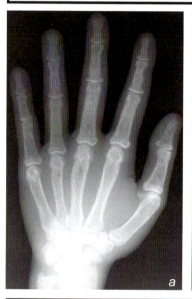

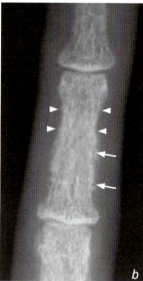

Fig.1a *Frontal view of the hand shows generalized osteopenia and cortical thinning.*

Fig.1b *Magnified view of the third middle phalanx shows a lace-like cortex due to bone resorption and enlargement of the Haversian canals (latter seen as the numerous holes in the cortex, [arrows]). There is also subperiosteal bone resorption (arrowheads).*

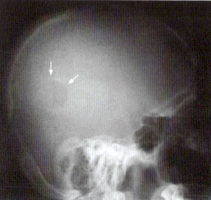

Fig.1c *Lateral view of the skull shows blurring of inner and outer tables of the skull (normally of distinct borders). There is also a generalized mottled appearance which is due to widespread granular bone resorption. This is termed a salt and pepper skull. There is a well-defined lucent lesion in the parietal bone indicating a Brown tumour (arrows)*

Case 2

A 67-year-old woman with no known primary malignancy, complained of generalized bone pain for 3 months. She appeared pale on physical examination with tenderness on deep palpation over the lumbar spine. Examination of other systems was unremarkable. Laboratory investigations revealed normochromic normocytic anaemia and raised ESR. Serum electrophoresis demonstrated the presence of abnormal M-paraprotein. In view of the laboratory results, a blood dyscrasia was suspected and radiographs of the skull, ribs and femur were performed (Fig. 2a-c).

Questions

(1) What abnormalities do you see on these selected radiographs ?

    Skull :   Multiple well-defined lucent lesions affecting the cranial vault

    Ribs :   Osteopenia and rib fractures

    Femur : Osteopenia, cortical thickening and focal cortical lucencies

(2) What is the diagnosis ?

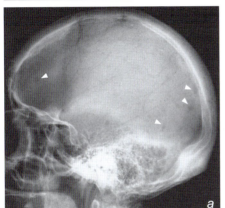

Fig.2a *Lateral view of the skull shows multiple small punched-out (well-defined) lucent lesions (arrowheads).*

Fig.2b *Oblique view of right lower ribs shows generalized osteopenia and rib fractures (arrows)*

Fig.2c *Lateral view of the proximal right femur shows generalized osteopenia with tunneling (arrowheads). More discrete lesions are also seen (arrows)*

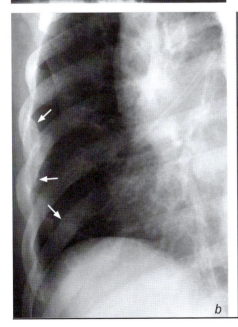

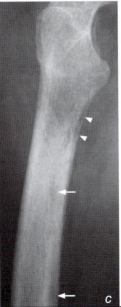

Case 3

A 46-year-old man presented with insidious onset right knee pain which progressively deteriorated over a four week period. He had a low grade fever for the past 3 days. There was no recent history of trauma. On examination, the knee was swollen with local erythema, tenderness and limited range of movement. Laboratory investigations revealed leucocytosis and a raised ESR. An infection was suspected and radiographs of the right knee (Fig.3a, b) were performed, followed by an ultrasound of the right knee (Fig. 3c).

Questions
(1) What abnormalities do you see on imaging ?
    Radiographs: Fullness of the suprapatellar pouch (arrowheads)
                Osteopenia on both sides of the knee joint
                Marginal bone erosion at medial tibial condyle (arrow)
(2) Abnormal: longitudinal view of the suprapatellar pouch :
    Joint effusion (asterisk)
    Thickening of the synovium (between crosses)
(3) <u>What is the diagnosis ?</u>

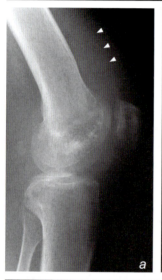
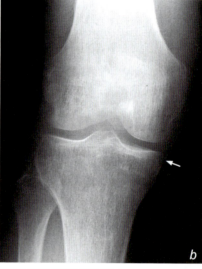

Fig.3a Lateral view of the knee joint shows fullness of the suprapatellar pouch (arrowheads). This may be due to a joint effusion and/or synovial thickening.

Fig.3b Frontal view of the knee shows mild periarticular osteopenia. This would suggest hyperaemia around the joint and is a non-specific indicator of increased blood flow. There is only bone erosion at the edge of the medial tibial condyle (arrow). This is an indicator of active synovial activity/inflammation.

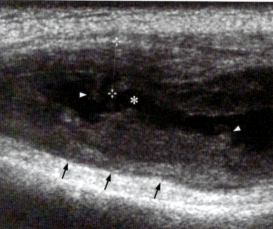

Fig.3c Longitudinal sonogram of the suprapatellar pouch. Black arrows indicate the anterior cortex of the distal femur. There is increased fluid (normally a thin film) within the supra-patellar pouch (asterisk). There is severe synovial thickening as marked by the crosses.

Case 4

A 39-year-old woman complained of multiple joint pain for six months, most severely affecting the small joints of both hands. There was morning stiffness which improved with movement. Physical examination showed swelling of both wrists associated with decreased range of movement. Laboratory investigations revealed raised ESR. White cell count was not elevated. In view of the patient's history, radiographs of both hands and wrists were performed (Fig. 4a).

Questions

(1) What abnormalities do you see on this radiograph ?

    Overall: Bilateral symmetrical distribution of disease

    Wrists: Loss of joint space most markedly affecting the radiocarpal joint

              Erosion of the carpal bones and distal radial articular surface

    Hands: Periarticular osteopenia

              Loss of joint space in some of the metacarpophalangeal (MCP) joints

              Soft tissue swelling around the third proximal interphalangeal (PIP) joints

              Loss of joint space of the third PIP joints and marginal erosions

(2) What is the diagnosis ?

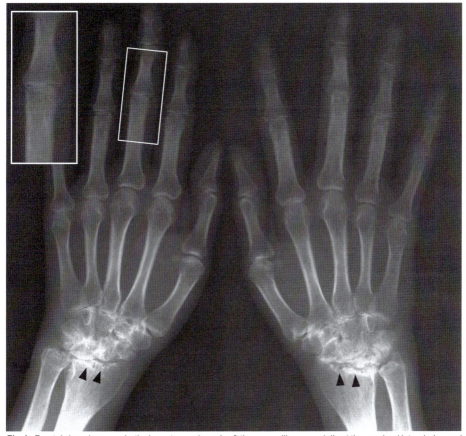

Fig.4a *Frontal view shows periarticular osteopenia and soft tissue swelling especially at the proximal interphalangeal joints. There is loss of joint space with erosions (arrowheads) which is most marked in the carpus, especially the radiocarpal articulation.*

Case 5

A 60-year-old retired construction site worker complained of right knee pain for 1 year. The pain was aggravated by movement. There was no associated morning stiffness. Physical examination showed mild varus deformity of the knee with reduced range of movement. Local tenderness was elicited over the medial joint space and crepitus felt upon flexion and extension of the right knee. Laboratory investigations were normal. Frontal and lateral radiographs of knee were performed (Fig. 5a, b).

Questions

(1) What abnormalities do you see on these radiographs ?

Frontal view: Loss of joint space (worse in medial tibiofemoral compartment)
Subchondral sclerosis
Marginal osteophytes
Intra-articular bodies superimposed over lateral tibial condyle

Lateral view: Loss of joint space, subchondral sclerosis best seen at dorsal surface of the patella
Intra-articular bodies form a chain behind the lateral tibial condyle

(2) <u>What is the diagnosis ?</u>

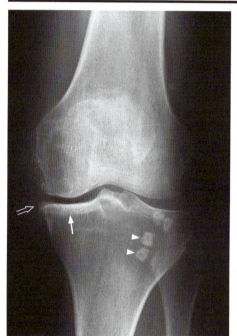 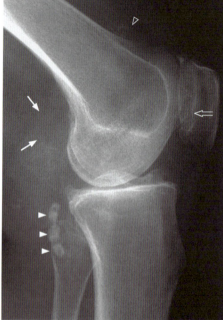

Fig.5a Frontal view of the knee shows loss of joint space, subchondral sclerosis (arrow) and marginal osteophytes (open arrow) affecting most severely the medial tibio-femoral compartment. There are multiple ossified densities representing loose bodies (arrowheads).

Fig.5b Lateral view of the knee shows loss of joint space, marginal osteophytes and subchondral sclerosis of the patellofemoral joint (open arrow). There is a large calcified body (arrows) in the popliteal fossa, most likely within a Baker's cyst. Intra-articular bodies in an outpouching probably from the proximal tibiofibular joint (arrowheads), and in the suprapatellar pouch (open arrowhead).

Case 6

A 32-year-old man with good past health complained of insidious onset of low back pain and stiffness for 1 year, particularly in the morning. Physical examination showed restricted range of movement of lumbar spine and local tenderness was elicited over both sacro-iliac regions. Examination of eyes revealed evidence of bilateral uveitis. Laboratory investigations were unremarkable apart from raised ESR level. In view of the symptoms, radiographs of the lumbar spine and pelvis were performed (Fig. 6a, b).

Questions

(1) What abnormalities do you see on these radiographs ?

       Pelvis: Ankylosis of both sacro-iliac joints

                         Partial ankylosis of the pubic symphysis

                         Loss of joint space, erosions and secondary sclerosis of the right hip

       Lumbar spine: Squaring of vertebral bodies

                         Syndesmophyte formation

                         Ankylosis of intervertebral facet joints

                         Ossification of interspinous and supraspinous ligaments

(2) <u>What is the diagnosis ?</u>

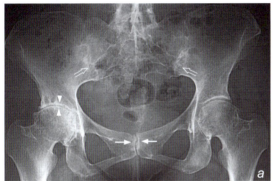

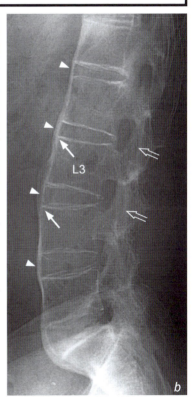

Fig.6a *Frontal view of the pelvis shows ankylosis of the sacro-iliac joints (open arrows). There are also erosive changes and loss of joint space at the pubic symphysis (arrows) indicating symphysitis. There is loss of joint space in the right hip joint (arrow heads). This loss of joint space involves the whole joint (as opposed to the superolateral weight-bearing area in osteoarthrosis). There are also subchondral cysts (lucent foci) sclerosis and marginal osteophytosis related to secondary degenerative changes, in the right hip joint.*

Fig.6b *Lateral view of the lumbosacral spine shows thin ossification of the anterior aspect of the intervertebral discs and the anterior longitudinal ligament (arrowheads). The vertebrae are square (arrows) in outline ('square vertebrae') and the facet joints are ankylosed (open arrows).*

Case 7

A 35-year-old woman with a known history of systemic lupus erythematosus was treated with oral corticosteroids for 2 years. She has been suffering progressive hip pain for the past 3 months. There was no fever or history of trauma. Physical examination showed decreased range of movement in left hip and slight limb shortening. Local tenderness was elicited over both hips. Laboratory investigations including ESR and WCC were unremarkable. In view of the symptoms a radiograph of the pelvis was performed (Fig. 7a).

Questions

(1) What abnormalities do you see on this radiograph ?

Mixed sclerosis and lucencies of the superior part of the femoral heads (worse on the left)

Flattening of the femoral heads

Superolateral subluxation of the left femoral head

(2) What is the diagnosis ?

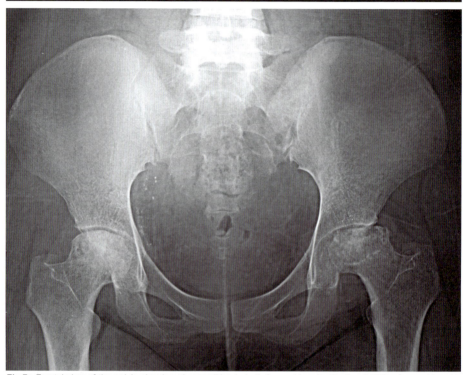

Fig.7a Frontal view of the pelvis showing abnormalities in both femoral heads. On the right the femoral head is flattened and there is sclerosis within the femoral head. On the left, the flattening (with bone loss) is worse and the femoral head is subluxed superiorly and laterally.

Case 8

A 60-year-old man, a heavy drinker for 30 years, complains of severe pain over the right big toe for 2 days. Similar attacks of pain have occurred intermittently over the past 10 years. Physical examination showed a hot, red and swollen metatarso-phalangeal joint of the big toe with marked tenderness. Hard subcutaneous whitish masses were also noted in this area. A radiograph of his foot was performed (Fig. 8a).

Questions

(1) What abnormalities do you see on this radiograph ?

    Soft tissue swelling over the medial aspect of the first metatarso-phalangeal (MTP) joint

    Bony defect in distal metatarsal head

    Loss of joint space of the first MTP joint

    Lateral subluxation of the first proximal phalanx

(2) What is the diagnosis ?

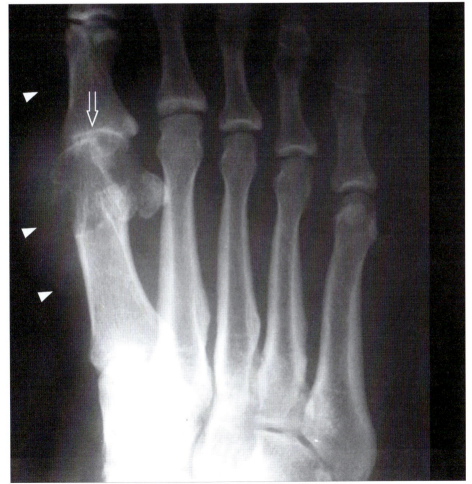

Fig.8a *Frontal view of the first MTP joint shows a large soft tissue swelling (arrowheads) with some calcification indicating a tophus. There is adjacent bone erosion and loss of joint space (open arrow).*

Case 9

A 13-year-old boy complained of malaise, weight loss and a progressive painful swelling over the distal left thigh for 3 months. There was no fever or history of recent trauma. Physical examination showed a hard mass over the distal thigh with mild localized tenderness. The left knee was unremarkable. Laboratory investigations revealed raised ESR and normal WCC. In view of the history, radiographs of the distal femur were performed (Fig. 9a, b).

Questions

(1) What abnormalities do you see on this radiograph ?

A mixed osteolytic and sclerotic lesion with ill-defined margins

Cortical thinning and disruption

Spiculated new bone formation

Overlying soft tissue mass

(2) <u>What is the diagnosis ?</u>

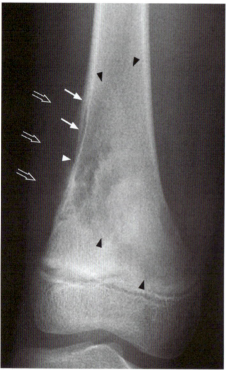

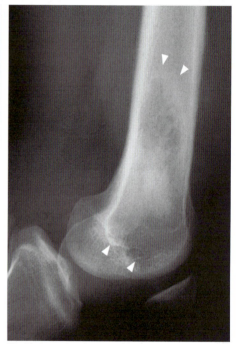

Fig.9a Frontal radiograph of the distal left femur shows a mixed sclerotic and lytic lesion in the metaphyseal region. The margins (black arrowheads) of this lesion are ill-defined, especially the proximal border which shows a wide zone of transition. There is thinning of the medial cortex due to tumour infiltration (white arrowhead). The penetration of tumour through the cortex has resulted in spiculated new bone formation (arrows) and a soft tissue mass (open arrows). The perpendicularly orientated (with respect to the cortical surface) periosteal new bone formation is considered to represent a fast expanding lesion (not enough time for sufficient calcification/ossification to establish a horizontal layer).

Fig.9b Lateral radiograph shows the margins of this lesion (arrowheads) slightly better.

Case 10

A 15-year-old boy complained of malaise, weight loss and a progressively painful swelling over the right ankle for 3 months. There was a history of recent trauma. Physical examination showed swelling over the malleolus with mild localized tenderness. The opposite ankle joint was unremarkable. Laboratory investigations revealed raised ESR and normal WCC. In view of the history, radiographs of the distal fibula and tibia were performed.

Questions

(1) What abnormalities do you see on this radiograph (Fig. 10a) ?
- An ill-defined area of lucency with a moth-eaten pattern of bone destruction and cortical disruption.
- No obvious fracture seen
(2) What is the diagnosis?

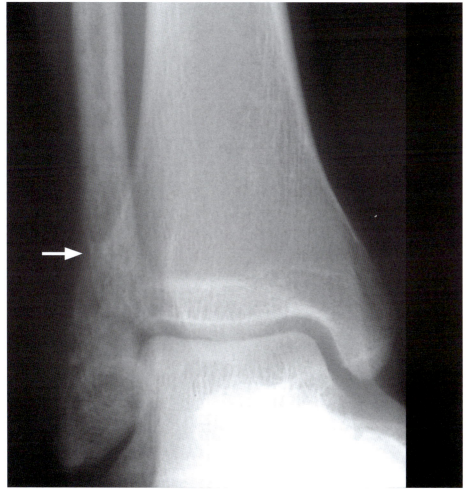

Fig.10a *Frontal radiograph of the distal tibia and fibula shows a mixed lytic and sclerotic lesion in the distal fibular metadiaphysis. The cortex is thinned (arrow) and the proximal border of the lesion is difficult to define (i.e. wide zone of transition).*

Case 11

A 63-year-old man, with known history of carcinoma of lung, complained of generalized bone pain for 3 months. The pain was dull in nature and progressive over this period. Physical examination showed tenderness over the left sided ribs, lower thoracic spine and left iliac bone. In view of the history and the diffuse nature of symptoms, a bone scan was performed (Fig. 11a).

Questions

(1) What abnormalities do you see on this bone scan ?
   - Multiple foci of increased tracer uptake mainly in the axial skeleton (spine, pelvis and ribs)
   - Lesions also seen in the appendicular skeleton, right femoral shaft and left femoral head and neck
(2) What is the diagnosis ?

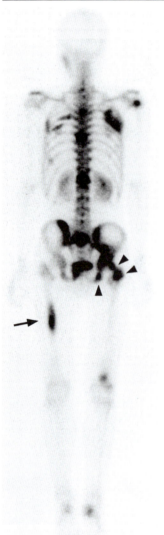

Fig.11a   *Whole body bone scan of this patient demonstrates multiple foci of increased radionuclide uptake (hot spots), especially in the axial skeleton (spine, ribs and pelvis). The appendicular skeleton is also involved, most notably in the right femoral shaft (arrow) and around the left hip joint (arrowheads).*

Case 12

A 24-year-old man with a history of Haemophilia A, presents with a painful left knee swelling. Frontal and lateral radiographs were performed (Fig. 12a and b).

Questions

(1) What abnormalities do you see on these radiographs ?

Frontal view: Loss of joint space especially in the medial tibiofemoral compartment

Subchondral cortical bone irregularities and sclerosis

Enlarged intercondylar groove

Periarticular osteopenia

Lateral view: The joint capsule is distended as indicated by bulging of the suprapatellar pouch and popliteal fullness.

There is also a subtle increase in density of the entire joint space

The extent of subchondral cortical bone irregularity is more clearly seen, and also involves the patella aside from both femoral and both tibial condyles.

(2) What is the diagnosis ?

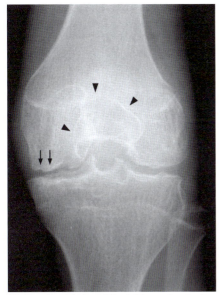

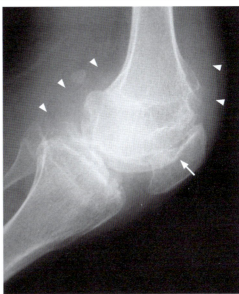

Fig.12a *Frontal view of the left knee showing loss of joint space, worse in the medial tibiofemoral compartment. There are multiple subchondral cortical bone irregularities with underlying sclerosis (arrows). The intercondylar groove is markedly enlarged (arrowheads) as a result of bone erosion by pannus. There is periarticular osteopenia (a patient of this age should normally have thicker cortices and more dense trabeculae).*

Fig.12b *Lateral view of the left knee shows a distended joint as indicated by the bulging suprapatellar pouch and the popliteal fullness (arrowheads). There is also a subtle diffuse increase in density of the joint capsule due to deposition of iron. On the lateral view, the front to back extent of subchondral cortical bone irregularity is more clearly seen. This involves the patella (arrow) aside from both femoral and tibial condyles.*

Case 13

A 4-year-old previously healthy child complained of progressive back pain for 2 weeks. She also developed fever, chills and rigor over the recent 2 days. General examination revealed a febrile, lethargic looking child. On physical examination, there was localized tenderness over the lower lumbar spine and decreased range of movement. The right hip was held in flexion. Laboratory investigations showed leucocytosis. Urinalysis was normal. A radiograph of the lumbar spine was performed (Fig.13a, b), followed by a CT scan of the abdomen (Fig. 13c).

Questions

(1) What abnormalities do you see on these images ?

    Radiograph: L3/4 disc space narrowing - due to destruction of cartilage by bacteria

                  Bony erosion at adjoining end-plates (loss of the dense line of endplate cortex)

                  Vertebral body sclerosis indicating osteomyelitis, i.e. involvement of vertebral body as well as intervertebral disc.

    CT scan: Rim enhancing low density lesion in the enlarged right psoas muscle.

                  Low density collection with rim enhancement in the spinal canal (anterior epidural space)

                  Destruction of the posterior aspect of the L3 vertebral body.

(2) What is the diagnosis ?

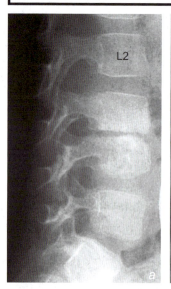 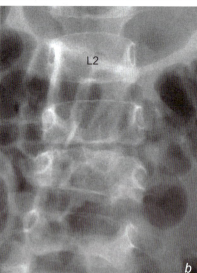

Fig.13a, b *Lateral and frontal views of lumbar spine show loss of disc height at the L3/4 level. There is destruction of the adjacent endplates (loss of the endplate bony cortex) and sclerosis in the bone underlying the endplate.*

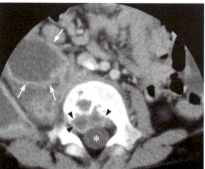

Fig.13c *Axial CECT at the L3 level. The bone destruction and epidural abscess (arrowheads) are well demonstrated. The dural sac (asterisk) is only mildly distorted. There is an associated right psoas abscess (arrows).*

Case 14

A 57-year-old poorly controlled diabetic presents with a discharging sinus from his leg. He claims to have had this problem off and on for the last 10 years. On examination, there is skin erythema, a discharging sinus and granulation tissue over the proximal tibia. A swab was sent for culture and radiographs of the leg were performed (Fig. 14a, b).

Questions

(1) What abnormalities do you see on these radiographs ?

Frontal view: Extensive mixed sclerosis and lysis with mild expansion of the tibia.

Thick periosteal reaction.

Calcification of proximal tibial vessels.

Lateral view: Cortical destruction in the proximal tibia.

(2) What is the diagnosis ?

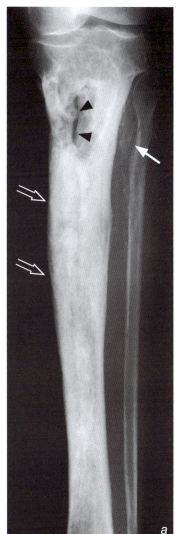

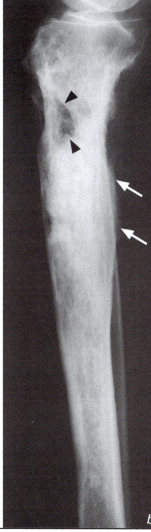

Fig.14a Frontal radiograph of the tibia shows a well-established periosteal reaction (thick, continuous and inseparable from original cortex) (open arrows). This covers most of the tibia. In the metaphyseal region there is evidence of a cortical break (arrowheads). There is vascular calcification (arrow) which is commonly seen in diabetic patients.

Fig.14b Lateral radiograph of the tibia shows the same thick and smooth periosteal reaction (arrows). The cortical break can now be placed in the anterior surface of the tibial metaphysis and its configuration is that of a large sinus tract (cloaca) leading into the medullary cavity.

a

b

183

Case 15

A 46-year-old woman newly diagnosed with disseminated carcinoma of breast, complained of an insidious onset of lower-thoracic spine pain for one month and recent weakness of both legs. The pain radiated to the periumbilical region. There was no fever or recent trauma. Physical examination showed tenderness over lower thoracic vertebrae. There was decreased muscle power in both lower limbs and sensory deficit in the T9 and T10 dermatomes. Both ankle and knee jerks were brisk. Laboratory investigations were unremarkable. Radiographs of the thoracolumbar spine were performed (Fig. 15a and b).

Questions

(1) What abnormalities do you see on these radiographs ?

    Lateral: Mild wedging of the T10 vertebral body

            Sclerosis of T10 vertebral body

    Frontal: Sclerosis of T10 left pedicle

            Left paraspinal soft tissue bulge at the T10 level and reduced vertebral height

            N.B. Intervertebral disc space is preserved

(2) What is the diagnosis ?

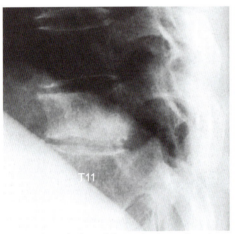

Fig.15a *Lateral view of thoracolumbar spine shows wedging of the body of T10. There is no destruction of the endplates. The vertebral body, especially its postero-inferior aspect, is sclerotic compared to the adjacent vertebra.*

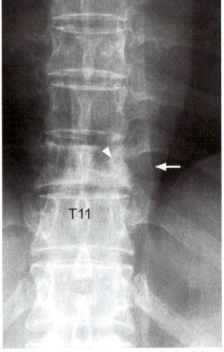

Fig.15b *Frontal view of the corresponding level shows decreased height of the T10 vertebral body. The adjacent disc spaces are well preserved. The left pedicle is sclerotic and not well defined (arrowhead). There is a focal bulge of the paravertebral soft tissue (arrow), suggesting paravertebral extension of the pathological process.*

Case 16

A 46-year-old manual worker complained of severe low back pain radiating to left buttock and leg shortly after lifting a heavy object. Physical examination showed localized tenderness at lumbosacral region with limited flexion and extension. No abnormal decrease in muscle power or sensation was demonstrated. No fractures were seen on radiographs of the lumbosacral spine or pelvis. An MRI of the lumbosacral spine was performed for further evaluation.

Questions

(1) What abnormalities do you see on these sagittal and axial MRI images (Fig. 16a, b and c) ?

Sagittal image: Loss of lumbar lordosis

Disc desiccation of lower lumbar levels (L3/4, L4/5, L5/S1)

Corresponding loss of disc height

Posterior disc protrusion

Compression on cauda equina

Partial effacement of the left neural exit foramen

Axial image: Central, paracentral, left paraforaminal and lateral disc protrusion

Left multifidus muscle atrophy

(2) <u>What is the diagnosis ?</u>

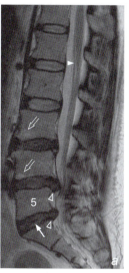
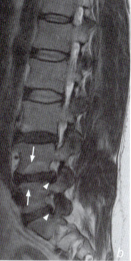

Fig.16a *Median sagittal T2W MRI image of the lumbar spine shows straightening of the normal lumbar lordosis suggesting muscle spasm (from pain). The lower three discs (L3/4, L4/5 and L5/S1) demonstrate the typical findings of degeneration: disc desiccation (decreased signal = decreased fluid content); possible cleft of gas (arrow); loss of disc height (due to loss of nucleus pulposis from desiccation and/or prolapse); posterior disc protrusion (open arrowheads) which compress the cauda equina. Note that the spinal cord (arrowhead) ends at the L1/2 level in this patient (which is the usual level for most). There is also signal change (termed Modic change) in the bone marrow adjacent to the endplates (open arrows) believed to be a response to altered stress as a result of disc degeneration.*

Fig.16b *Left lateral sagittal T2W MRI image of the lumbar spine shows partial effacement of the left L4 and L5 nerve root exit foramina as a result of the paraforaminal disc protrusion (arrowheads). This impingement may cause nerve root symptoms. Modic changes are present (arrows).*

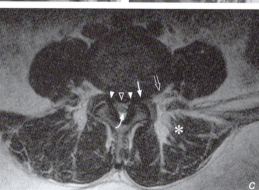

Fig.16c *Axial T2W MRI image at the L5/S1 level. There is posterior central (open arrowhead), bilateral paracentral (arrowheads), left paraforaminal (arrow) and left lateral (open arrow) disc protrusion. There is significant canal stenosis and the cauda equina is compressed (curved arrow). There is partial fatty replacement of the left multifidus muscle (asterisk) as a result of the 'denervation'.*

Hyperparathyroidism

Hyperparathyroidism (Fig. 1a-c)

Discussion:
This is a disease due to over-activity of the parathyroid gland. It may be: primary, due to a parathyroid adenoma; secondary, due to chronic renal disease leading to loss of calcium and phosphorus; tertiary, parathyroid glands acting independent of calcium homeostasis after prolonged secondary hyperparathyroidism. Increased parathormone (PTH) results in increased osteoclast activity, leading to increased bone resorption and increased serum calcium levels. The radiographic findings reflect some of the pathology, including:

- Subperiosteal outer cortical bone resorption - most prominent in middle phalanx of 2nd and 3rd fingers (Fig. 1a)
- Cortical tunneling – bony resorption within Haversian canals of cortex.
- Lace-like appearance of bone cortex due to a combination of the above signs (Fig. 1a, b and d)
- Apparent joint-space widening due to bone resorption
- Brown tumour (osteoclastoma) - well-defined cystic lesion in affected bone, representing a focal mass of osteoclasts and fibrous tissue (Fig. 1c). Commonly in skull, femur and pelvis.

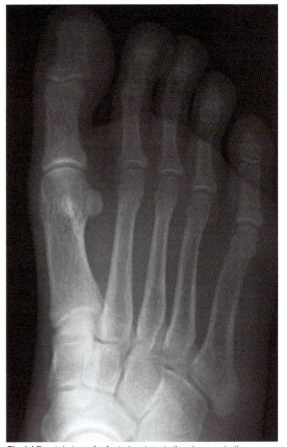

Fig.1d *Frontal view of a foot showing similar changes to those seen in the hands with lace-like cortex and bone resorption.*

Hyperparathyroidism

- Insufficiency fractures as a result of the weakened bones (Fig. 1e, f)
- Soft tissue/vascular calcification - due to high serum calcium levels
- Chondrocalcinosis - calcification within cartilages

Bone scan may show a 'superscan' (Fig. 1g) where there is diffuse increase in uptake in the entire skeleton due to increased bone activity.

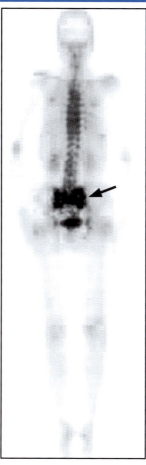

Fig.1e Bone scan of a different patient shows increased tracer uptake in both sacral alae and the sacral body forms an 'H' configuration (arrow). This has been termed the 'Honda' sign and signifies sacral insufficiency fractures.

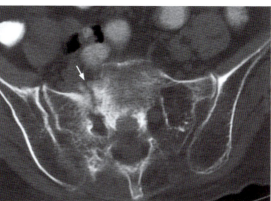

Fig.1f CT of the pelvis (bone window) shows a fracture of the right sacral ala (arrow). The underlying bones are osteopenic. This is a common site for insufficiency fractures.

Discussion Case 1

Hyperparathyroidism

Parathyroid adenoma is the underlying cause in majority (~80-90%) of cases (Fig. 1h). Other less common causes include parathyroid hyperplasia and parathyroid carcinoma.

Ultrasound of neck is sensitive in detecting parathyroid and helps the surgeon to accurately localize the lesion before surgery. If an ultrasound cannot detect a parathyroid lesion in a patient with biochemical evidence of hyperparathyroidism, radionuclide MIBI scan should be used to detect a hyperfunctioning adenoma.

Role of imaging in patients with hyperparathyroidism

- Demonstrate bone and soft tissue changes radiographically as a baseline for monitoring progress
- Demonstrate complications such as Brown tumours or insufficiency fractures
- Identify/localize a parathyroid adenoma

Note:

(1) Hyperparathyroidism is a clinical diagnosis, based on biochemical tests.

(2) Subperiosteal, outer cortical and peri-articular bony resorption are characteristic radiograph findings, most commonly demonstrated on plain radiograph of hands.

(3) Ultrasound neck or radionuclide MIBI scan help pre-operative localization of a parathyroid adenoma.

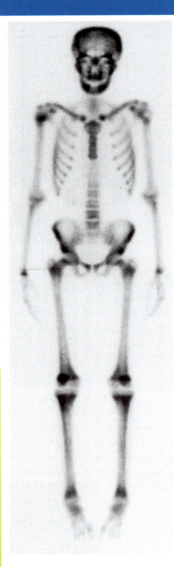

Fig.1g Bone scan shows a diffuse increase in activity in all bones secondary to hyperparathyroidism. This is also called a superscan. The way to diagnose this is to look at the renal activity relative to the bones. In this patient and in others, the bone activity is much, much higher compared to the renal activity (see other examples of a bone scan in other cases in this chapter for comparison).

Discussion Case 2
Multiple myeloma

Multiple myeloma (Fig. 2a-c)

Discussion:
Multiple myeloma (diffuse malignant plasma cell proliferation) is the most common primary malignant bone tumour and occurs mostly in patients over 50 years of age.

Bones containing red marrow are particularly vulnerable and are targeted in a radiographic 'skeletal survey'.

- These bones include: flat bones (skull, pelvis, ribs etc.), lower thoracic lumbar spine and proximal femur and humerus. Radiographs show evidence of bone marrow infiltration such as:
- Multiple lucent lesions in bones (Fig. 2a, b, g).
- Destruction of cortex (Fig. 2c, d)
- Generalized osteopenia (Fig. 2e, f).

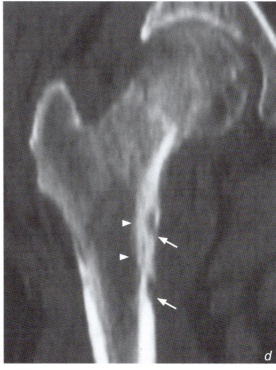

Fig.2d Reformatted CT of the right proximal femur in the coronal plane shows focal thickening as a result of periosteal and endosteal reaction (arrowheads) and tunneling (due to tumour infiltration). More discrete cortical lesions are also present (arrows).

Fig.2e Lateral view of the lumbosacral spine shows generalized osteopenia (generalized increased lucency of the vertebral body). The cortical bone is relatively less affected by osteoporosis than medullary bone.

Fig.2f Frontal view of the lumbar spine shows generalized osteopenia. Note the bones demonstrate a generalized mottled (multiple tiny lucencies) appearance.

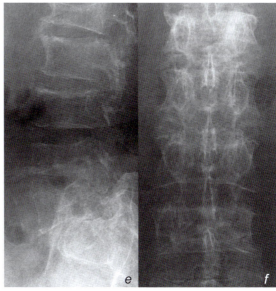

Discussion Case 2
Multiple myeloma

Multiple myeloma and metastases are the two most common causes of multiple bone lesions in elderly patients. Multiple myeloma is a neoplastic process of plasma cells and involves bone marrow. However, in most cases, it does not elicit much osteoblastic response. Therefore a bone scan in these patients is usually normal (no hot spots) and thus it is not used for evaluating disease extent (as opposed to the evaluation of bone metastases). This lack of osteoblastic response is less common with other neoplastic/metastatic diseases.

As a haematological neoplasm, complications may arise due to thrombocytopenia (i.e. haemorrhage) (Fig. 2h), hyper-coagulability (i.e. infarction, Fig. 2i, j) or leucopenia (i.e. infection).

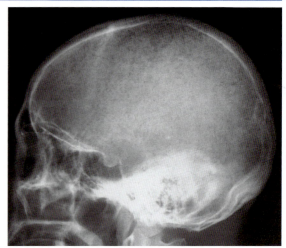

Fig.2g *Lateral skull view of another patient with multiple myeloma. Here the skull lesions were more extensive with multiple small lucencies. This is termed a 'raindrop' skull.*

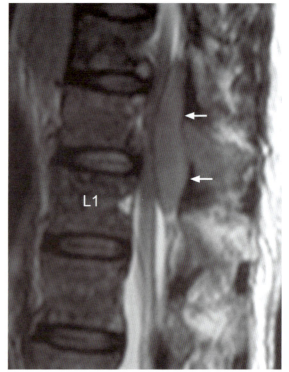

Fig.2h *Sagittal MRI, T2W (cerebrospinal fluid and fat are bright) image of the thoracolumbar region of another patient. There is diffuse marrow replacement (for an elderly patient this part of the spine normally contains bright fatty marrow) by myelomatous infiltration. There is a posterior epidural haematoma (arrows) compressing the lower spinal cord and conus medullaris.*

Discussion Case 2
Multiple myeloma

Fig. 2i *Sagittal MRI, T2W image of the thoracolumbar region of another patient. There is diffuse marrow replacement by myelomatous infiltration. There is a focal area of conal enlargement with high signal (arrow). This was later shown to be an area of spinal cord infarction (probably a consequence of hyperviscosity and occlusion of vessels).*

Fig. 2j *Axial MRI, T2W image (T12 level) shows enlargement and increased signal (oedema) within the conus medullaris.*

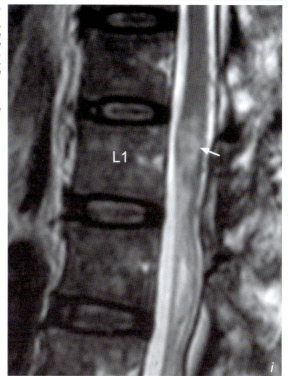

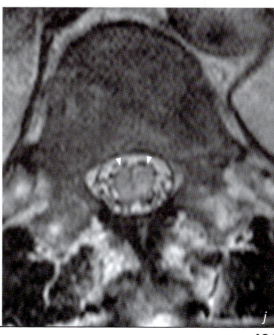

Discussion Case 2
Multiple myeloma

Plasmacytoma is a focal form of malignant plasma cell proliferation. It tends to produce a large lesion affecting a single bone/area (Fig. 2k).

Role of imaging in patients with multiple myeloma
- Radiographs as a survey to monitor disease extent and complications (fracture)
- MRI and/or CT for complications (haemorrhagic, infections, etc.)

Note:

(1) Multiple myeloma should be considered in elderly patients with multiple osteolytic lesions.

(2) Diagnosis is based on combination of laboratory and bone marrow biopsy results.

(3) Radiographic skeletal surveys help support the diagnosis and assess the extent of skeletal involvement.

(4) Generalized osteopenia and multiple osteolytic lesions are the typical radiologic features.

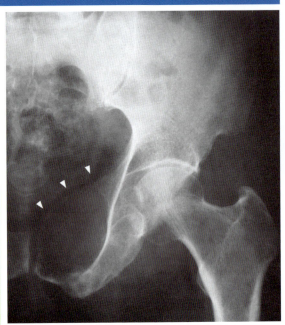

Fig. 2k *Frontal view of the left hip, of another patient, shows expansion and destruction of the left pubic body and superior ramus by a plasmacytoma (arrowheads).*

Septic arthritis

Septic arthritis (Fig. 3a-c)

Discussion:

Septic arthritis is an infection of the synovial membrane (hyperaemic and thickened) which produces an exudative effusion. Proteolytic enzymes are released which damage chondrocytes leading to articular cartilage loss and the infection may enter the underlying bone (osteomyelitis). At the joint margins (capsular insertions), the infected synovium may erode into the adjacent bone and also cause osteomyelitis. In the early stages of septic arthritis, radiographs may be normal (except for perhaps evidence of a joint effusion). Therefore, alternative imaging investigations are essential (due to the possible serious consequences). Sonography is the modality of choice (Fig. 3c). It is readily available and good at demonstrating the presence of a joint effusion (which may not be clinically apparent in the hip or in obese patients). It also allows image-guided aspiration of the effusion for microbiological evaluation.

As the disease becomes more established, bony radiographic changes may be seen. These include (Fig. 3a, b):

- Periarticular osteopenia, especially in the subarticular zone (under the subchondral cortex), due to hyperaemia.
- Marginal erosions by the synovium
- Loss of joint space due to cartilage destruction.

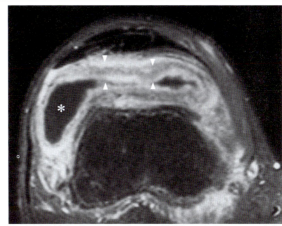

Fig.3d *Axial fat-saturated, post-contrast MR image of the suprapatellar pouch (fluid is dark, contrast enhancement is bright). The effusion within the suprapatellar pouch gravitates to the lateral recess (asterisk). The hypertrophied (reactive) synovium enhances and is markedly thickened (between arrowheads). Same patient as in Fig. 3a, b, c.*

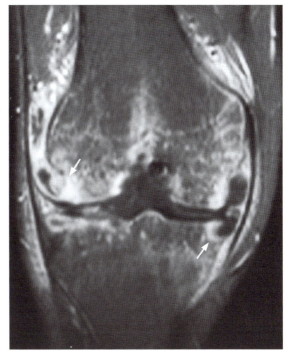

Fig.3e *Coronal fat-saturated, post-contrast MR image of the knee (fluid is dark, contrast enhancement is bright). Contrast enhancement extends into the femoral and tibial condyles indicating bone involvement by the infection (osteomyelitis) (arrows). This is due to erosion by the inflamed/hyperaemic synovium. The medial tibial condylar erosion seen on the frontal radiograph can be seen to contain some non-enhancing fluid. Same patient as in Fig. 3a-d.*

Discussion Case 3
Septic arthritis

These changes are not specific and may be seen in other forms of inflammatory arthropathy such as rheumatoid arthritis. Definitive diagnosis is based on microbiology results.

If there is extension of the infection into bone, radiographic changes due to osteomyelitis may be present (refer to case 14 for further information on osteomyelitis)

- Ill-defined, permeative bony destruction by the infection at the metaphysis
- Periosteal reaction as the infection spreads outwards through the Haversian canals in the cortex and lifts up the periosteum
- Cortical disruption due to destruction

In these cases, MRI will show both the synovial and bony inflammation, and is therefore good at providing a global view of the extent of the disease (Fig. 3d, e).

In poorly treated or resistant cases of septic arthritis, possible sequelae include degenerative joint disease (Fig. 3f, g) and ankylosis (Fig. 3h).

Role of imaging in patients with septic arthritis

- Exclude other causes of a swollen joint such as a fracture or neoplastic lesion usually with radiographs
- Confirm the presence of a joint effusion, usually with ultrasound, and guide aspiration for microbiological culture
- Look for signs of osteomyelitis (MRI more sensitive)
- To monitor progress and follow-up for complications

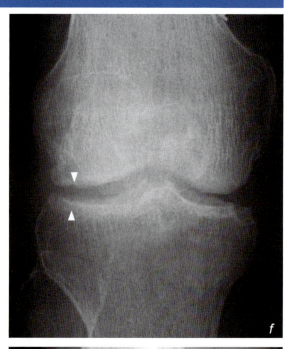

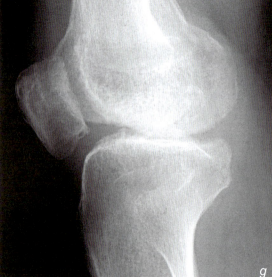

Fig.3f,g *Same patient as in Fig. 3a-e. Three months later, frontal and lateral views of the knee show loss of joint space, particularly in the lateral compartment (between arrowheads). There is associated subchondral bone sclerosis.*

Septic arthritis

Note:
(1) In the presence of a hot, painful and swollen joint, septic arthritis must be excluded.
(2) Early radiographs may be normal. Ultrasound is good for demonstrating a joint effusion.
(3) MRI is better at demonstrating bone involvement.

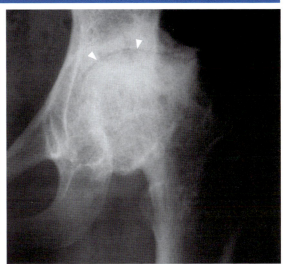

Fig.3h *Frontal view of the left hip of another patient shows the aftermath of a previous septic arthritis. The joint space is almost completely obliterated, there is marginal new bone formation and periarticular sclerosis (arrowheads).*

Rheumatoid arthritis

Rheumatoid arthritis (Fig. 4a)

Discussion:

Rheumatoid arthritis is a connective tissue disorder which targets synovial tissue (pannus formation). There is a 3:1 female predilection and most commonly begins between 20 and 40 years of age.

Imaging of the wrists and hands reflect the pathological features of rheumatoid arthritis (Fig. 4a and b):

- Bilateral symmetrical distribution affecting mainly the radiocarpal, MCP and PIP joints
- Periarticular osteopenia - due to periarticular hyperaemia in response to synovial inflammation.
  N.B. hyperaemia of any cause leads to increased bone resorption and osteopenia
- Periarticular soft tissue swelling - due to synovial thickening and joint effusion.
- Periarticular bony erosion - pannus attacks the margins of the joint first (due to proximity)
- Subchondral cysts - pannus invades into subchondral bone
- Joint space narrowing - due to cartilaginous destruction
- Joint subluxation leading to deformities (swan-neck, boutonierre, etc.)

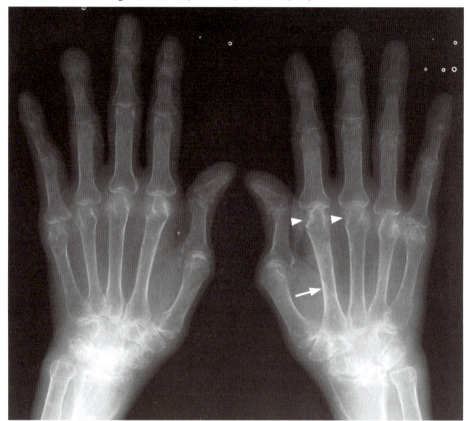

Fig.4b *Radiograph of the right hand in a 64-year-old woman with rheumatoid arthritis. Changes are more advanced in this patient than those in Fig. 4a. Joint subluxation is present in the first interphalangeal joint. There is also generalized osteopenia (marked cortical thinning, arrow). Marginal erosions are best seen at the metacarpal heads (arrowheads).*

Rheumatoid arthritis

Normal appearing radiographs do not exclude the diagnosis of rheumatoid arthritis. Radiographs are only one of the many criteria for diagnosing the disease.

Any synovial joint may be affected (Fig. 4c)

Late radiological features of rheumatoid arthritis include:
- Fibrous or bony ankylosis of affected joints
- Secondary degenerative changes

Role of imaging in patients with rheumatoid arthritis
- Confirm clinical suspicion of disease
- Determine site and severity of disease
- Monitor progress of joint involvement and treatment response.

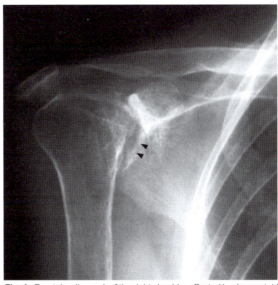

Fig. 4c Frontal radiograph of the right shoulder affected by rheumatoid arthritis, showing loss of joint space and glenoid marginal erosions (arrowheads). There is superior migration of the humeral head indicating associated rotator cuff tendon tear.

Note:
(1) Bilateral symmetrical erosive arthropathy predominantly involving proximal small joints of hand and wrist.

(2) Diagnosis of rheumatoid arthritis is based on a combination of clinical, laboratory and radiological investigations.

04 MUSCULOSKELETAL

Discussion Case 5
Degenerative joint disease

Degenerative joint disease (Fig. 5a, b)

Discussion:
This is the most common form of arthropathy. It is non-inflammatory and the primary pathology is cartilage loss.

The characteristic features of degenerative joint disease reflect the consequences of cartilage loss:
- Joint space narrowing due to loss of cartilage. This is typically worse in the medial tibiofemoral compartment and may result in a varus angulation of the knee joint (genu varum)
- Marginal osteophytes
  - reactive new bone formation in response to altered stress on the articular surface
- Subchondral sclerosis
  - reactive bone formation in response to stress
- Subchondral cyst formation
  - synovial fluid driven into defects of the subchondral bone under pressure
- Joint subluxation.
- Intra-articular bodies
  - cartilage fragments are nourished by synovial fluid within the joint, they grow and may calcify or ossify.
- Joint effusion
  - seen as increased density in suprapatellar pouch in lateral view

Knee joint is one of the commonest sites of involvement in osteoarthritis (Fig. 5c). Other common sites include weight-bearing joints (such as hip joints, lumbar and cervical spine (Fig. 5c, d)) and hands (typically the distal interphalangeal joints and first carpometacarpal joint).

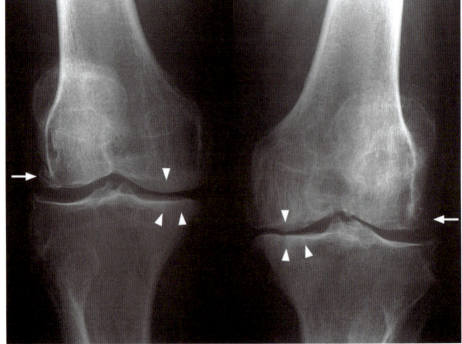

Fig. 5c *Radiograph of both knees, showing loss of joint space (especially in the medial tibiofemoral compartments) indicating cartilage loss. There is subchondral sclerosis (arrowheads) and marginal osteophytes (arrows), which are reactive changes.*

Degenerative joint disease

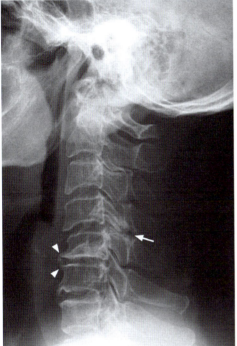

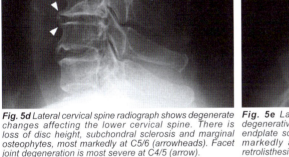

Fig. 5d *Lateral cervical spine radiograph shows degenerate changes affecting the lower cervical spine. There is loss of disc height, subchondral sclerosis and marginal osteophytes, most markedly at C5/6 (arrowheads). Facet joint degeneration is most severe at C4/5 (arrow).*

Fig. 5e *Lateral lumbar spine radiograph shows degenerative changes. There is loss of disc height, endplate sclerosis and marginal osteophytes, most markedly at L1/2 and L4/5. There is also mild retrolisthesis (posterior subluxation) of the L2 and L3 vertebral bodies.*

Radiologic features helpful in distinguishing DJD from inflammatory arthropathy (e.g. rheumatoid arthritis (RA)) include:
- Bone density - preserved in DJD (juxta-articular osteopenia in RA)
- Peri-articular erosion - absent in DJD (periarticular bony erosion in RA)
- Reactive bone changes (sclerosis and osteophytes) - present in DJD (absent in RA, peri-articular osteopenia in RA)
- Distribution of joint involvement - DJD usually affects weight-bearing joints or DIP and CMC joints of hands (RA usually bilateral symmetrical and can involve any joint).

Role of imaging in patients with degenerative joint disease
- Confirm clinical suspicion
- Exclude other pathology (inflammatory arthropathy, septic arthritis or fracture)
- Determine site and severity of disease (compartments involved, intra-articular bodies, varus/valgus deformity)

> **Note:**
> (1) Degenerative joint disease (osteoarthritis) is a common cause of joint pain particularly in elderly patients.
> (2) Joint space narrowing, marginal osteophytes, subchondral sclerosis and cyst formation are characteristic radiological features of osteoarthritis.

Discussion Case 6
Ankylosing spondylitis

Ankylosing spondylitis (Fig. 6a, b)

Discussion:

This is a chronic inflammatory condition involving mainly the axial skeleton. There is a male predilection with symptoms usually beginning between 15 and 35 years of age.

The calcification and ossification of connective tissue dominates this disease (as compared with joint space loss or erosions).

Frontal and lateral radiographs of lumbar spine and sacro-iliac joints in these patients show characteristic features of ankylosing spondylitis:

- Squaring of vertebral bodies: due to osteitis of the corners of vertebral bodies
- Syndesmophyte formation: ossification of annulus fibrosis of intervertebral discs
- Ankylosis of intervertebral facet joints: better seen in lateral view
- Ossification of interspinous and supraspinous ligaments
  The above signs in combination give the bamboo-like appearance (Fig. 6c, d)
- Ankylosis of both sacro-iliac joints: due to long-standing inflammatory sacro-iliitis

Early changes of ankylosing spondylitis occur in the lumbo-sacral region and sacro-iliac joints (Fig. 6e). Later it may extend upward to involve thoracic or even cervical spine (Fig. 6f, g).

Apart from spine, the other common sites of joint involvement are large joints (hip, knee and shoulder), which is different from rheumatoid arthritis (small joints).

Once the diagnosis is established, the possibility of extra-articular complications (such as uveitis, upper lobe pulmonary fibrosis, aortitis/aortic aneurysm) should be considered.

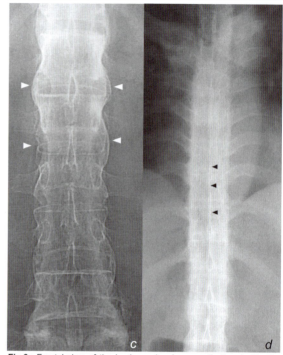

Fig.6c *Frontal view of the lumbar spine (same patient as in Fig. 7a, b) shows syndesmophytes at the margins of the intervertebral discs (arrowheads).*

Fig.6d *Frontal view of the thoracic spine in a patient with more advanced syndesmophyte formation (termed a 'bamboo spine'). The interspinous ligaments are also calcified/ossified (arrowheads), giving a total of three longitudinal lines (together with the intervertebral disc syndesmophytes (termed the 'trolley tracking' sign).*

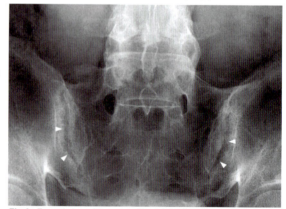

Fig.6e *Frontal view of the sacro-iliac joints of another patient showing early changes (pre-ankylosis) of sacro-iliitis. The cortices of both sides of the joints are poorly defined (loss of the continuous white line) and there are also erosions. These changes are usually better seen on the iliac side rather than the sacral side of the joint (arrow heads).*

Ankylosing spondylitis

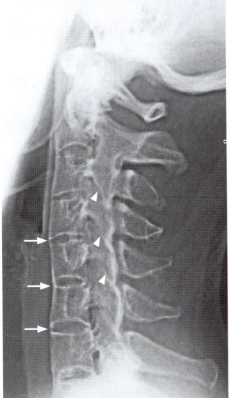

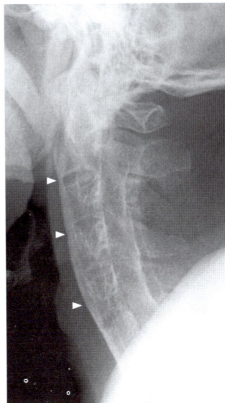

Fig.6f   Lateral view of the cervical spine shows syndesmophytes (arrows). The facet joints are difficult to discern as facet joint ankylosis is present (arrowheads).

Fig.6g Lateral view of the cervical spine with more advanced disease. The individual vertebral bodies are difficult to discern as the veil-like calcification/ossification obscures all margins (arrowheads). This spine is stiff (like a stick of chalk) and prone to fracture.

Role of imaging in patients with ankylosing spondylitis

- Confirm clinical suspicion of ankylosing spondylitis
- Determine site, extent and severity of disease (number of segments, amount of calcification/ankylosis)

Note:
(1) Ankylosing spondylitis should be considered in young males with chronic low back pain and signs of sacro-iliitis.
(2) Bilateral symmetrical sacro-iliitis, syndesmophyte formation, ligamentous ossification and articular ankylosis are characteristic radiological features.
(3) The calcification and ossification of connective tissue forms a large component of this disease.

Discussion Case 7
Avascular necrosis of the femoral head

Avascular necrosis of the femoral head
(Fig. 7a)

Discussion:

Avascular necrosis is a form of osteonecrosis (death of the osteocytes in marrow) usually used for describing the disease in the epiphysis. AVN may be primary (idiopathic) or secondary to trauma, alcoholism, corticosteroids, haemoglobinopathy, collagen vascular diseases, etc.

The bone undergoes three pathological phases:

(1) Avascular: ischaemic death of osteocytes;

(2) Revascularization: dead bone invaded by new vessels, resulting in bone resorption and immature new bone deposition (weak and prone to stress fracture);

(3) Remodelling: new bone matures

Radiographs of avascular necrosis reflect the pathological progression:

- Mottled trabeculae (sclerotic and lucent foci) in femoral head - sclerotic foci containing thickened, infarcted trabeculae (with new bone laid on) mixed with lucent foci of reparative bone resorption.

- Homogeneous sclerotic area - central area of dead bone with collapse (Fig. 7b)

- Flattening of the normally hemispherical cortical outline - micro-fracture or plastic remodelling (Fig. 7b)

- Collapse of femoral head - in severe disease (Fig. 7c)

- Secondary osteoarthritis - late sequelae due to altered mechanical stress on joint (Fig. 7c)

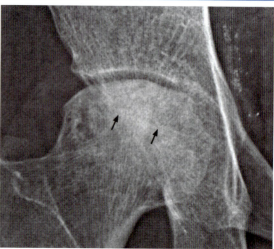

Fig.7b *Magnified frontal view of the right hip shows that contour flattening occurs primarily in the superior aspect of the femoral head (the weight-bearing portion). The joint space is preserved. There is sclerosis within the femoral head (arrows).*

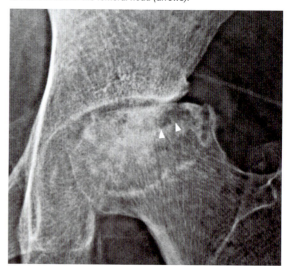

Fig.7c *Magnified frontal view of the left hip shows loss of bone of the superior one third of the femoral head. There is superolateral subluxation of the femoral head. There is also some loss of joint space and cystic areas (arrowheads) in the femoral head (secondary degenerative changes).*

Avascular necrosis of the femoral head

- Subchondral crescent of lucency (Fig. 7d) may sometimes be present as an intermediate stage before collapse. This lucent rim represents subcortical undermining of bone.

Radiographs are usually normal in early cases of avascular necrosis. If there is a high index of clinical suspicion, further evaluation by MRI or radionuclide marrow and bone scan helps in detection of early disease.

MRI (Fig. 7e) is an extremely sensitive method for detecting AVN. It is particularly useful in early AVN when radiographs are normal.

Osteonecrosis occurring outside the epiphysis is usually called bone infarction. These tend to remodel well and have no major sequelae (compared to the joint degeneration of AVN)

Role of imaging in patients with avascular necrosis
- Confirm clinical suspicion of avascular necrosis
- Determine site and severity of disesase
- Allow progress to be closely monitored

> **Note:**
> (1) Collapse of the femoral head with patchy sclerotic change is a typical radiological finding in avascular necrosis of femoral head.
> (2) MRI is the imaging modality of choice for confirmation and detection of early disease when radiographs are usually normal.

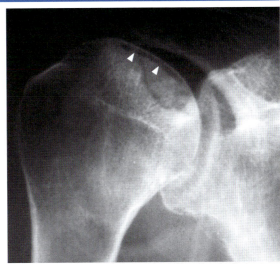

Fig.7d *Frontal view of a left shoulder (different patient) showing a lucent subcortical crescent (arrowheads) representing subchondral bone resorption. The contour of the overlying cortex is very slightly flattened (not as spherical as the rest of the humeral head).*

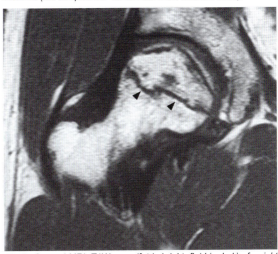

Fig.7e *Coronal MRI, T1W scan (fat is bright, fluid is dark) of a right hip of a different patient. There is a geographic area outlined by a dark band (arrowheads). This geographic area is an area of avascular necrosis and the dark band marks the area boundary between dead (inside band) and viable bone (outside). At this early stage, there is no flattening or collapse of the femoral head as evident from the preserved superior spherical contour.*

Discussion Case 8
Gouty arthritis

Gouty arthritis (Fig. 8a)

Discussion:

This is an inflammatory arthritis secondary to sodium mono-urate crystal deposition (i.e. one type of crystal arthropathy). There is a marked male predilection usually affecting patients 40-60 years old. The lower extremity is commonly involved, especially the first MTP joint, but it occasionally affects the intertarsal and knee joints. Acute gouty arthritis is a clinical diagnosis and the radiographs may be normal. Definitive diagnosis can be made by the presence of positively birefringent urate crystals in synovial (joint) fluid under fluorescence microscopy.

In chronic (tophaceous) gout, tophi (large amorphous deposits of urate) build up over many (5-7) years. These tophi tend to be deposited at the extremities and less vascular tissues such as the ear, tendons, skin of the hands and feet.

Radiographic features of chronic tophaceous gout comprise (Fig. 8b, c):

- Peri-articular soft tissue swelling - due to joint effusion (inflammation)
- Eccentric subcutaneous soft tissue mass with/without calcification - representing gouty tophi
- Bony erosion: (a) at articular margin due to inflamed synovium; (b) periarticular, due to pressure erosion by adjacent tophi; (c) intraosseous, due to intraosseous tophus
- Joint space narrowing - represents cartilaginous destruction and occurs late in the disease.

Fig.8b Magnified view of the first MTPJ shows signs of inflammatory arthropathy, as indicated by loss of joint space (arrow) and marginal erosion (arrowhead). The large bony defect (asterisk) in the head and neck of the first metatarsal is the result of bone resorption due to the formation of a large tophus within the bone. This has breached the cortex and extended into the surrounding area, causing the soft tissue swelling. Despite the destruction, the margin of the lesion is well defined by a sclerotic rim (open arrows).

Fig.8c Radiograph of both feet of another patient showing marked soft tissue swelling (arrowheads) around the first MTP joints.

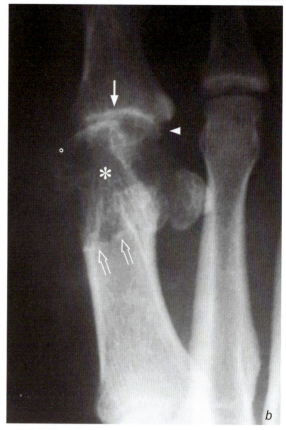

b

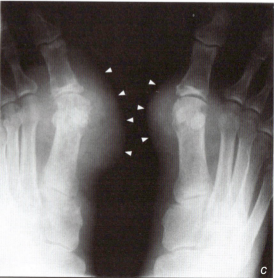

c

Discussion Case 8
Gouty arthritis

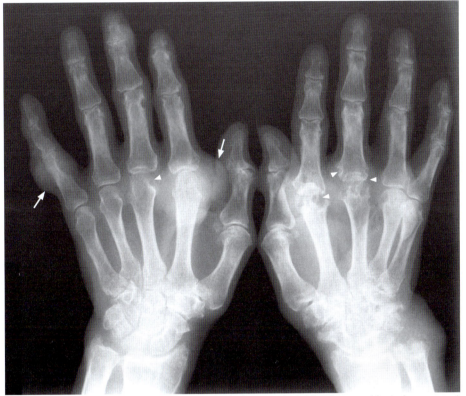

Fig.8d *Frontal view of both hands (of another patient) shows marked deformity caused by tophaceous gout. Large soft tissue swelling (with some calcification) are present indicating tophi (arrows). There is associated adjacent bone erosion. Signs of inflammatory arthropathy are evident as loss of joint space and marginal erosions (arrowheads)*

With severe disease more joints are affected resulting in significant deformity (Fig. 8d).

If clinically indicated, abdominal ultrasound may be performed in patients with chronic gouty arthritis for detection of renal stone and renal nephropathy as pure urate calculi are radiolucent and not detectable by radiography.

Role of imaging in patients with gouty arthritis

- Exclude other causes for symptoms (fracture, infection, etc.)
- Document extent of disease in tophaceous gout
- Guide joint aspiration (if required, and usually with ultrasound) for definitive diagnosis

---

Note:

(1) Recurrent arthritis affecting metatarsophalangeal joint of big toe in a middle aged male is the typical clinical presentation of acute gout. Radiographs may be normal at this stage.

(2) Chronic tophaceous gout is visible on radiographs as a combination of soft tissue swelling, erosions and joint derangement

---

205

Discussion Case 9
Osteosarcoma

Osteosarcoma (Fig. 9a, b)
A subsequent bone scan did not demonstrate any other lesion. On biopsy the femoral lesion was found to be an osteosarcoma.

Discussion:

Osteosarcoma is the most common primary bone tumour in children and young adults. It has a bimodal age distribution (10 to 25 years and over 60 years).

In the older age group it is usually in bones with pre-existing abnormalities such as Paget's disease, multiple exostosis or multiple enchondromata. It commonly affects the metaphyseal region of long bones, and the distal femur is the most common site.

The radiographic and macroscopic appearances depend on the degree of ossification.

The more sclerotic lesions have higher serum alkaline phosphatase levels.

On radiographs, half of all osteosarcomas are sclerotic, a quarter are lytic, and the remainder mixed.

Radiographs, CT and MRI reflect different aspects of the pathological features (Fig. 9c, d and e)

Fig.9c Frontal radiograph of the distal femur of another patient shows a mixed sclerotic and lytic lesion (borders outlined by arrowheads). There is a focal area of cortical thinning with overlying periosteal reaction medially (arrow).

Fig.9d Reformatted CT coronal view of the same region gives a similar though clearer image of the lesion (arrowheads). The periosteal reaction is also better demonstrated (arrow).

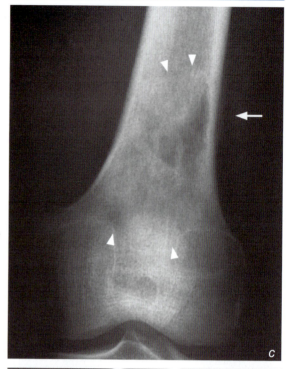

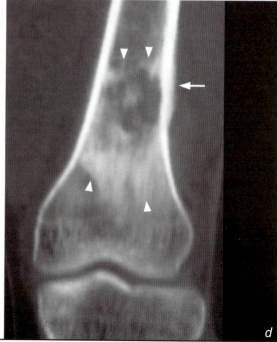

Discussion Case 9
Osteosarcoma

- Mixed osteolytic and sclerotic lesion with ill-defined margins representing areas of destruction by the tumour (lytic area) and areas of new bone formation (sclerotic area)
- Cortical thinning, break through and disruption
- Periosteal new bone formation as it is lifted by tumour. This may be:

Disrupted periosteum elevation (Codman's triangle) adjacent to the primary tumour (Fig. 9f)

Spiculated (sunburst appearance) which indicates rapid growth (in turn suggesting an aggressive lesion) (Fig. 9g, h)

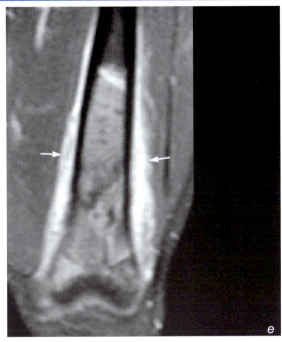

Fig.9e *Coronal, fat-saturated, post-contrast T1-weighted image (high signal indicates contrast enhancement, fat and fluid are dark) in the same patient as in Fig. 9c,d . The true extent of the lesion is better demonstrated (longer in extent than appreciable on the corresponding radiograph or CT). Also, the circumferential nature of the periosteal reaction (arrows) is seen.*

Fig.9f *Frontal radiograph of the distal femur of another patient with an osteosarcoma. Lamellar continous reaction is present over one cortex (arrows). On the other side the periosteal reaction is disrupted in its centre, leaving behind the edges of the periosteal reaction (which form triangles, Codman's triangle, arrowheads).*

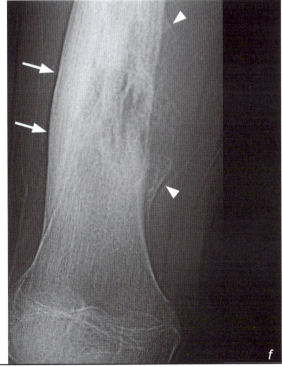

Osteosarcoma

- Overlying soft tissue mass
  - represents soft tissue oedema which
    may be due to sympathetic oedema
    or tumour invasion (Fig. 9g, h)

Many of the imaging findings are
non-specific and may be seen in other
forms of neoplasm and also in infection.
Final diagnosis depends on biopsy results.

Fig.9g *Frontal radiograph of the proximal fibula of another patient shows a sclerotic lesion centred in the neck of the fibula with a large ossified soft tissue component around it (arrows show outer aspect).*

Fig.9h *Lateral radiograph of the same region as in Fig. 9g shows the ossified soft tissue component. There are sun-ray spicules of bone (arrows).*

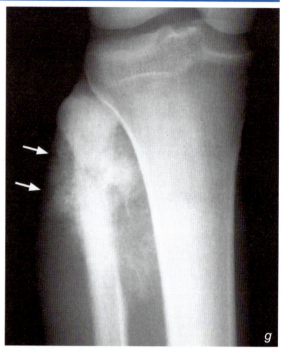

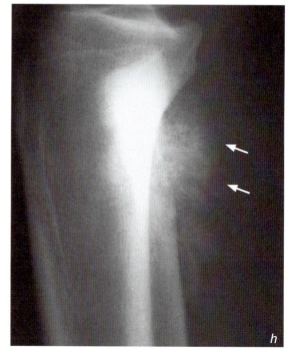

Osteosarcoma

MRI is better at
- Delineating the extent of tumour within the bone and adjacent soft tissue.
- Neurovascular bundle and intra-articular tumour involvement.

The complications of osteosarcoma are: pathological fracture (Fig. 9i, j) and metastasis. Bone metastases are effectively screened by bone scans, and lung metastases are best screened using CT.

Role of imaging in patients with osteosarcoma
- Confirm clinical suspicion
- Determine site and extent of lesion
- Direct biopsy
- Post-chemotherapy/follow-up for progress.

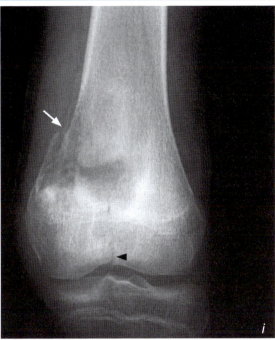

Fig.9i Frontal radiograph of another distal femur showing a pathological fracture extending from the medial cortex (arrow) to the intercondylar region (arrowhead).

Fig.9j Coronal proton density MRI (fat, fluid and tumour of different shades of grey) of the same region as in Fig. 9i. The eccentric tumour is well demonstrated, as is the pathological fracture extending through the tumour from the medial cortex (arrow) to the intercondylar region (arrowhead).

> **Note:**
> (1) Osteosarcoma is the commonest primary malignant bone tumour in children and adolescents.
> (2) Mixed osteolytic and sclerotic lesion with ill-defined margin, spiculated periosteal reaction and overlying soft tissue involvement are typical radiological features.
> (3) MRI is necessary for pre-treatment staging.

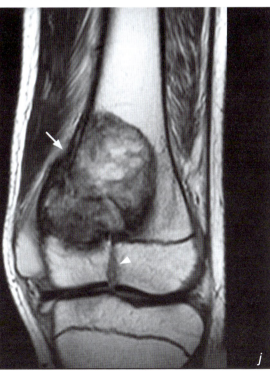

Ewing's sarcoma

Ewing's sarcoma (Fig. 10a). Aggressive lesion of the distal fibula. A biopsy of the lesion revealed a Ewing's sarcoma.

Discussion:

Ewing's sarcoma is a malignant bone neoplasm of primitive cell type (may have derived from stem cells in the bone marrow). Most patients are under 30 years old.
It usually affects the long bones (peripheral skeleton) in younger patients and flat bones (axial skeleton) in older patients. The diaphyseal or metaphyseal marrow is involved.

Radiographic features include:
- Mixed osteolytic and sclerotic lesion with ill-defined margins, representing areas of   destruction by the tumour (lytic area) and areas of new bone formation (sclerotic area) (Fig. 10a, b and c). Diffuse sclerosis may be seen in flat bone lesions (Fig. 10d). Pure lytic lesions are rare.
- The lesion is described as permeative, i.e. wide zone of transition.
- Periosteal reaction is commonly thin and continuous (Fig. 10b) and may be laminated (onion-skin-like)
- Cortical thinning, penetration and disruption
- Overlying soft tissue mass: may represent either soft tissue oedema or infiltration

Many of the imaging findings are non-specific and may be seen in other forms of neoplasm and also in infection. Final diagnosis depends on biopsy results.

Fig.10b *A coned down frontal radiograph of the radial shaft of another patient shows a mixed lytic and sclerotic lesion in the diaphysis. The distal part of the lesion shows cortical thinning and disruption (open arrow). There is a thin continuous lamellar periosteal reaction (arrowheads). The proximal and distal borders are ill-defined (arrows). Biopsy confirmed an Ewing's sarcoma.*

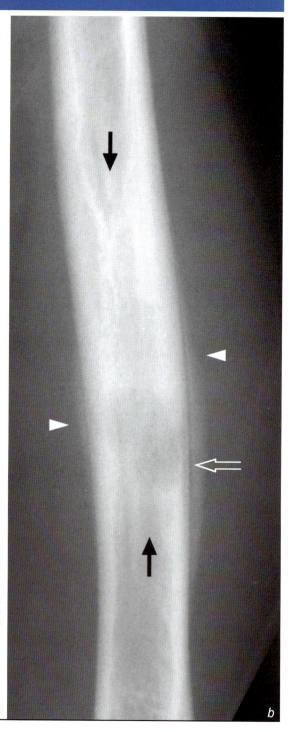

b

Ewing's sarcoma

Role of imaging in patients with Ewing's sarcoma
- Confirm clinical suspicion
- Determine site and extent of lesion
- Direct biopsy
- Post-therapy/follow-up for progress.

Fig.10c Frontal radiograph of the right pelvis of another patient shows a large mixed lytic and sclerotic lesion. The borders of this lesion (arrowheads) are poorly defined. There is cortical destruction medially (arrows). Biopsy confirmed an Ewing's sarcoma.

Fig.10d Frontal radiograph of the right pelvis of another patient shows a diffusely sclerotic lesion (arrowheads). Biopsy confirmed an Ewing's sarcoma.

> **Note:**
> (1) Ewing's sarcoma is a common primary malignant bone tumour in young patients.
> (2) Mixed osteolytic and sclerotic lesions with ill-defined margin, thin continuous periosteal reaction and overlying soft tissue mass are typical but non-specific radiological features.

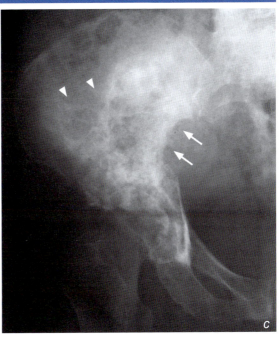

c

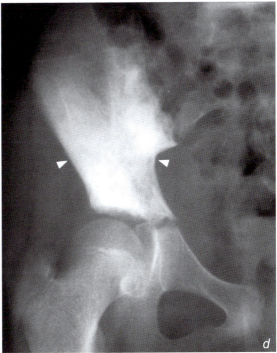

d

04 MUSCULOSKELETAL

Discussion Case 11
Multiple bone metastases

Multiple bone metastases (Fig. 11a)

Discussion:
Whole body radionuclide bone scan features of bone metastases include:
- Multiple 'hot' spots affecting the skeleton, representing local increased osteoblastic activity in response to metastatic infiltration.
- Predominant involvement of the axial skeleton

The advantages of radionuclide bone scan for detecting suspected bony metastases include:
- More sensitive than radiograph, diagnosis can be made before radiographic changes occur
- Allow imaging of the whole bony skeleton with a single injection (rather than taking multiple radiographs)

Radionuclide bone scan involves intravenous injection of a radiopharmaceutical which is taken up by skeletal tissue. The extent of uptake reflects the local blood supply and osteoblastic activity. Bone scan is, however, not specific for bone metastases, and any form of bony lesion with increased osteoblastic activity (such as fracture, infection, etc.) will appear as 'hot' spot. Therefore correlation with radiographic and clinical information is necessary to refine the diagnosis. Radiograph of pelvis in this patient showed features of bone metastases (Fig. 11b):
- Bony destruction (lytic) of right femoral cortex corresponds to bone scan hot spot (Fig. 11b)
- However, there were no radiographic lesions in the left femoral head and neck and left inferior pubic ramus corresponding to these areas of increased activity on bone scan (Fig. 11b)
- Sclerotic T7 vertebral body (Fig. 11c)

The radiological appearances are not entirely specific for bone metastases. Multiple myeloma or infection could have the same appearance. Clinical history of known malignancy supports the diagnosis. An MRI of the thoracolumbar spine confirmed the presence of the lesions and also provides information regarding important adjacent structures such as the spinal cord (Fig. 11d, e).

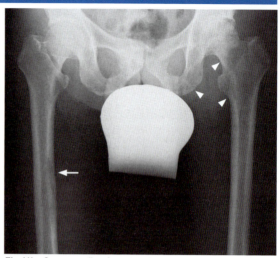

Fig.11b *Corresponding frontal radiograph of the hips and femora shows a long lytic (destructive) lesion involving the medial cortex of the right femoral shaft (arrow) which corresponds to the hot spot on bone scan. No lesion, lytic or sclerotic, is seen around the left hip joint. Radiographs are not sensitive for detecting bone metastasis. It is estimated that approximately 50% of normal bone has to be destroyed before a destructive lesion is visible on radiographs (Fig. 11a-g belong to the same patient).*

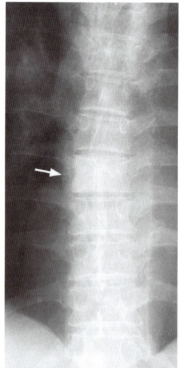

Fig.11c *Frontal radiograph of the lower thoracic spine of the same patient. The entire T7 vertebral body is sclerotic 'ivory vertebra' indicating diffuse osteoblastic activity as a response to infiltration by metastatic cells. An ivory vertebra is seen in Paget's disease, tuberculosis and many types of neoplastic/ metastatic diseases (Fig. 11a-g belong to the same patient).*

Discussion Case 11
Multiple bone metastases

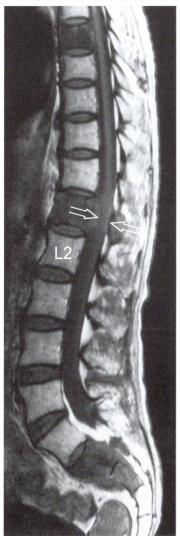

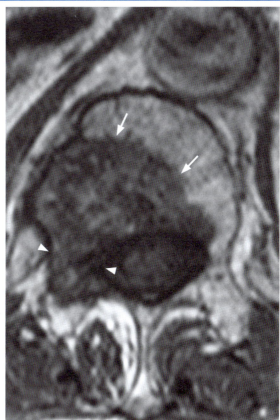

Fig.11e *Axial T2W MRI of the L1 vertebra of a different patient with bony metastasis. There is metastatic involvement of the vertebral body (arrows) which extends to the right pedicle (arrowheads). Pedicular involvement is highly suggestive of neoplasm (not infection).*

Fig.11d *Sagittal T1W scan (fat is bright, fluid is black) of the thoracolumbar spine. For a patient of this age, the vertebral bodies should show diffuse marrow replacement by fat (bright or largely bright signal). In this patient, the T7, L1, S2 and S3 vertebral bodies show a dark grey signal indicating disease involvement. At the L1 level, the spinal cord is surrounded by neoplastic tissue (arrows) which has breached the vertebral cortex and extended into the spinal canal (Fig. 11a-g belong to the same patient).*

Discussion Case 11
Multiple bone metastases

Computed tomography, due to its high resolution, is frequently used to look for a primary lesion in patients found to have bone metastasis (Fig. 11f, g).

Note:

(1) Radionuclide bone scan is the initial imaging modality of choice for detection of bone metastases.

(2) A bone scan is sensitive but non-specific for bone metastases. Correlation with radiographs and clinical history is necessary.

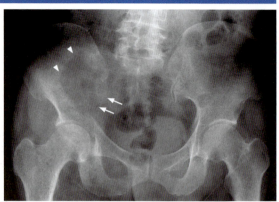

Fig.11f Frontal radiograph of another patient (62-year-old male) who presented with right hip pain. There is bone destruction which has resulted in loss of the inferior iliac cortical margin (arrows) and has extended superiorly to the iliac wing (arrowheads). A bone scan was performed and revealed this to be a solitary bone lesion.

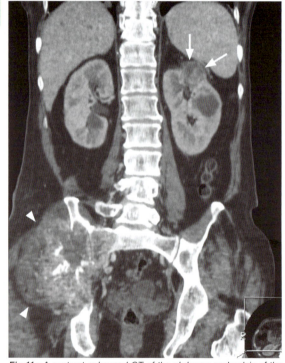

Fig.11g A contrast enhanced CT of the abdomen and pelvis of the patient in Fig. 11f was performed to look for a primary lesion. A reconstructed coronal image is shown in this figure. The destructive lesion in the right iliac bone can be seen to harbour a large soft tissue mass which has extended outwards into the gluteal region (arrowheads). There is a small (2.5 cm) soft tissue density lesion in the upper pole of the left kidney (arrows). This lesion turned out to be a primary renal cell carcinoma. Bone metastases from the kidney and thyroid are classically large and expansile.

Haemophilic arthropathy

Haemophilic arthropathy (Fig.12a, b)

Discussion:

Haemophilia A is an X-linked recessive disease characterized by a deficiency of Factor VIII (Factor IX for Haemophilia B) and hence a bleeding tendency. Recurrent episodes of haemarthrosis results in synovial hypertrophy (pannus formation). The pannus then erodes the cartilage adjacent to it and sets off a cycle of cartilage loss, subchondral bone erosion and repair (sclerosis) and degenerative joint disease.

The typical joints involved are the knee, elbow and ankle.

The radiological findings reflect the joint pathology:

- Distended joint capsule (haemarthrosis and synovial hypertrophy)
- Loss of joint space (loss of cartilage)
- Subchondral cortical irregularity (erosion of the subchondral bone and subchondral cyst formation)
- Degenerative joint disease
- Widened intercondylar notch of femur (bone erosion by pannus)
- Subtle increase in density of the joint capsule (iron deposition from recurrent haemarthroses)
- Periarticular osteopenia (bone resorption due to periarticular hyperaemia and disuse)

With chronic haemophilic arthropathy, there will be gross joint deformity (Fig. 12c).

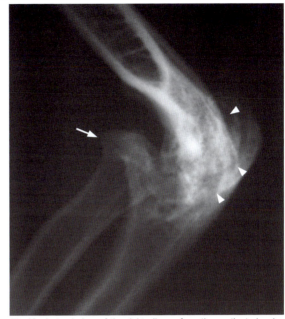

Fig.12c *Lateral view of the right elbow of another patient showing gross joint deformity. The head of the radius (arrow) is dislocated anteriorly. The small trochlea is sitting in an enlarged olecranon (both the result of erosion and remodelling). There are degenerative changes with loss of joint space, sclerosis and subchondral cysts (arrowheads).*

Note:

(1) Haemophilic arthropathy is characterized by pathology combining both synovial hypertrophy (joint distension and erosions) and degenerative joint disease (loss of cartilage and resultant bone reparation)

(2) Radiographic changes therefore bear resemblance to both inflammatory arthropathy and degenerative joint disease.

Vertebral discitis/osteomyelitis

Psoas abscess and vertebral discitis/ osteomyelitis (Fig.13a-c)

Discussion:

Pathology involving the psoas muscles, due to their deep retroperitoneal location, are relatively occult clinically and radiologically/sonographically. Vertebral/discal infection may extend to involve its surrounding structures (paraspinal muscles, mediastinum, retroperitoneal structures, etc.). In the lumbar region, the psoas muscle is commonly involved due to its proximity. Owing to the course of the psoas muscle (lumbar spine to lesser trochanter), the patient may complain of groin pain and movement of the hip may aggravate the pain.

Psoas abscesses may occur without lumbar vertebral or discal infection. Although the imaging appearance is not organism specific, abscesses due to tuberculosis tend to have extensive soft tissue spread and large collections (Fig. 13e, f). Nonetheless, needle aspiration (usually under image guidance) is required for organism identification. Another common cause for a psoas mass is a psoas haematoma (Fig. 13g). These usually occur in patients on anti-coagulants or with a bleeding diathesis. The patient usually presents with back pain or loin pain and laboratory tests may show anaemia. The size of the haematoma may be clinically deceptive due to its retroperitoneal position.

Role of imaging in patients with discitis/spinal osteomyelitis

- Confirm clinical suspicion of a psoas abscess.
- CT/MRI to determine the extent of infection.
- Image-guided aspiration for organism identification.
- Image-guided drainage for treatment.

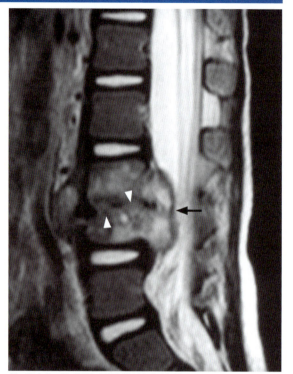

Fig.13d *Sagittal MRI, T2W (fluid is bright) image of the lower lumbar spine. There is destruction of the endplates (arrowheads) on both sides of the L3/4 disc. The signal in the L3 and L4 vertebral bodies is increased indicating oedema (inflammation) which in this clinical setting implies osteomyelitis. There is also destruction of the side walls of these vertebra, through which the infection has spread to form paraspinal abscesses. The arrow shows the epidural component, which is indenting the dural sac.*

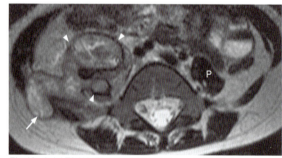

Fig.13e *Axial T2W MRI at the L5 level shows the right psoas muscle being expanded by an abscess (arrowheads). The normal left psoas (P) could be used for comparison. The psoas abscess has extended laterally through the right oblique abdominal muscles to become subcutaneous in location (arrow).*

Vertebral discitis/osteomyelitis

Note:

(1) Presence of back pain and clinical evidence of sepsis raises the suspicion of infective discitis.

(2) Disc space narrowing with adjacent end-plate destruction are characteristic radiological features.

(3) MRI is the imaging modality of choice for detection of complications such as abscess.

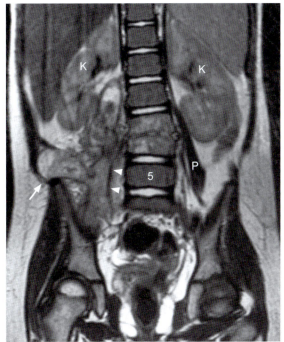

Fig.13f *Coronal T2W MRI shows the vertical extent of the right psoas abscess (arrowheads), its medial relation with the infected L3 & L4 vertebrae, and its lateral extension into the subcutaneous fat (arrow). P=normal left psoas, K=kidney. Same patient as in Fig. 13e.*

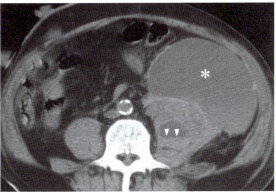

Fig.13g *Axial non-contrast CT showing a large haematoma outside (asterisk) and within the left psoas muscle. There is a blood-fluid level (haematocrit, arrowheads) for the haemorrhage inside the left psoas.*

Chronic suppurative osteomyelitis

Chronic osteomyelitis of tibia
(Fig. 14a, b)

Discussion:

Chronic osteomyelitis represents a continuation of unresolved acute infection (due to poor response to treatment or other associated conditions such as an immunocompromised state, foreign body).

The extremities are most commonly affected and the metaphysis is the usual site of initial infection.

The pathological process (and some of the radiographic changes) are:
- The infecting organism is deposited within the medullary cavity (haematologically or direct spread from a wound or penetrating injury).
- Inflammatory reaction occurs around the focus of infection.
- Resultant oedema and exudate increase, raising the intramedullary pressure.
- Raised pressure compromises blood supply resulting in bone, haematopoietic tissue and marrow fat infarct.
- New periosteal bone forms a thick wall around the infected area (involucrum Fig. 14c).
- Sinus tract formation (cloaca Fig. 14d) as pus pushes through the involucrum.
- Dead bone (sequestrum), from the infarct.

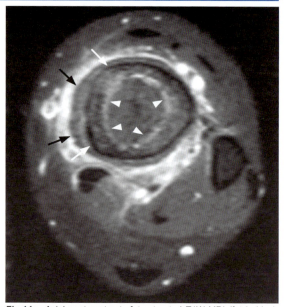

Fig.14c *Axial post-contrast fat-saturated T1W MRI (fat is black, fluid is black, contrast enhancement is bright) of the tibia of another patient with chronic osteomyelitis. There are 3 concentric rings surrounding the medullary cavity. The innermost thin ring is a layer of endosteal reaction (arrowheads point out the contrast enhancing endosteum). The outermost layer is a thick layer of periosteal new bone (black arrow). In between these two layers is the original cortical bone (outer surface indicated by arrows).*

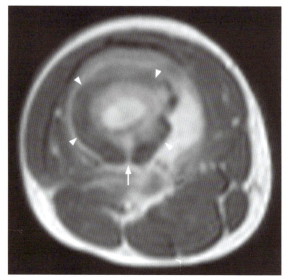

Fig.14d *Axial T2W MRI (fat is bright, fluid is bright, cortical bone is black) of the distal femur of another patient with chronic osteomyelitis. There is a thick and undulating layer of periosteal new bone (arrowheads). The infection has decompressed through a cloaca (arrow).*

Chronic suppurative osteomyelitis

One variation is Brodie's abscess (Fig. 14e, f) which is a smoldering and indolent bone infection in childhood. Here the bone reaction manages to wall off most of the infection (thus aptly named an abscess). The gross spread and remodelling (Fig. 14g) seen in suppurative chronic osteomyelitis is not seen. Imaging does not identify the causative organism. Needle aspiration under CT guidance helps to obtain infective material for microscopy and culture if clinically necessary.

MRI accurately assesses the extent of bone and soft tissue involvement (Fig. 14c, d, f).

Role of imaging in patients with suppurative osteomyelitis
- Confirm clinical suspicion of infection.
- Determine site and configuration of infection.
- MRI to assess extent of infection, especially the soft tissue involvement.
- Guide biopsy to obtain material for culture.

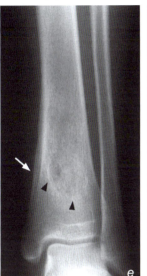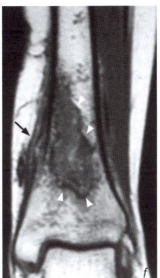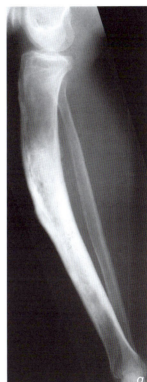

Fig.14e Frontal radiograph of a young patient with a Brodie's abscess in the distal tibia. There is a thin rim of sclerosis (arrowheads) around the infected region. A thick periosteal reaction (arrow) is present medially.

Fig.14f Coronal T1W MRI of the distal tibia of the patient in Fig.14e. The abscess is surrounded by a dark rim (arrowheads) of sclerotic bone. The lesion is closest to the cortical surface superomedially. There is extension of the infection outwards to produce a focal periosteal reaction (arrow).

Fig.14g Lateral radiograph of the tibia of another patient with chronic osteomyelitis. There is extensive and well-established periosteal reaction around the tibia. This new bone is structurally weak and vulnerable to remodelling, resulting in a bowing deformity.

Note:
(1) Chronic osteomyelitis is characterized by local bone reaction to wall-off and limit the infection.
(2) Classic features are a sequestrum, involucrum, cloaca.

Pathological spinal fracture

Pathological spinal fracture (Fig. 15a, b) T10 pathological fracture (probably due to metastasis) causing spinal cord compression.

CT-guided biopsy of the T10 vertebral body confirmed metastatic involvement.

Discussion:

MRI thoracic spine of this patient showed features of vertebral metastasis with spinal cord compression (Fig. 15c-f):

- Replacement of the normal fatty marrow signal in the vertebral body represents metastatic deposit (Fig. 15c, d).
- Loss of height of T10 vertebral body, due to pathological fracture of the weakened bone.
- Bulging of the posterior vertebral body contour, due to destruction of the posterior cortex and intra-spinal, epidural protrusion of the metastatic mass (Fig. 15c, d).
- Posterior displacement and kinking of the spinal cord by the epidural mass (Fig. 15c, d, e).
- Preservation of intervertebral disc helps to distinguish metastases from infective discitis.
- Coronal view shows the vertical extent of the tumour mass (Fig. 15f), involvement of the left pedicle and extension of tumour across the left neural exit foramina. The latter probably causes compression.
- Involvement of left T9 and T10 nerve roots resulting in symptoms along their respective dermatomes (Fig. 15f).

The vertebrae are commonly involved in disseminated bone metastases. Extension of metastatic tumour mass from the vertebral body into the adjacent epidural space causes compression of the spinal cord and nerve roots.

Early detection is important as neurological damage is potentially reversible after surgical decompression or radiotherapy.

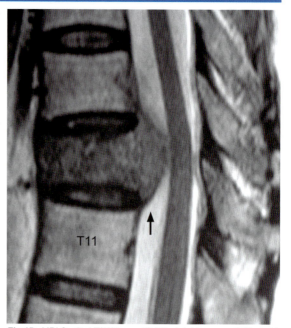

Fig.15c *MRI Sagittal T2W image (fluid is bright, marrow fat is dark). There is abnormal low signal in the compressed T10 vertebral body indicating marrow replacement. The intervertebral disc and endplates are preserved. The posterior cortex is destroyed and there is an epidural mass (arrow) displacing the spinal cord posteriorly.*

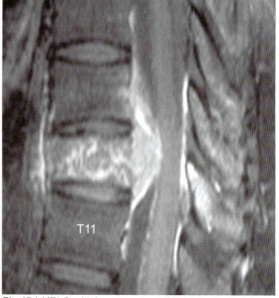

Fig.15d *MRI Sagittal post-contrast T1W fat-saturated image (enhancement is bright, fluid and fat are dark). Both the intravertebral and epidural components of the mass enhance after contrast.*

Discussion Case 15
Pathological spinal fracture

Fig.15e MRI axial T1W images at the T10 level. The epidural mass is indented centrally at either side of the posterior longitudinal ligament (arrowhead) forming two bulges pushing the spinal cord (arrow) posteriorly against the laminae.

Fig.15f MRI coronal post-contrast T1W fat-saturated image (enhancement is bright, fluid and fat are dark). The epidural mass has a roughly H shape configuration as a result of tumour extension (arrowheads) through the exit foramina. There is also involvement of the T10 left pedicle (arrow).

Note:
(1) Spinal cord compression should be considered in patients with disseminated malignancy presenting with spinal neurological symptoms.
(2) MRI spine is the imaging modality of choice.
(3) Early diagnosis and treatment is important for good neurological recovery.

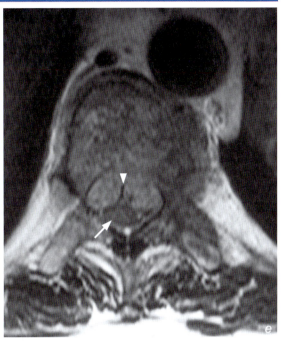

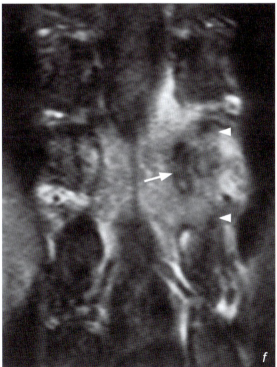

04 MUSCULOSKELETAL

221

Discussion Case 16
Degenerative disc disease

Degenerative intervertebral discs with prolapse and spinal canal stenosis (Fig. 16a-c)

Discussion:

Degenerative disc disease is one of the commonest causes of low back pain with/without sciatica, especially in older patients, manual labourers and contact sport players. The pain may be due to pathology in a variety of related structures:

- Disc protrusion with/without macroscopic annular tear (the annulus fibrosus is innervated and damage to it causes pain)
- Nerve root compression (by protruded disc, and/or hypertrophied ligamentum flavum and/or facet joints)
- Facet joint degeneration (these are synovial type joints and may undergo the typical degenerative changes, i.e. loss of cartilage/joint space/ subchondral sclerosis and osteophytosis
- Anterior or posterior vertebral subluxation due to abnormal translatory movement. The lower lumbar spine (especially the L4/5 and L5/S1 levels) are most commonly affected. MRI is the most sensitive imaging modality for detection of complications related to degenerative disc disease, including (Fig. 16a-g):
- Spinal stenosis (cord or cauda equina compression)
- Effacement of the lateral recess(es) (compression of the subjacent nerve root)
- Effacement of the neural exit foramen (compression of the exiting nerve root)

Fig.16d & e *Sagittal and axial T2W MRI of the lumbar spine of a normal patient for comparison. The nucleus pulposis is of normal high signal and contained within the annulus fibrosis. The axial image shows the normally separate nerve roots of the cauda equina suspended in CSF. The deep muscles of the back are symmetrical.*

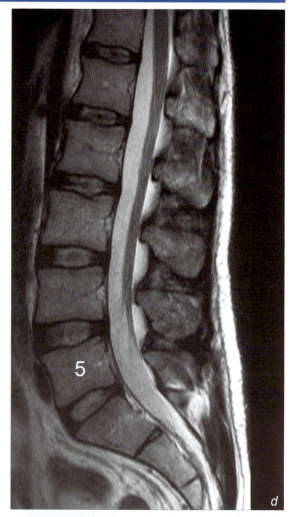

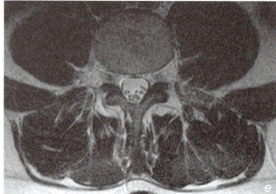

Degenerative disc disease

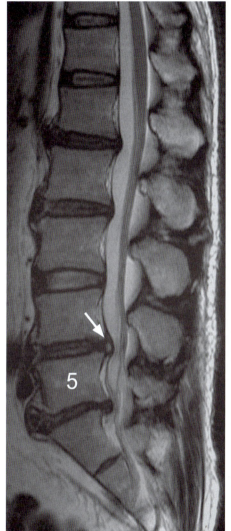

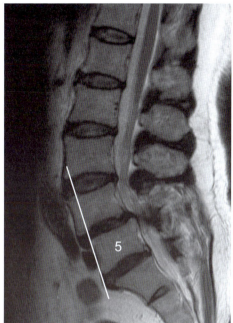

Fig.16g *Median sagittal T2W MRI image of the lumbar spine of a different patient shows changes of disc degeneration. Here there is anterior subluxation (anterolisthesis) of the L4 vertebral body. The amount of subluxation can be demonstrated by drawing a line along the anterior or posterior cortex of the subjacent vertebral body and assessing how much the suprajacent vertebra has slipped. Here it is less than 25% of the AP diameter of the L4 vertebral endplate and thus classified as a grade I anterolisthesis. It would be considered grade II if it was between 25% and 50%, grade III if between 50% and 75% and so on.*

Fig.16f *Median sagittal T2W MRI image of the lumbar spine of a different patient shows a variety of changes of disc degeneration. There is posterior disc protrusion at the L4/5 and L5/S1 levels. There is a focus of high signal indicating an annular tear (arrow) in the posterior aspect of the L4/5 disc. There are also less severe changes at the L1/2 and L2/3 levels.*

Discussion Case 16
Degenerative disc disease

Radiographs of the lumbo-sacral spine are usually performed for a quick evaluation (Fig. 16h) of the status of the vertebrae and discs. Reformatted CT images provide similar but more detailed information (Fig. 16i).
Similar degenerative disc changes may also occur in the cervical levels.

Role of imaging in degenerative disc disease:
- Rule out other causes of back pain: vertebral fracture, discitis/osteomyelitis etc.
- Define and locate site/sites of abnormality
- Estimate extent of canal stenosis and/or neural exit foraminal narrowing
- Follow-up imaging for progress after treatment

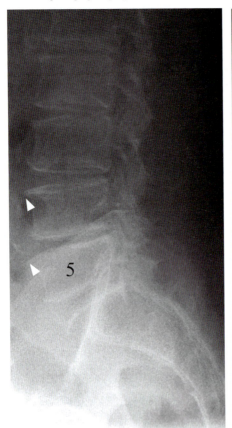

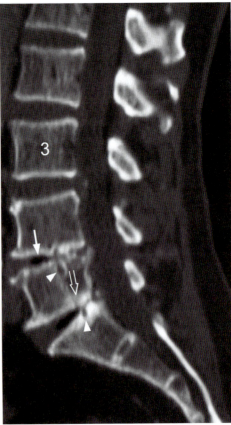

Fig.16h Lateral radiograph of the lumbo-sacral spine of a different patient shows loss of disc height at the spine L4/5 and L5/S1 levels. There are also anterior endplate osteophytes (arrowheads).

Fig.16i Median sagittal reformatted CT image of a different patient shows the bony architecture in exquisite detail. There is loss of disc height and intra-discal gas (arrow) of the L4/5 and L5/S1 discs due to disc desiccation. The intra-discal gas is a vacuum phenomenon which occurs when there is a joint space enlargement (due to a distraction movement) and dissolved nitrogen diffuses to fill this void. There is endplate irregularity and small pits from disc herniation (arrowheads). There is reactive subchondral bony sclerosis (open arrow).

Degenerative disc disease

Note:
(1) Low back pain with/without sciatica is commonly caused by degenerative disc disease.
(2) MRI is the imaging modality of choice.
(3) Complications such as spinal cord, nerve root or cauda equina compression can be assessed by MRI.

TRAUMA

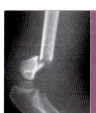

Contributors:

**Gregory E. Antonio, James F. Griffith,
David P.N. Chan, Anil T. Ahuja**

Questions

Case 1 - 11   228 - 238

Discussion

Colles' fracture   239 - 240
Fracture of the femoral neck   241 - 242
Anterior shoulder dislocation   243 - 245
Fractures of osteoporotic spine   246
Pathological fracture   247 - 248
Incomplete fracture   249 - 250
Supracondylar fracture   251 - 252
Tibial plateau fracture   253
Cervical spine fracture   254 - 256
Post-traumatic cord compression   257 - 258
Atlanto-axial subluxation/dislocation   259 - 260

Chapter 05

Case 1

A 75-year-old woman, with a known history of osteoporosis, complained of severe pain of the distal left forearm after falling on an outstretched hand. On physical examination, there was a swelling over the distal forearm with localized tenderness and a fracture was suspected. Radiographs of the wrist were performed (AP and lateral) (Fig. 1a and b).

Questions

(1) What abnormalities do you see on these radiographs ?
   Frontal view: Cortical disruption of the distal radius
                      Discontinued white band in distal radius
   Lateral view: Dorsal angulation of distal radial fragment and carpus
                      - Soft tissue swelling over the wrist
(2) What is the diagnosis ?

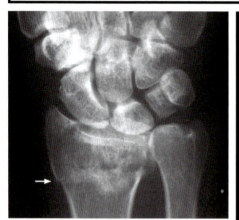

Fig.1a *Frontal view of the wrist shows cortical disruption (arrow), and a white band (due to overlapped bone) across the distal radial metaphysis.*

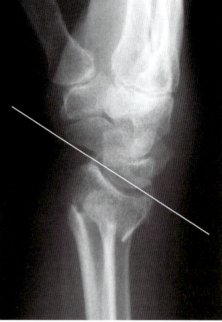

Fig.1b *Lateral view shows that the distal radial articular surface (white line) is dorsally angulated (approximately 30 degrees) with respect to the radial shaft (there is normally a 10-15 degree volar angulation). This angulation results in the classical 'dinner fork' sign.*

Case 2

An 88-year-old woman, with a known history of osteoporosis, fell from her bed and could not stand afterwards. She had severe pain over the right hip region. Physical examination showed shortening of the lower limb which was also held in external rotation. Marked localized tenderness was present over the hip joint. As a fracture was suspected, radiographs of the left hip were performed (Fig. 2a and b).

Questions

(1) What abnormalities do you see on these radiographs ?

Lucent line through base of neck of femur

Discontinuity of cortex of the femoral neck

Medial angulation of the femoral shaft resulting in a varus deformity

(2) What is the diagnosis ?

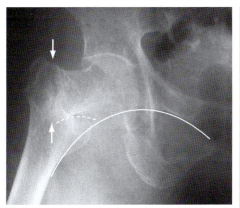

Fig.2a Frontal view shows a lucent (fracture) line (running between the arrows) and an angulated femoral neck cortex (interrupted white line) of a basicervical fracture with angulation. There was a resultant varus deformity and disruption of Shenton's line (white continuous line). Shenton's line is a line drawn on the frontal radiograph, along the inferior margin of the superior pubic ramus and inferomedial cortex of the femoral neck. This should be a smooth curve, a disruption of this line is seen in hip dislocations, femoral neck fractures and slipped femoral epiphysis. In this patient, the neck of the inferomedial surface of the femoral neck (broken line) does not form a smooth curve with the superior pubic ramus.

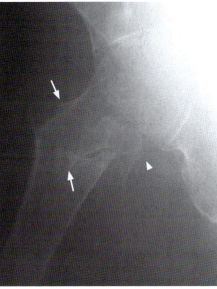

Fig.2b Lateral view shows the fracture line (arrows) and also a trochanteric fracture (arrowhead)(separate fracture of the greater trochanter). The latter component was not well demonstrated in the frontal view.

Case 3

A 45-year-old man was hit on the back of the right shoulder during a football game and complained of severe shoulder pain subsequently. On physical examination he could not actively move the right upper limb. The lateral outline of the shoulder was flat and a bulge was felt just below the lateral portion of the clavicle (in the clavipectoral triangle). In view of the history, radiographs of the right shoulder were performed (Fig. 3a and b: frontal and Y views).

Questions

(1) What abnormalities do you see on these radiographs ?

      Frontal view: Loss of contact between the humeral head and glenoid

                   Humeral head lies inferior to the glenoid

      Y view: Humeral head lies anteroinferior to glenoid

(2) <u>What is the diagnosis ?</u>

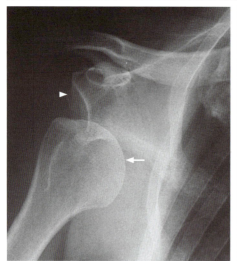

Fig.3a *Frontal view shows inferior dislocation of the humeral head (arrow) with respect to glenoid fossa (arrowhead).*

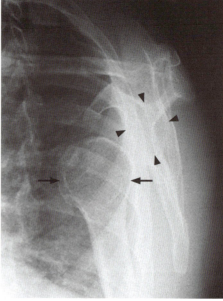

Fig.3b *The Y view shows the glenoid fossa en face (arrowheads) and sitting at the center of the Y shaped profile of the scapula. The humeral head (arrows) is dislocated anteriorly and inferiorly.*

Case 4

An 88-year-old woman with multiple medical problems complained of low back pain for two months. There was no fever or history of significant trauma. Physical examination revealed localized tenderness over the lumbar spine and increased kyphosis, without neurological deficit. Laboratory investigations showed normal white cell count, serum calcium and phosphate levels. Serum alkaline phosphatase level was also within normal limits. Radiographs of the thoraco-lumbar spine (Fig. 4a and b) were performed in view of the history.

Questions

(1) What abnormalities do you see on these radiographs ?

    Frontal view: Biconcave-shaped T12 vertebral body

               Loss of height of L1

               Increased density of vertebral body (due to bone impaction)

               Preserved outlines of the pedicles

    Lateral view: Generalized decreased bone density

               Increased kyphosis centred at thoracolumbar junction

               Wedge-shaped T12 (worse) and L1 vertebral bodies

(2) What is the diagnosis ?

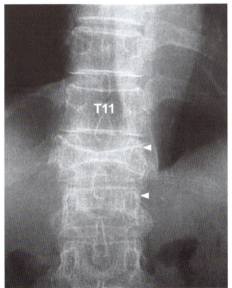

Fig.4a *Frontal view shows loss of height of the T12 (worse) and L1 vertebral bodies. The outlines of pedicles (arrowheads) are preserved, making metastatic disease less likely.*

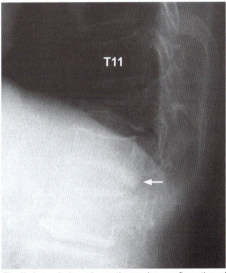

Fig.4b *Lateral view shows the wedge configuration of both fractures and the resultant exaggerated kyphosis at the thoracolumbar junction. The lower part of the posterior margin of the L1 vertebral body is bulging posteriorly (arrow) suggesting retropulsion. This view also shows the degree of osteoporosis of the spine. The vertebral bodies demonstrate generalized osteopenia with a thin bright cortical rim (relative to the darker osteopenic centre).*

Case 5

A 63-year-old woman, with a history of breast carcinoma, complained of right pelvic pain for 3 months. The pain was dull in nature and progressive over this period. Physical examination showed soft tissue swelling and local tenderness at right iliac bone. Laboratory investigations revealed a raised alkaline phosphatase. Parathyroid hormone level was normal. Radiographs of the pelvis were performed in view of the clinical history (Fig. 5a and b, frontal and oblique radiographs).

Questions

(1) What abnormalities do you see on these radiographs ?

Frontal view: Patchy sclerosis of the right iliac bone mixed with mottled lucencies

Break in the cortex of the iliac bone with the fracture line extending into the iliac body

Diastasis of the right sacro-iliac joint

Oblique view: Lucent line traversing the iliac bone

(2) What is the diagnosis ?

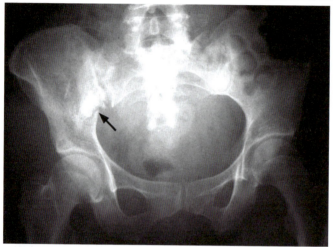

Fig.5a *Frontal view of the pelvis shows patchy sclerosis and lucencies in the right iliac bone. There is a break in the cortex of the iliac bone (arrow). There is diastasis (widening) of the right sacroiliac joint, compared to the left.*

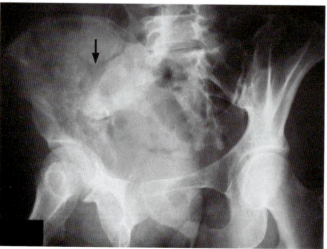

Fig.5b *Oblique (45 degree) view of the pelvis shows that the fracture line extends deep into the iliac body and also branches (arrow). The underlying bone shows mixed sclerosis and lucency indicating pathology (neoplasia or infection, inflammatory, ischaemia)*

Case 6

A 4-year-old boy complains of severe left forearm pain shortly after falling off his bicycle. Physical examination shows swelling and marked localized tenderness over the distal left forearm. Range of movement is severely limited by pain. A fracture was suspected and radiographs of the forearm were performed (Fig. 6a frontal, b lateral view).

Questions

(1) What abnormalities do you see on these radiographs ?
   - On the frontal view, fracture lines are present extending partially across the ulnar and radial shafts
   - On the lateral view, cortical disruption of the distal ulnar shaft is present on one side but intact on the other. Similar but more subtle changes are seen in the radial shaft.
(2) What is the diagnosis ?

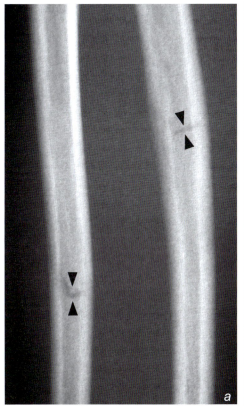

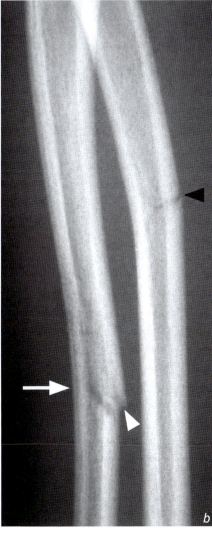

Fig.6a *Frontal view of the forearm shows fracture lines extending partially across the ulnar and radial shafts (arrowheads). There is no displacement or angulation present in this view.*

Fig.6b *Lateral view of the forearm shows cortical disruption of the ulnar shaft on one side (white arrowhead) but apparently intact on the other (arrow). There is mild bowing/angulation of the ulnar shaft (concavity facing the arrow). Similar but more subtle signs are present in the radial shaft (black arrowhead).*

Case 7

An 8-year-old boy presented with a painful right elbow after falling on an outstretched hand. Physical examination showed localized pain and swelling just above the right elbow. The range of movement was limited by severe pain. Radiographs of the elbow were performed for further evaluation (Fig. 7a lateral, frontal view was non-contributory).

Questions

(1) What abnormalities do you see on these radiographs ?
     Frontal view: There is no evidence of a fracture
     Lateral view: The anterior and posterior fat pads are elevated
               There is a break in the anterior cortex of the humerus

(2) What is the diagnosis ?

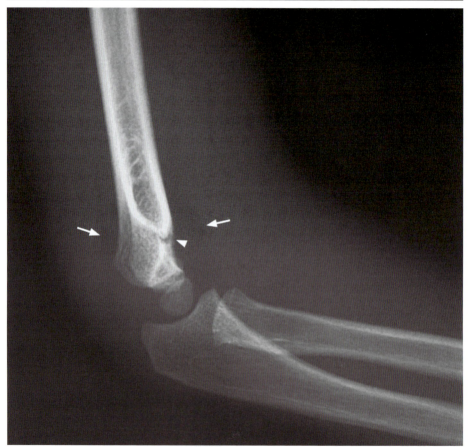

Fig.7a *Lateral radiograph shows elevation of both the anterior and posterior fat pads (arrows). These fat pads are elevated by increased joint capsule content (by blood in this case) indicating pathology. Non-displaced supra-condylar fracture (arrowhead) is present (Image courtesy of Dr Yolanda Lee, Department of Diagnostic Radiology and Organ Imaging, The Chinese University of Hong Kong).*

Case 8

A 30-year-old man was in a motor vehicle accident and sustained an injury to his right knee. On examination, there was a swelling around the knee with generalized tenderness. Frontal and lateral radiographs were performed for further evaluation (Fig. 8a lateral view and b coned frontal view).

Questions
(1) What abnormalities do you see on these radiographs ?
   Lateral view: Swollen suprapatellar pouch
   Frontal view: Fracture line extending inferiorly from the lateral tibial plateau
(2) What is the diagnosis ?

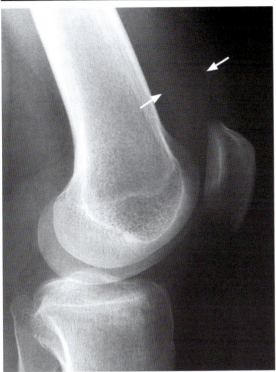

Fig.8a *Lateral radiograph of the knee shows a distended suprapatellar pouch (arrows). No bony abnormalities are seen.*

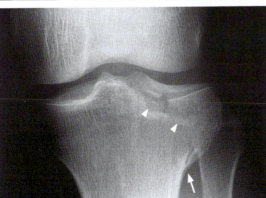

Fig.8b *Frontal view of the knee centred on the tibial plateau. There is a fracture line extending from the lateral tibial plateau inferiorly (arrowhead). There is another cortical irregularity in the lateral tibial metaphysis (arrow).*

Case 9

A 43-year-old man was brought in by ambulance after being knocked down by a car. He was alert and haemodynamically stable on general examination. There was marked localized tenderness over the mid cervical region. Muscle power was globally reduced in all four limbs. A lateral cervical spine radiograph (Fig. 9a) was performed as part of a trauma radiographic series.

Questions

(1) What abnormalities do you see on this lateral cervical radiograph ?

Small triangular (teardrop) fractured fragment of bone in the anteroinferior aspect of the C3 vertebral body.

Prevertebral soft tissue swelling associated with this fracture.

Widening of the space between spinous processes of C3 and C4.

Loss of normal cervical lordosis.

(2) What is the diagnosis ?

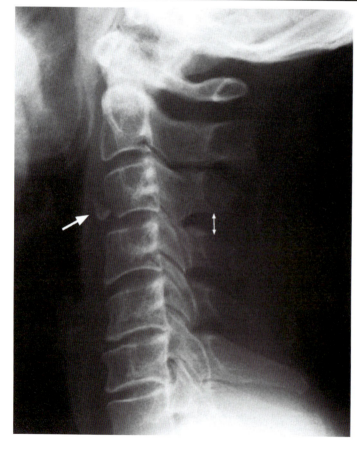

Fig.9a Lateral cervical spine radiograph shows a triangular-shaped (teardrop) fracture at the anteroinferior aspect of the C3 vertebral body. Soft tissue swelling is present at this level due to a small associated haematoma. There is an increased separation of the distance between the C3 and C4 spinous processes (double headed arrow) indicating a hyperflexion mechanism injury and injury to the inter-spinous ligament. Note the loss of normal cervical lordosis.

Case 10

A 36-year-old man was brought in by ambulance shortly after falling onto his back from a height of 10 metres. Physical examination revealed localized tenderness in thoracolumbar region, and a T11 spinal level paraparesis. The abdomen was soft, chest and neck non-tender, and blood pressure was normal.

A frontal radiograph of the thoracolumbar spine was performed as part of a trauma series (Fig. 10a).

Questions
(1) What abnormalities do you see on this radiograph ?
    Loss of height of the T12 vertebral body
(2) What is the diagnosis ?

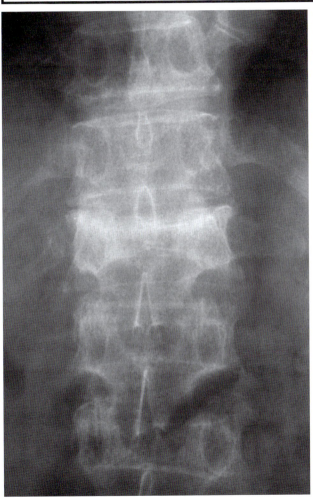

Fig.10a *Frontal radiograph of the thoracolumbar junction shows loss of height of the T12 vertebral body and sclerosis. The pedicles are intact.*

Case 11

A 37-year-old woman with a known history of rheumatoid arthritis, presented with two months of neck pain aggravated by rotating the head. There was no history of recent trauma or fever. Physical examination showed localized tenderness over the upper cervical spine in the sub-occipital region. The range of rotation was limited by pain while neck flexion and extension were unaffected. Laboratory investigations revealed an elevated ESR and a normal white cell count. A lateral cervical spine radiograph (Fig. 11a) was done as part of a cervical spine series.

Questions

(1) What abnormalities do you see on this lateral cervical radiograph ?
    Increased joint space between anterior arch of C1 and odontoid process of C2
    Indistinct outline of odontoid process (due to cortical erosion)

(2) What is the diagnosis ?

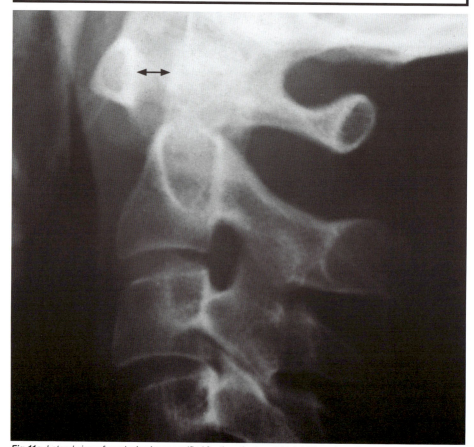

Fig.11a *Lateral view of cervical spine magnified for the atlanto-axial joint. There is an increase in the atlanto-axial distance (distance between posterior aspect of anterior arch of C1 and anterior aspect of odontoid process of C2, double head arrow). In normal adults this should measure 3 mm or less. The cortex of the odontoid process is poorly defined due to erosion secondary to the underlying inflammatory disorder.*

05 TRAUMA

Colles' fracture (Fig. 1a, b)

Discussion:

Colles' fracture is the commonest fracture to occur in an osteoporotic elderly patient falling onto an outstretched hand. Radiographs in two orthogonal projections help detect displacement, angulation and impaction of the fracture. These are important considerations when planning reduction.

Features of Colles' fracture seen in this patient's radiograph (Fig. 1a, b):

- Transverse fracture of distal radius - usually about 2-3cm proximal to the distal radial articular surface
- Impaction (overlapping) of the trabeculae/cortices produces discontinued/continuous white line (fracture line)
- Lateral view shows dorsal angulation of distal fragment resulting in the classic clinical "dinner fork" deformity (normally there is approximately 10 degrees volar angulation of the distal radial articular surface)
- Soft tissue swelling over dorsal aspect of distal forearm
- Generalized decrease in bone density indicating underlying osteoporosis

Aside from dorsal angulation, the wrist and hand may be markedly displaced (Fig. 1c) and soft tissue damage (neurovascular or tendon injury) may be significant.

The fracture may also extend to involve the distal articular surface (Fig. 1d) which may result in a step deformity of the distal articular surface and predispose to premature degenerative joint disease.

Fig.1d Frontal view of the wrist of another patient shows a fracture line extending to the distal radial articular surface (arrow). If a large step or gap is present, the resultant irregular articular surface may result in local premature degenerative joint disease.

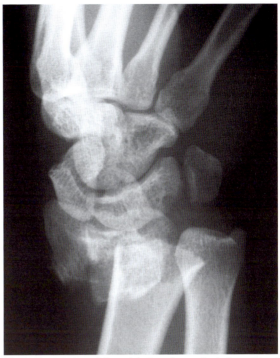

Fig.1c Frontal view of the wrist of another patient shows lateral displacement (almost full radial shaft width) of the distal radial fragment together with the wrist and hand en bloc.

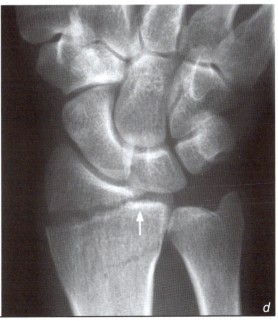

d

Management is usually by means of closed reduction and immobilization. A post-reduction radiograph is usually performed to check for alignment. In patients with signs of trauma around the wrist one must be aware of other common traumatic lesions at the site, e.g. fracture of the scaphoid (Fig. 1e) and scapholunate dissociation (Fig. 1f).

Role of imaging in patients with wrist fractures

- Confirm clinical suspicion of a fracture
- Determine site and configuration of fracture (number of fragments, displacement/angulation, articular surface involvement)
- Post-reduction/follow-up radiographs to confirm satisfactory alignment.

Note:

(1) Colles' fracture is the commonest fracture in an osteoporotic elderly patient who falls on an outstretched hand.

(2) Frontal and lateral radiographs of affected wrist are the imaging modality of choice.

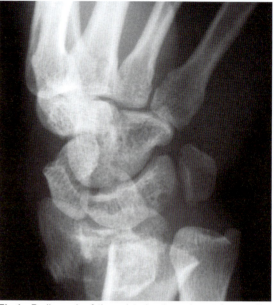

Fig.1e *Radiograph of the wrist showing a lucent fracture line through the waist of the fracture. Note that the blood supply of the proximal pole of scaphoid enters at the waist and curves backwards (proximally). A fracture here or more proximally may disrupt this supply, resulting in avascular necrosis of the proximal fragment.*

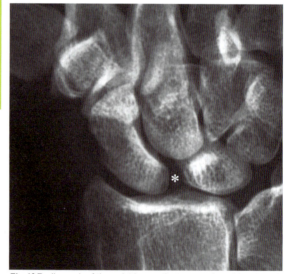

Fig.1f *Radiograph of the wrist in a patient presenting with wrist pain after a fall. There is a wide gap (asterisk) of over 3 mm between the scaphoid and lunate (scapholunate dissociation). This indicates that the scapholunate ligamant is torn (Image courtesy of Dr Yolanda Lee, Department of Diagnostic Radiology and Organ Imaging, The Chinese University of Hong Kong).*

Fracture of the femoral neck

Fracture of the femoral neck (Fig. 2a, b)

Discussion:
Some cases of femoral neck fracture may be difficult to detect on radiographs. A careful search of disruption of the continuity of bony trabeculae within the femoral neck is required. Drawing Shenton's line is also a quick method to check for subtle changes in alignment (Fig. 2a).

The major descriptive terms are:
- Location of fracture (Fig. 2c):
  (1) sub-capital (Fig. 2d);
  (2) mid-cervical (Fig. 2e);
  (3) basi-cervical (Fig 2a);
  (4) inter-trochanteric (Fig. 2f);
  (5) sub-trochanteric.
- Number of large (over 2 cm) fragments
- Angulation of the femoral shaft with respect to the femoral head

Surgical internal fixation is usually the treatment of choice and allows early mobilization.

Role of imaging in patients with hip fractures
- Confirm clinical suspicion of a fracture
- Determine site and configuration of fracture (number of fragments, displacement/angulation, articular surface involvement)
- Radiographs of the affected hip on follow-up are necessary to detect complications including:
  (1) avascular necrosis of femoral head – sclerosis of femoral head. Collapse of the subchondral cortex in more advanced cases. Risk of avascular necrosis increases as the fracture line gets closer to the femoral head.
  (2) non-union
  (3) osteoarthritis – joint space narrowing, subchondral cyst/ sclerosis and osteophyte formation.

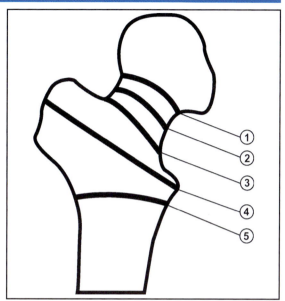

Fig.2c Drawing showing the nomenclature for the location of neck of femur fractures: (1) sub-capital; (2) mid-cervical; (3) basi-cervical; (4) inter-trochanteric; (5) sub-trochanteric.

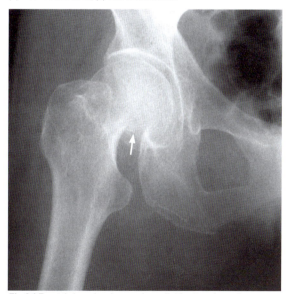

Fig.2d Frontal view showing a sub-capital fracture (arrow).

05 TRAUMA

Discussion Case 2
Fracture of the femoral neck

- Radiographically occult fractures may require diagnosis by either MRI, CT or bone scan.

Note:
(1) Fracture of neck of femur should be considered after fall in elderly patient with symptoms and signs localized to hip joint.

(2) Frontal and lateral radiographs of the affected hip would confirm the diagnosis.

(3) Description should include the fracture location, number of fragments and degree of angulation.

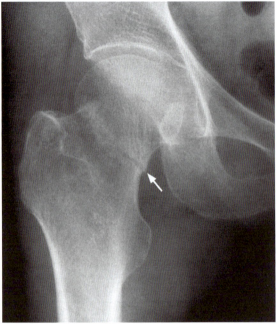

Fig.2e Frontal view showing a mid-cervical fracture(arrow)

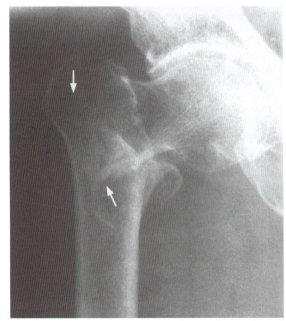

Fig.2f Frontal view showing an inter-trochanteric fracture (arrows)

Anterior shoulder dislocation

Anterior shoulder dislocation (Fig. 3a, b)

Discussion:

In some cases of anterior shoulder dislocation, a fracture may be present aside from shoulder dislocation (Fig. 3c) Additional views (the Y view) are performed to ascertain the antero-posterior location of the humeral head with respect to the glenoid. The dislocation is anterior, in over 90% of shoulder dislocations. Another view which helps to evaluate the antero-posterior relation, is the axillary view (Fig. 3d).

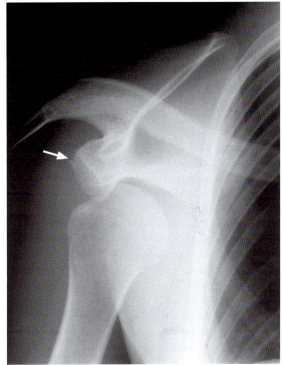

Fig.3c *Frontal view of a different patient with antero-inferior displacement of the humeral head. There is a small fracture fragment just lateral to the glenoid (arrow).*

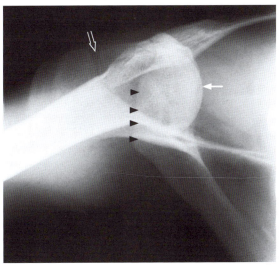

Fig.3d *Axillary view of the same patient in Fig. 3c shows anterior displacement of the humeral head (arrow) with respect to the glenoid (outlined by arrowheads). The acromio-clavicular joint is indicated by an open arrow.*

Anterior shoulder dislocation

Treatment for anterior dislocation is usually by closed reduction. Radiograph of the affected shoulder should be taken after reduction to check for successful reduction.

Due to the impaction of the superolateral aspect of the humeral head against the antero-inferior edge of the glenoid a fracture of the humeral head (Hill-Sachs defect) occurs in 60% of cases (Fig. 3e). Similarly there may be damage to the glenoid labrum due to the dislocation (Fig. 3f). Labral damage in anterior dislocation is considered a risk factor predisposing to recurrent dislocation.

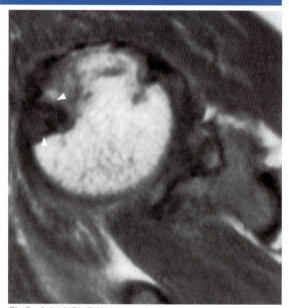

Fig.3e *Axial MRI, T1W image of another patient with a previous dislocation showing a triangular-shaped fracture (arrowheads) in the superior aspect of the humeral head. This is a Hill-Sachs defect and lies in the classic posterolateral location (exact location will depend on the site of impact with the edge of the glenoid).*

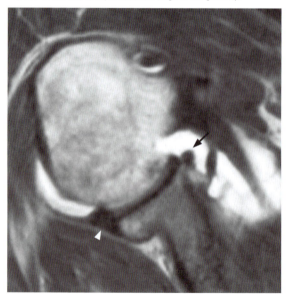

Fig.3f *Axial MR arthrogram, T1W image (contrast is bright, glenoid labrum, tendons and ligaments dark) in a patient with previous shoulder dislocation. The antero-inferior labrum (arrow) was avulsed off the edge of the glenoid and has moved medially (compare this with the intact posterior labrum, which is marked with arrowhead).*

Anterior shoulder dislocation

In older patients, there may also be an associated rotator cuff tendon tear (Fig. 3g).

Posterior shoulder dislocation is much less common (Fig. 3h).

The appearance is rather characteristic, with the humeral head internally rotated, giving it a 'light-bulb' appearance.

Role of imaging in patients with shoulder dislocation

- Confirm clinical suspicion of a dislocation
- Determine location of the dislocated humeral head
- Demonstrate fractures if present
- Post-reduction radiograph to confirm satisfactory alignment
- MRI for soft tissue, especially labral injury.

Note:

(1) Diagnosis of anterior shoulder dislocation can usually be made clinically.

(2) Radiographs of shoulder in frontal and axial (or lateral) views confirm the diagnosis.

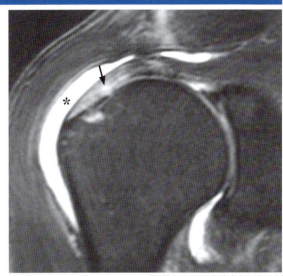

Fig.3g Coronal MR arthrogram, T1W (contrast is bright, glenoid labrum, tendons and ligaments dark) in a patient with previous shoulder dislocation. There is leakage of intra-articular contrast into the subacromial-subdeltoid bursa (asterisk) as a result of a tear in the supraspinatus tendon. The tendon tear in this patient extends within the substance of the tendon (arrow) rather than showing sharp retracted ends.

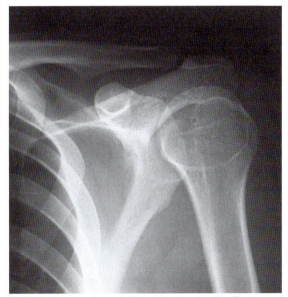

Fig.3h Radiograph of a posteriorly dislocated shoulder. The humeral head is force placed into internal rotation because of the dislocation, giving appearance of the 'light-bulb' sign (Image courtesy of Dr Tom Cheung, Department of Diagnostic Radiology and Organ Imaging, The Chinese University of Hong Kong).

Discussion Case 4
Fractures of osteoporotic spine

Fractures of osteoporotic spine (Fig. 4a, b)

Discussion:

In elderly patients presenting with low back pain, the differential diagnosis includes lumbar spondylosis (degeneration), osteoporotic fractures, discitis/osteomyelitis, neoplastic infiltration of the spine or adjacent retroperitoneal structures.

In osteoporosis, there is reduced bone mass. However, it is of normal composition (compared with osteomalacia where the bone is of abnormal composition).

T11 and 12 are the most common sites for thoracic fractures (higher levels are supported by rib cage). The typical findings of osteoporosis in vertebral bodies are (Fig. 4b):

- Generalized decreased bone density
- 'Picture framing' appearance of vertebral bodies, the cortex is the major weight-bearer hence the last to be resorbed. The cortical bone stands out against the osteopenia of the trabecular bone.

A flexion mechanism results in wedge-shaped vertebral body fracture. If there is a significant component of compression in the mechanism of injury, a burst-type configuration results. In this patient (Fig. 4b) the latter is present and there is bulging of the L1 posterior vertebral body cortex seen on the lateral view. This retropulsion may push into the spinal canal resulting in canal stenosis.

MRI (Fig. 4c) better delineates the spinal canal and status of its contents if there are lower limb neurological symptoms or if surgical intervention is contemplated.

Role of imaging in patients with osteoporotic spinal fractures

- Confirm clinical suspicion of a fracture
- Determine site and configuration of fracture (wedge or burst type, retropulsion of posterior wall)
- Act as baseline for future reference (worsening of the fracture or development of new fractures)
- MRI for status of the spinal canal

> **Note:**
> (1) Osteoporosis is commonly seen in elderly female patients.
> (2) Decreased bone density, cortical thinning and loss of trabeculae are typical radiological features of osteoporosis.

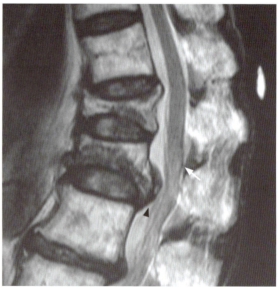

Fig.4c Sagittal MRI, T2W image (fluid and marrow fat are bright) of the thoracolumbar junction. The fractures of T12 and L1 are seen. There is a retropulsed fragment in the inferior aspect of the L1 vertebral body (arrowhead). This is pushing onto the cauda equina at its origin (note the conus (arrow) ending just above this level). Same patient as in Fig. 4a, b.

Pathological fracture

Pathological fracture (Fig. 5a, b)
The radiological appearances seen
in this case are not specific for bone
metastases. Multiple myeloma, primary
benign or malignant bone tumour (such
as chondrosarcoma) or infection could
have a similar appearance and result in
a pathological fracture. However, the
clinical history of known malignancy
supports the diagnosis.

Discussion:

The iliac bone is a common site to
harbour clinically 'silent' lesions. These
can grow to a large size or cause fractures
before the patient presents. CT scan
allows better appreciation of the size and
configuration of the lesion affecting the
iliac bone (Fig. 5c).

Once there is suspicion of bone
metastasis, the presence of other
lesions will need to be sought for and a
radionuclide bone scan may be helpful.
Performing a bone scan has the following
advantages:
- More sensitive than plain
   radiograph, diagnosis can be made
   before radiographic changes occur.
- Convenience: allows imaging of
   the whole bony skeleton in a
   single examination.

Whole body radionuclide bone scan in
patients with multiple bone metastasis
typically shows multiple 'hot' spots,
representing areas of increase in
osteoblastic activity in response to
the metastatic deposit. The extent of
uptake reflects the local blood supply
and osteoblastic activity. These lesions
predominantly affect the axial skeleton.
However, in this patient (Fig. 5a, b, c) the
pelvic lesion was largely 'cold' (arrow)
except for the fracture (Fig. 5d). This is
probably because the fractured fragment
is relatively avascular.

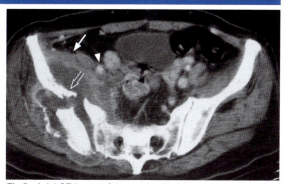

Fig.5c *Axial CT image of the pelvis with intravenous contrast (soft tissue window settings) shows a large soft tissue mass on both sides of the fractured bone (open arrow). This mass does not enhance much. The iliacus muscle (arrow) is elevated and there is medial displacement of the iliac vessels (arrowhead). Note the diastasis of the right side joint.*

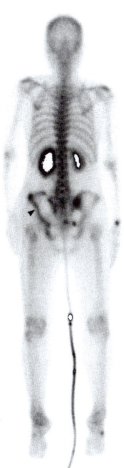

Fig.5d *Bone scan of this patient shows photopenia (lack of radionuclide uptake) in the posterior aspect of the iliac bone (indicating ischaemia to the area or a pure osteolytic lesion) as compared to the left side. There is a band of increased radionuclide uptake (arrowhead) in the anterior aspect of the iliac bone coinciding with the fracture site and margin of the tumour anterior to it.*

05 TRAUMA

Discussion Case 5
Pathological fracture

Role of imaging in patients with suspected pathological fractures
- Confirm clinical suspicion of a fracture
- Determine site and configuration of fracture (number of fragments, displacement/angulation, articular surface involvement)
- Assess the appearance of the underlying bone (osteolytic (Fig. 5e), osteosclerotic or diffusely infiltrated, etc.)
- Detect other sites of involvement (bone scan)

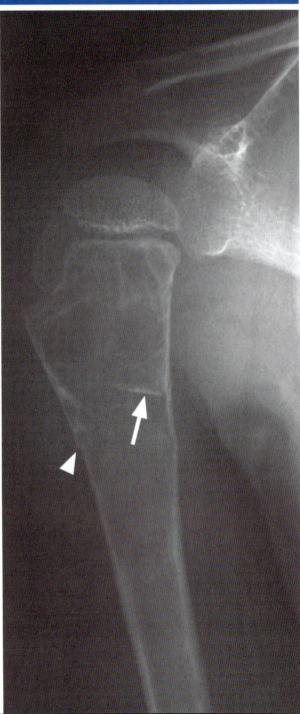

***Fig.5e** Radiograph of the proximal humerus shows a fracture through a lytic expansile bone lesion after minor trauma. Aside from a breach of the cortex (arrowhead), a fractured fragment (arrow) has collapsed into the lytic lesion. The underlying lesion is a bone cyst. It is not uncommon for bone pathology to be discovered only after a fracture through it. Often only trivial trauma is required to fracture through the underlying lesion.*

Note:

(1) In a patient with a known history of cancer, underlying bony abnormalities associated with a fracture should raise the suspicion of metastatic involvement.

(2) Iliac bone is a common site for silent lesions.

(3) Bone scans may not always be 'hot' for metastatic deposit(s).

Discussion Case 6
Incomplete fracture

Incomplete fractures of radius and ulna (Fig. 6a, b)

Discussion:

Incomplete fractures are defined by a disrupted cortex on one side of the bone and the other side is buckled or bent. There are two types of such fractures: greenstick and torus fractures.

In a greenstick fracture, the bone is bent, the convex side (effect of tensile force) is disrupted (Fig. 6b) and the concave side (compression force) intact.

In a torus fracture, one or both cortices bulge out (Fig. 6c) due to a compression force.

These incomplete fractures tend to occur in children as young bones are more deformable (plastic) when subjected to a compression force. Hence the compressed side either bends or buckles rather than breaks cleanly. The relatively more robust periosteum probably also plays a role. Incomplete fractures may be subtle (Fig. 6c and d). A careful search for subtle buckling is necessary in children with high level of clinical suspicion of a fracture (Fig. 6e).

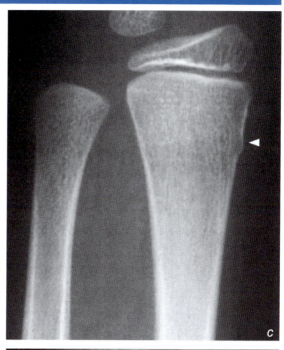

c

Fig.6c Frontal view of the distal forearm of another skeletally immature patient shows a torus fracture in the lateral aspect of the distal radial meta-diaphysis (arrowhead). There is no extension of the fracture to the other cortex of the bone. The ulna appears unremarkable on this view.

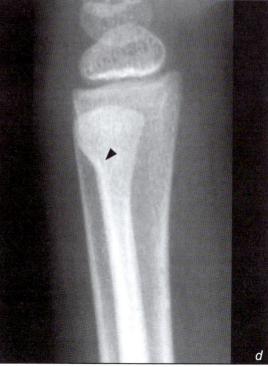

d

Fig.6d Same patient as in Fig. 6c. Lateral view of the distal forearm shows an incomplete fracture involving the dorsal cortex of the distal ulnar metaphysis (arrowhead). The radial fracture is not seen on this view. This case illustrates the value of obtaining orthogonal views (frontal and lateral) to screen for fractures. It also reinforces the principle that ring structures (such as paired bones) fracture in two places, so look carefully for a second lesion if one lesion is discovered.

Incomplete fracture

Role of imaging in patients with incomplete fractures

- Confirm clinical suspicion of a fracture
- Determine site and configuration of fracture
- Follow-up radiographs to confirm satisfactory alignment.

> **Note:**
> (1) Incomplete fractures are common in children.
> (2) Focal cortical disruption (bent or buckled) with intact cortex on opposite side are the typical radiological features.

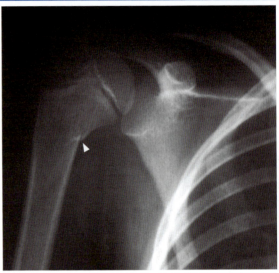

Fig.6e *Frontal view of the proximal humerus of a skeletally immature patient showing an incomplete fracture (arrowhead).*

Supracondylar fracture

Supracondylar fracture (Fig. 7a)

Discussion:
This is the most common elbow fracture in children (compared to adults, in whom radial head fractures are the most common [Fig. 7b]).

Occasionally, there is only slight displacement of the distal fragment or the fracture may be impacted. In such cases, the fat pad sign (Fig. 7a, b) may be the only clue to a fracture.

The fat pad sign indicates that there is distension of the elbow capsule (resulting in displacement of the fat pad which normally resides in the coronoid and olecranon fossae). The anterior fat pad, which is partially seen in many normal elbows, is only considered abnormal if it is triangular (sail) in shape. The posterior fat pad is normally not visible.

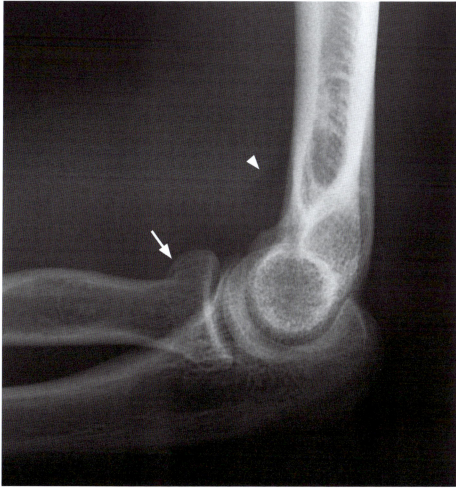

Fig.7b *Lateral radiograph showing an elevated anterior fat pad (arrowhead) and a break in the cortex of the radial head (arrow) (Image courtesy of Dr C.M.Chu, Department of Diagnostic Radiology and Organ Imaging, The Chinese University of Hong Kong).*

Discussion Case 7
Supracondylar fracture

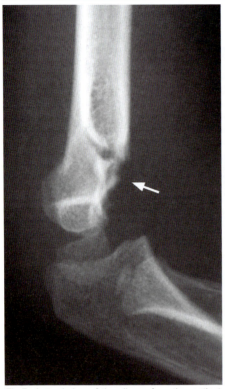

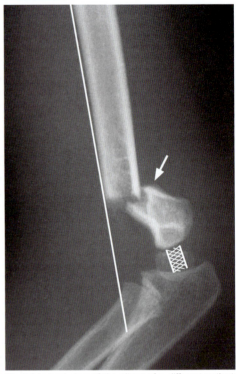

Fig.7d *Lateral view of the elbow of a different patient. The anterior humeral line (white line) drawn along the anterior cortex of the distal humeral shaft should normally pass through the middle third (cross-hatched) of the capitellum. If it doesn't, this would indicate angulation or displacement of the capitellum as a result of a fracture (arrow).*

Fig.7c *Lateral view of the elbow of another patient, the fracture (arrow) is obvious as the distal fragment is more posteriorly angulated.*

More commonly, the distal fragment is posteriorly angulated and/or displaced (Fig. 7c, d).

Repeated radiographs after reduction are necessary to ensure no residual angulation or rotational deformity. A line drawn along the anterior cortex of the distal humerus cortex should normally pass through the middle third of the capitellum (Fig. 7d). Deviation from this indicates angulation or displacement of the capitellum with respect to the humeral shaft and thus a fracture or poor post-reduction alignment.

Role of imaging in patients with supracondylar fractures
- Confirm clinical suspicion of a fracture
- Determine site and configuration of fracture (number of fragments, displacement/angulation, intra-articular involvement)
- Post-reduction/follow-up radiographs to confirm satisfactory alignment.

Note:
(1) Supracondylar fractures are common in children falling on an outstretched hand
(2) The fracture line may be difficult to detect in both the frontal and lateral radiographs. The fat pad sign may be helpful in these situations.

Tibial plateau fracture

Fracture of the lateral tibial plateau
(Fig. 8a, b)

Discussion:
Tibial plateau fractures occur commonly in motor vehicle accidents. The lateral plateau is most commonly affected (approximately three quarters of cases). Associated abnormalities include collateral and cruciate ligament injury. Tibial plateau fractures may result in degenerative disease of the knee joint due to a step deformity or gap in the articular surface. The fracture configuration, relationship (displacement, angulation and rotation) between fragments and sub-articular cortex irregularities are best demonstrated with CT (Fig. 8c and d).

Role of imaging in patients with tibial plateau fractures
- Confirm clinical suspicion
- Determine site and configuration of fracture
- Detect other sites of involvement
- Post-treatment follow-up
  radiographs for progress.

Note:
(1) Tibial plateau fractures occur commonly in motor vehicle accidents.
(2) CT is usually required to delineate the fracture and its fragments clearly.

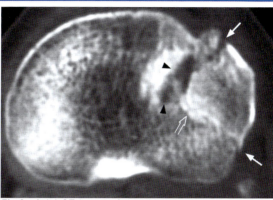

Fig.8c *Axial CT image of the tibial plateau shows a defect (arrowheads) created by separation of fracture fragments. The posterior part of this fracture is impacted (open arrow). The cortical disruptions (arrows) are well demonstrated (same patient as in Fig. 8a,b).*

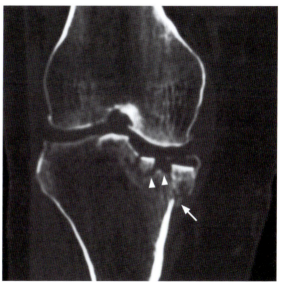

Fig.8d *Reformatted coronal CT image shows the depressed subchondral cortex (arrowheads), indicating that there is a step deformity of the articular surface. The metaphyseal cortical break (arrow) is better demonstrated than on the radiograph (same patient as in Fig. 8a, b, c).*

05 TRAUMA

Cervical spine fracture

Teardrop fracture of C3 vertebral body
(Fig. 9a)

Discussion:

Teardrop fractures occur in the antero-inferior aspect of a cervical vertebral body. They may be caused by a hyperextension or hyperflexion injury. The small size of the fracture belies the associated soft tissue damage. The spinal ligaments are often disrupted and the spinal cord stretched during the injury (it takes significant force to cause the bony fracture). However, after the initial displacement, the spine usually reverts to a more normal alignment. The radiographic appearance is the end result after the spine has 'snapped back' into a more normal-appearing alignment.

Several fractures are unique to the cervical spine, these include:
- 'Dens' (odontoid process of C2) fracture (Fig. 9b)
- 'Hangman's' (C2 pedicle) fracture (Fig. 9c)

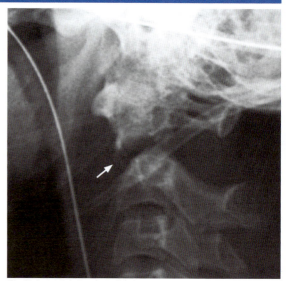

Fig.9b *Lateral radiograph of the upper cervical spine shows a fracture (arrow) of the body of the odontoid process of the axis (C2). The C1 and fractured C2 fragment have moved anteriorly with respect to the rest of the cervical spine. See Fig. 9f on how to draw the spinal lines to check for alignment.*

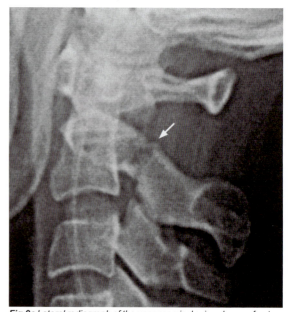

Fig.9c *Lateral radiograph of the upper cervical spine shows a fracture (arrow) of the pedicle of the C2. This is called a Hangman's fracture despite the fact it is the hangee who gets the injury. This fracture is usually due to a hyperextension injury, as seen in a motor vehicle accident.*

05 TRAUMA

Discussion Case 9
Cervical spine fracture

- 'Clay shoveler's' (spinous process avulsion) fracture (Fig. 9d)

Cervical fractures are usually not difficult to detect. On the other hand, subluxations and dislocations may be subtle and overlooked (Fig. 9e). The four spinal lines (Fig. 9f) should be checked to ensure proper alignment and to allow detection of subtle abnormalities.

Role of imaging in patients with cervical spine trauma:
- Confirm clinical diagnosis
- Localize injured segment
- Lateral radiographs act as a guide for further imaging

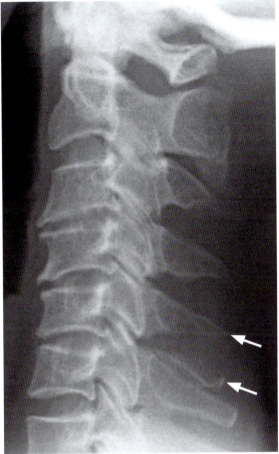

Fig.9d *Lateral radiograph of the cervical spine showing a fracture of the spinous process. This is an avulsion injury caused by a strenuous pull of the latissimus dorsi, trapezius and rhomboid muscles. It used to be seen in labourers (farmers or builders) hence its name (also called a coal-miners fracture).*

05 TRAUMA

Discussion Case 9
Cervical spine fracture

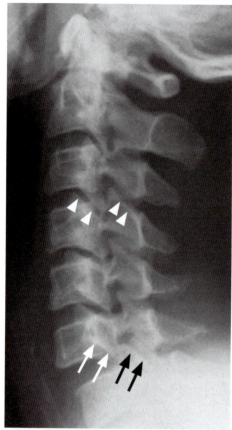

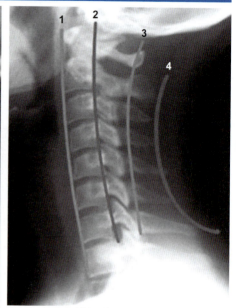

Fig.9f *A normal lateral cervical radiograph with four spinal lines drawn on it.*
1. *Anterior vertebral line: drawn along the anterior margins of the vertebral bodies*
2. *Posterior vertebral line: drawn along the posterior margins of the vertebral bodies*
3. *Spinolaminar line: connecting the spinolaminar junction of the vertebral bodies*
4. *Posterior spinal line: drawn along the tips of the spinous processes, also called interspinous line*
All of these should form a gentle curve. Abnormal alignment is indicated by a step in a line or an increased or decreased separation between the segments along any line. With this knowledge, go back to Fig. 9a to e and see if these lines are disrupted.

Fig.9e *Lateral radiograph of the cervical spine of a patient with neck pain after a motor vehicle accident. The abnormality is subtle and is at the C6/7 level. The cervical spine above the C7 level is rotated, as evident by the obliquity (non-overlapping) of the facet joints (arrowheads). Both facet joints should roughly overlap each other in a straight lateral view. At the C7 level, there is overlapping of the two superior articular facets (black arrows). One of the inferior articular facets of C6 (white arrows) is naked (not articulating with its counterpart) and is anterior to the superior facet of C7. This condition is termed a unilateral facet joint dislocation.*

Note:
(1) Cervical spinal injury should be considered in any trauma patient with pain, localized tenderness, severe head injury or localizing neurological signs of cervical spinal cord.
(2) Lateral radiograph of cervical spine is the radiological investigation for initial assessment.
(3) Disruption of cervical spinal lines, fracture and to a lesser extent prevertebral soft tissue swelling are the important radiological signs.

256

Post-traumatic cord compression

Fracture of T12 (Fig. 10a)

A CT of the spine would better assess the fracture, evaluate integrity of spinal canal and the presence and location of fracture fragments.

MRI will better evaluate spinal cord integrity.

Discussion:

In a major trauma setting, radiographs may be limited. Keen observation and a high index of suspicion are required to make the diagnosis.

CT (Fig. 10b, c, d) of the same patient as in Fig. 10a with sagittal reformat better evaluates the fracture and shows:

- Fracture of the T11 and T12 vertebral bodies with cortical disruption of the anterior cortex (this suggests a flexion mechanism of injury)
- Disruption of the T12 posterior wall with retropulsion of fragments, indicates that this is also a burst fracture (which suggests a significant axial compression mechanism). This retropulsion results in narrowing of the spinal canal and impingement of spinal cord
- Anterolisthesis (anterior subluxation between vertebra) of T11 and an increase in kyphosis, as shown on sagittal reformats, all add to the narrowing of the spinal canal.

Neurological deficit is relatively common in burst fracture. The severity depends on the vertebral level affected (spinal cord usually ends at the L1 or L2 level), the degree of displacement of bony fragments into spinal canal, superimposed anterolisthesis and kyphosis.

MRI (Fig. 10e) provides more information on the contents of the spinal canal, especially the integrity and extent of cord involvement.

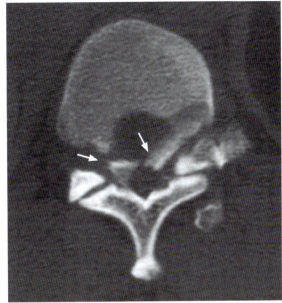

Fig.10b *Axial CT through the inferior aspect of T11. The endplate is fractured and there are bone fragments (arrows) displaced into the spinal canal.*

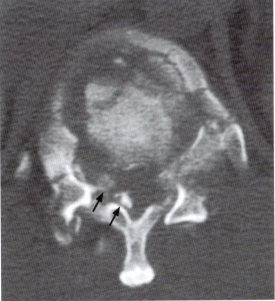

Fig.10c *Axial CT through the superior aspect of T12. The vertebral body fracture is severely comminuted and there are bone fragments (arrows) within the spinal canal.*

Post-traumatic cord compression

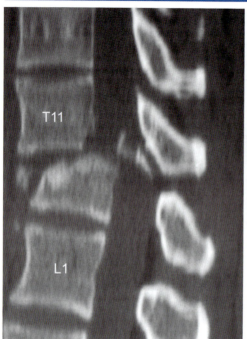 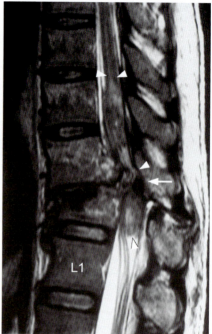

Fig.10d Reformatted sagittal CT image shows the full extent of the fracture. Aside from the T11 and T12 fractures and a retropulsed fragment within the spinal canal, there is anterolisthesis (anterior subluxation) of T11. The latter further increases the degree of spinal stenosis and the likelihood of spinal cord injury, and contributes to an exaggerated kyphosis at this level.

Fig.10e Sagittal MRI, T2W image (fluid and blood are bright). In addition to the T11 and T12 fractures and anterolisthesis, resulting in the narrowing of the spinal canal, extensive cord damage as evidenced by the swelling and high signal (fluid or blood) within the cord from the T10 to T12 levels (arrowheads). At the T11/12 level, the cord is compressed (arrow).

Role of imaging in patients with spinal injury

- Confirm clinical suspicion of a fracture with radiograph
- Determine site and configuration of fracture (number of fragments, displacement/angulation, spinal alignment). More bone information is obtained by CT.
- MRI for spinal canal/cord pathology

Note:

(1) Burst fracture of lumbar vertebrae should be suspected in patient after a fall with localized bony tenderness and lower limb neurological deficit.

(2) The diagnosis is usually apparent on radiographs.

(3) CT or MRI helps assess degree of narrowing of spinal canal and spinal cord compression.

Atlanto-axial subluxation/dislocation

Atlanto-axial subluxation/ dislocation secondary to rheumatoid arthritis (Fig. 11a)

Discussion:

Rheumatoid arthritis is one of the commonest causes of atlanto-axial subluxation. The presence of bony erosion of odontoid process helps to differentiate it from other causes (e.g. congenital/traumatic causes).
Up to 20-25% of patients with severe rheumatoid arthritis have this complication.
Atlanto-axial subluxation is important to recognize because of the potential complication of spinal cord compression. MRI of cervical spine is indicated for better assessment of underlying bony erosion, degree of subluxation and to evaluate cervical spinal cord compression (Fig. 11b, c).

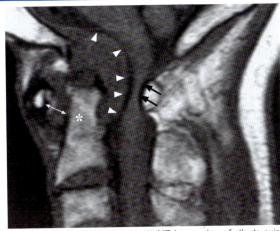

Fig.11b *Sagittal T1W (fluid is black) MR image view of atlanto-axial joint. There is a large soft tissue mass (arrowheads) around the odontoid process (asterisk) of C2. There is widening of the atlanto-axial joint (double head arrow). The whole of C1 has subluxed forward and the spinal canal is stenosed, severely compressing the spinal cord (arrows).*

Features of atlanto-axial subluxation due to rheumatoid arthritis include:
- Widening of atlanto-axial distance (Fig. 11a) (i.e. the distance between posterior aspect of anterior arch of C1 and anterior aspect of odontoid process of C2).
- In normal adults this should measure 3 mm or less.
- Step between posterior arch of C1 and posterior element of C2.
- Erosion of odontoid process (due to synovitis in rheumatoid arthritis).
- Degree of subluxation often changes with movement (becoming worse on flexion).

Role of imaging in patients with rheumatoid arthritis involving the atlanto-axial joint
- Confirm clinical diagnosis
- Detect complications such as cord compression, myelomalacia etc.
- Baseline for follow-up/serial change.

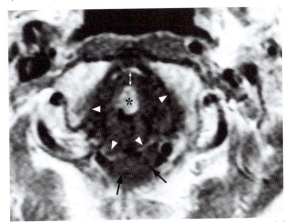

Fig.11c *Axial T1W (fluid is black) MR image view of atlanto-axial joint. There is a large soft tissue mass (arrowheads) around the odontoid process (asterisk) of C2, widening of the anterior atlanto-axial joint (double head arrow). The spinal cord (arrows) is compressed.*

Atlanto-axial subluxation/dislocation

Note:

(1) Patients with rheumatoid arthritis are prone to develop atlanto-axial subluxation.

(2) Widening of atlanto-axial distance on lateral cervical radiograph is the diagnostic radiological finding.

(3) Radiographs in neutral and flexion positions should be performed since the alignment may appear normal in the neutral position in the early stages.

GASTROINTESTINAL SYSTEM

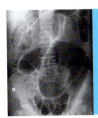

Contributors:
**Alex W.H. Ng, David P.N. Chan, K.T. Wong,
Gregory E. Antonio, Edmund H.Y. Yuen,
Anil T. Ahuja**

Questions

Case 1 - 11	262 - 272

Discussion

Pneumoperitoneum	273 - 275
Small bowel obstruction	276 - 278
Mechanical large bowel obstruction	279 - 280
Sigmoid volvulus	281 - 282
Gallstone ileus	283 - 284
Acute appendicitis	285 - 288
Acute mesenteric infarction	289 - 291
Carcinoma of the colon	292 - 296
Colonic diverticulosis	297 - 298
Carcinoma of the oesophagus	299 - 300
Crohn's disease	301 - 304

Chapter 06

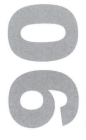

Case 1

A 56-year-old man, with a known history of peptic ulcer disease, complained of sudden onset of severe epigastric pain for one day. General examination revealed that the patient was afebrile but in severe pain. Abdominal examination showed generalized tenderness and guarding of the abdomen with 'board like' rigidity. Laboratory investigations were essentially normal. A clinical diagnosis of perforated peptic ulcer was made. An erect chest x-ray (CXR) (Fig. 1a) and a supine abdominal x-ray (AXR) (Fig. 1b) were performed as initial investigations.

Questions

(1) What abnormality can you see ?

    Figure 1a: 'Free gas under diaphragm' – indicates free peritoneal gas between the dome of the hemidiaphragm and superior surface of liver.

    Figure 1b: Supine abdominal radiograph showing signs of extraluminal gas including the Rigler's sign (also known as double wall sign) and triangular sign.

(2) <u>What is the diagnosis ?</u>

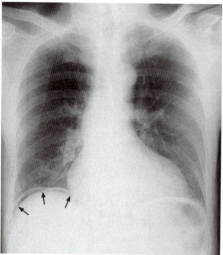

Fig.1a *Erect chest radiograph showing intraperitoneal free gas under the right hemidiaphragm – note the curvilinear lucency (arrows) between the right hemidiaphragm and liver.*

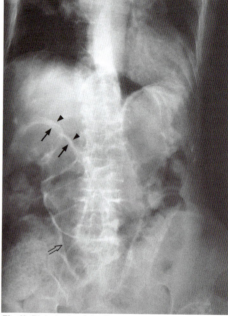

Fig.1b *Rigler's sign (also known as the double wall sign) - the inner mucosal surface of the bowel wall is delineated by intraluminal air (arrows) and the outer serosal surface of the bowel wall is also delineated by extraluminal intraperitoneal free air (arrow heads). Note the triangular collection of gas between adjacent loops of bowel (open arrow) - triangular sign.*

Case 2

A 69-year-old man with good past health complained of colicky abdominal pain, increasing abdominal distension, vomiting and constipation. On general examination he was afebrile, dehydrated and tachycardic. Abdominal examination showed a distended abdomen with visible peristalsis, and there was generalized abdominal tenderness but no mass could be palpated. Auscultation revealed tinkling and accentuated bowel sounds. There was no abdominal scar to indicate previous surgery. Laboratory investigations showed slightly elevated urea (probably related to dehydration) but were otherwise normal. A supine abdominal radiograph of this patient was performed (Fig. 2a).

Questions

(1) What radiological abnormalities can you identify on this radiograph ?
- There are multiple dilated bowel loops roughly central abdominal in location.
- Valvulae conniventes appearing as striations crossing completely across the width of the bowel loops.

(2) What is the diagnosis ?

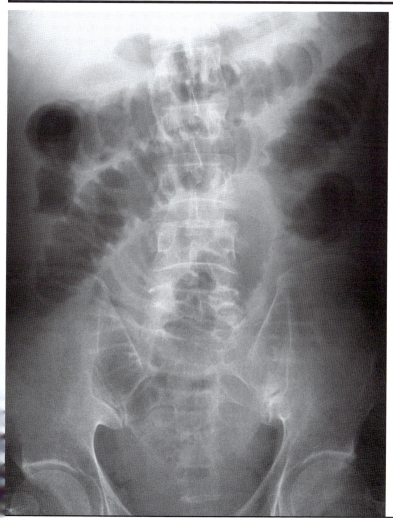

Fig.2a Supine abdominal radiograph showing multiple dilated small bowel loops in small bowel obstruction. Note the concentric linear 'bands' running through the bowel wall: valvulae conniventes, and the LUQ location, suggest that these are dilated jejunal loops.

Case 3

An 80-year-old man presented with colicky abdominal pain, constipation for three days, and repeated vomiting for 1 day. Physical examination showed a distended abdomen with hyperactive bowel sounds. No abdominal mass or organomegaly was detected. Laboratory investigations were unremarkable. The working diagnosis of mechanical intestinal obstruction was made and a supine AXR (Fig. 3a) was performed as an initial investigation.

Questions

(1) What radiological abnormalities can you see ?
- Gas-filled dilated bowel in the periphery of abdomen ('picture framing') - representing the location of the caecum, ascending, transverse and descending colon
- Widely-spaced incomplete bands along the walls of the dilated bowel - representing haustra (this is therefore large bowel)
- Absence of rectal gas

(2) <u>What is the diagnosis ?</u>

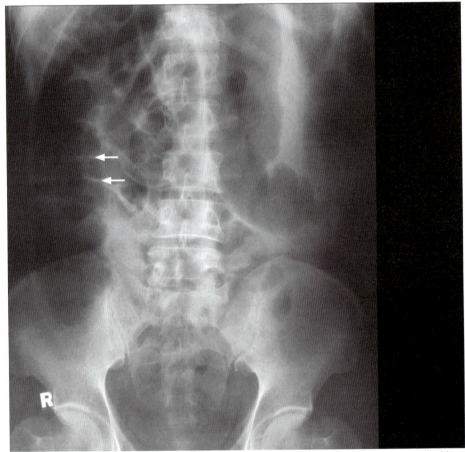

Fig.3a *Supine abdominal radiograph showing gas-filled dilated proximal large bowel and collapsed distal large bowel suggestive of mechanical large bowel obstruction. Gas-filled dilated bowel in the periphery of abdomen ('picture framing') - representing the location of the caecum, ascending, transverse and descending colon. Note the prominent haustra (arrows) - the widely spaced incomplete bands along the walls of the dilated bowel and absence of gas in the rectum.*

Case 4

An 86-year-old woman complained of sudden onset severe colicky lower abdominal pain for 4 hours. This was associated with vomiting and constipation. Physical examination showed that she was in agony with stable BP and pulse. The abdomen was distended, with marked local tenderness and guarding over the central lower abdomen. There was no physical sign of inguinal or femoral hernia. Laboratory investigations showed normal white cell count. An AXR (Fig. 4a) was performed as an initial investigation.

Questions

(1) What radiological abnormalities can you detect ?
- Massively distended bowel with inverted U-shaped configuration – representing a grossly dilated sigmoid colon.
- 'Coffee-bean sign' – distinct midline crease between the distended loop. It represents the two bowel walls in contact.
- Inferior convergence sign – the two limbs of the loop converge inferiorly, pointing to the left lower quadrant.

(2) <u>What is the diagnosis ?</u>

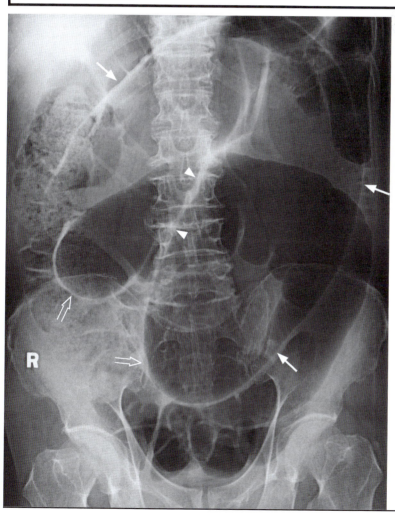

Fig.4a Supine abdominal radiograph showing grossly dilated sigmoid colon (arrows) with the 'coffee bean' sign (arrowheads) and inferior convergence sign of sigmoid volvulus (open arrows).

Case 5

A 70-year-old woman with a known history of gallstone disease, complained of colicky abdominal pain, vomiting, abdominal distension and constipation for three days. Physical examination showed a distended abdomen with hyperactive bowel sounds on auscultation. No focal peritoneal signs were present on palpation. Per rectal examination showed an empty rectum. Laboratory investigations were unremarkable. The clinical diagnosis of intestinal obstruction was made and a supine AXR performed (Fig. 5a).

Questions

(1) What radiological abnormalities can you see ?
  - Gas-filled distended stomach.
  - Paucity of distal bowel gas.
  - Gas within biliary ductal system (aerobilia).
  - A laminated, concentrically calcified nodule is present in the left lower quadrant.
  - Another densely calcified radio-opacity in the suprapubic region is likely to be a calcified fibroid.

(2) <u>What is the diagnosis ?</u>

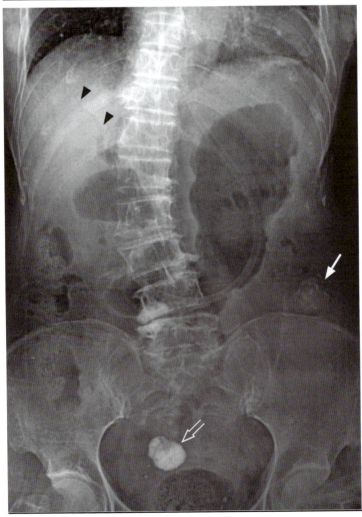

Fig.5a Supine abdominal radiograph showing gastric distension, a paucity of distal bowel gas, branching gas lucency in the centre (porta hepatis) of the liver suggesting aerobilia (arrowheads), laminated concentric calcification typical of gallstone in the left lower quadrant (arrow). A homogeneous, densely calcified fibroid is also present in the pelvis (open arrow).

Case 6

A 19-year-old female, with good past health, complained of abdominal pain, loss of appetite, nausea, vomiting and loose stools for 2 days. The pain started in the peri-umbilical region but shifted to the right lower quadrant in the past 10 hours. The pain was continuous and sharp in nature, and was aggravated by movement and cough. On physical examination she was febrile, pale, dehydrated with tachycardia. Examination of the abdomen showed tenderness, guarding and rebound tenderness over the lower abdomen with maximum tenderness localized to the McBurney's point. Per rectal examination revealed tenderness over the right pelvic region. Laboratory investigations revealed leukocytosis and raised ESR. A CT of the abdomen and pelvis was performed for further evaluation (Fig. 6a and b).

Questions

(1) What radiological abnormalities can you detect ?
- A distended, thick-walled and blind-ending tubular structure closely related to the caecum is present, which is consistent with an inflamed appendix.
- Adjacent fat streakiness and bowel wall thickening due to inflammatory change are also present.
- No evidence of free gas or fluid collection to suggest perforation.
- No appendicolith can be identified.

(2) <u>What is the diagnosis ?</u>

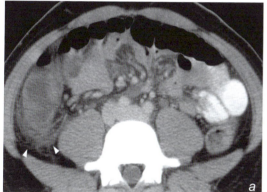
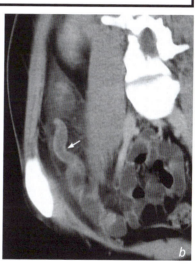

Fig.6a,b *Contrast enhanced computed tomography (CECT) demonstrates an inflamed, thick-walled and blind-ending tubular structure coming out from the caecum (arrow). Adjacent fat streakiness suggestive of inflammatory change are also present (arrowheads). The appearances are those of appendicitis.*

Case 7

A 72-year-old woman, with a known history of atrial fibrillation, complained of acute onset severe abdominal pain and rectal bleeding for one day. She was confused and in poor general condition with an irregularly irregular pulse. Examination of abdomen showed no focal peritonism. Digital examination was unremarkable. Laboratory investigations revealed mild leukocytosis. An urgent abdominal radiograph (Fig. 7a) was performed as an initial investigation.

Questions
(1) What radiological abnormalities can you detect on this abdominal radiograph ?
- Supine abdominal radiograph shows linear gas lucency projected in the periphery of the liver in the right upper quadrant (arrows). There is also dilatation of the small bowel in the abdomen.
(2) <u>What is the most likely diagnosis?</u>

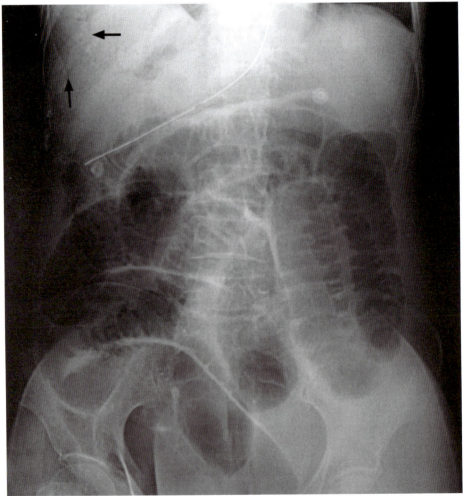

Fig.7a *Supine abdominal radiograph shows linear gas lucencies in the periphery of the liver in the right upper quadrant (arrows). The peripheral location suggests that these represent portal venous gas. There is also dilatation of the small bowel in the abdomen suggesting ileus.*

Case 8

A 78-year-old woman complained of per rectal bleeding, significant loss of weight and appetite for one month. Physical examination did not reveal any abdominal mass. No haemorrhoids were present on proctoscopy. Blood tests showed a hypochromic microcytic anaemia and raised CEA. Plain radiograph of abdomen was unremarkable. The working diagnosis of suspected colonic carcinoma was suggested and a contrast enema was performed (Fig. 8a).

Questions
(1) What radiological abnormality can you see in this image from a contrast enema series ?
  - Segmental colonic stricture with 'apple-core' appearance
  - Irregular mucosal pattern
  - Ulceration
(2) <u>What is the diagnosis ?</u>

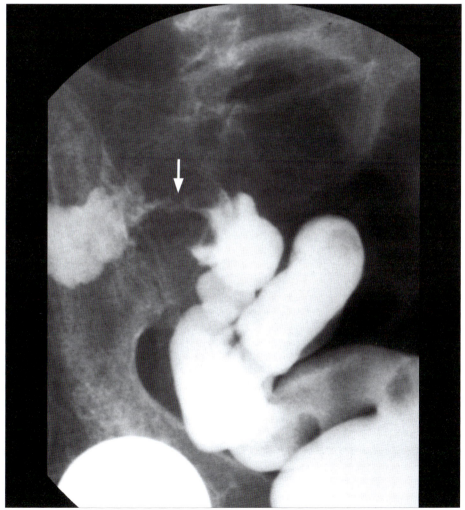

Fig.8a Contrast enema demonstrating a typical 'apple-core' lesion (arrow) of concentric colonic carcinoma.

Case 9

A 76-year-old woman presented with on and off left lower abdominal pain for 1 year. There were previous episodes of acute exacerbation with associated PR bleeding and fever which were treated with antibiotics. Physical examination showed no abdominal or pelvic mass. Laboratory investigations revealed normal haemoglobin and CEA level. A double contrast barium enema (Fig. 9a, b) was performed to exclude colonic pathology.

Questions

(1) What radiological abnormality can you identify on these images from a barium enema ?
- Multiple small outpouching from colonic wall - represent colonic diverticuli
- Smooth contour - inner wall lined by smooth mucosal surface
- Predominantly affecting transverse descending and sigmoid colon

(2) What is the diagnosis ?

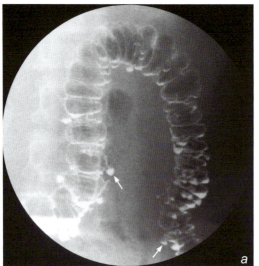

Fig. 9a, b *Double contrast barium enema demonstrating multiple colonic diverticuli appearing as small outpouchings (arrows) from the colonic wall.*

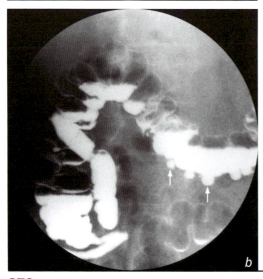

Case 10

An 83-year-old chronic smoker presented with painless progressive dysphagia for 3 months. He has also had significant weight loss and can currently only tolerate a liquid diet. Examination of the abdomen showed hepatomegaly with an irregular outline. Laboratory investigations revealed normochromic normocytic anaemia and low serum albumin. A working diagnosis of partial oesophageal obstruction was suspected and a barium swallow was performed (Fig. 10a) following an unsuccessful attempt at upper gastro-oesophageal endoscopy.

Questions
(1) What radiological abnormalities can you see on this barium swallow series ?
- Segmental stricture of lower oesophagus
- Mucosal irregularities of the involved segment
- Mucosal ulceration
- Dilatation of oesophagus proximal to the stricture

(2) What is the diagnosis ?

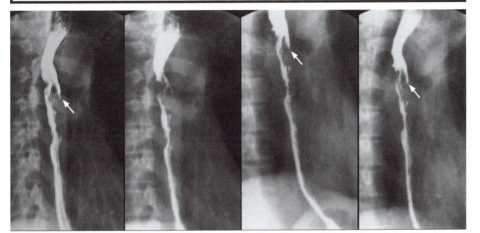

Fig.10a Barium swallow showing segmental oesophageal stricture with mucosal irregularity and ulcerations (arrows) causing obstruction and proximal dilatation - typical of malignant stricture from carcinoma.

Case 11

A 24-year-old man presented with recurrent episodes of diarrhoea, weight loss and colicky abdominal pain. Physical examination showed no abnormality. In view of clinical suspicion of pathology in the small bowel, a small bowel series was performed (Fig. 11a, b).

Questions

(1) What is seen on these images from a small bowel series ?
- Cobblestone mucosa with ulceration present in the terminal ileum
- Separation and displacement of small bowel loops
- Pseudodiverticula
- Pseudopolyps

(2) What is the diagnosis ?

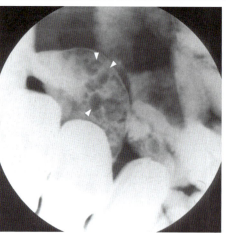 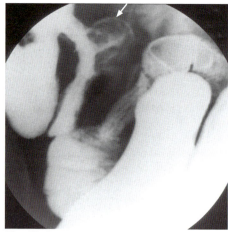

Fig. 11a Compression view with mucosal phase of the terminal ileum showing cobblestone mucosa with ulceration present in the terminal ileum (serpiginous longitudinal and transverse ulcers separated by areas of the oedema). There are several larger filling defects present in the terminal ileum suggestive of pseudopolyps (arrowheads) which are due to islands of hyperplasic mucosa between denuded mucosa.

Fig. 11b Compression view in collapsed phase of the terminal ileum showing separation and displacement of small bowel loops which is due to lymphoedematous wall thickening/increase in mesenteric fat and enlarged mesenteric lymph nodes. Pseudodiverticula (arrow) represent bulging area of normal wall opposite to the affected scarred wall on the antimesenteric side.

Discussion Case 1

Pneumoperitoneum

Pneumoperitoneum (Fig. 1a, b), probably secondary to perforated peptic ulcer

Discussion:
- Pneumoperitoneum (gas within the peritoneal cavity) may be due to many causes, including:
  - Gastro-intestinal tract perforation (peptic ulcer, diverticulum, ischaemic bowel, etc.)
  - Penetrating injury of the abdomen
  - Pneumomediastinum with peritoneal extension
  - Gas-forming intraperitoneal infection
  - Air entering via the female genital tract
- 30% of patients with perforated peptic ulcer do not have CXR finding of pneumoperitoneum
- An erect CXR is the initial imaging investigation of choice. The patient should be kept in the erect position for at least 10 minutes before the radiograph is taken to ensure adequate time for free gas to collect in a non-dependent portion of peritoneal cavity.
- If this is not possible, an AXR in the left lateral decubitus position (lying on the side with left side of body dependent) is an alternative. This way, any free gas will float to the non-dependent part of the peritoneal cavity (i.e. right side).
- Pneumoperitoneum, even if substantial, on supine AXR is sometimes difficult to detect. Radiographic signs include:
  1. Rigler's sign (Fig. 1b,c) - bowel wall outlined by intraluminal (normal) and peritoneal gas (abnormal)
  2. Triangular sign (Fig. 1b,c)
     - gas collecting between adjacent bowel loops

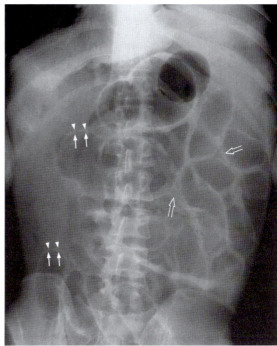

Fig. 1c *A different case of pneumoperitoneum showing typical signs including Rigler's sign - the inner mucosal surface of the bowel wall (arrows) and the outer serosal surface of the bowel wall (arrow heads), triangular sign (open arrows) and hyperlucency of the right sided abdomen which is due to increased free gas in the peritoneal cavity.*

3. Football sign
   - gas in peritoneum within a distended abdomen outlining intra-abdominal viscera (see figures in necrotising enterocolitis in paediatric section)
4. Gas outlining the falciform ligament (see figures in necrotising enterocolitis in paediatric section)
- If clinical suspicion remains high despite a negative CXR, a water soluble contrast examination of the bowel may help to confirm/rule out the diagnosis (by demonstrating contrast leakage from the site of perforation [Fig. 1d])
- A CT scan is better at demonstrating the extent of intraperitoneal free gas and detecting small amounts of gas (Fig. 1e). Note that hepatic interposition of the bowel (Fig. 1f) may mimic free gas under the diaphragm. This is called Chilaiditi's sign and is seen in asymptomatic patients. When it is associated with symptoms, either intermittent or persistent, it is known as Chilaiditi's syndrome.

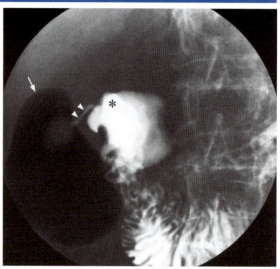

Fig.1d *Water soluble contrast examination showing a focal collection of free gas (arrow), a scarred duodenum (asterisk) and leak of contrast (arrowheads) from a duodenal perforation (Image courtesy of Dr Yolanda Lee, Department of Diagnostic Radiology and Organ Imaging, The Chinese University of Hong Kong).*

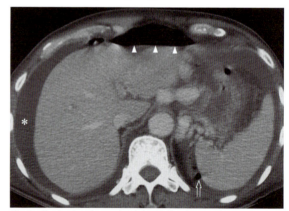

Fig.1e *Contrast enhanced axial CT showing another patient with free gas (arrowheads) present in the non-dependent position of the upper abdomen, anterior to the left lobe of liver and under the anterior abdominal wall. There are also several small locules of gas (open arrow) present on the right side of the spleen which can only be detected by CT scan. Free fluid is present in the right perihepatic space (asterisk).*

Pneumoperitoneum

Note:
(1) Erect chest radiograph is the initial radiographic examination of choice for suspected perforated peptic ulcer.
(2) The finding of 'free gas under diaphragm' in the appropriate clinical setting is diagnostic.

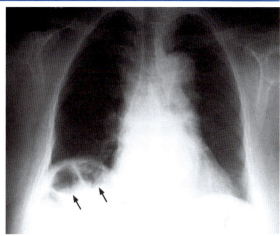

Fig.1f *Frontal radiograph showing hepatodiaphragmatic interposition of bowel (arrows) - Chilaiditi's sign. It may mimic pneumoperitoneum. When associated with symptoms it is called Chilaiditi's syndrome (Image courtesy of Dr Esther Hung, Department of Diagnostic Radiology and Organ Imaging, The Chinese University of Hong Kong).*

06 GASTROINTESTINAL SYSTEM

Small bowel obstruction

Small bowel obstruction at the jejunal level (Fig. 2a)

Discussion:

- Mechanical small bowel obstruction results in small bowel dilatation and the accumulation of both gas and fluid proximal to the point of obstruction. Distal to this point the calibre of small and large bowel is non-dilated/collapsed.
- Plain radiograph changes may appear as early as 3 to 5 hours after the onset of complete obstruction and are usually readily apparent after 12 hours. For incomplete obstruction the radiographic abnormalities may take many hours or even days to evolve.
- Dilated (maximal diameter of normal small bowel <3 cm) small bowel loops containing fluid and/or gas are readily identified on the supine radiograph.
- An erect film may show multiple fluid levels (Fig. 2b) which is non-specific and may be seen in paralytic ileus, gastroenteritis, jejunal diverticulosis, etc.
- The 'string of beads' sign refers to a linear chain of small gas bubbles (which are trapped between the valvulae conniventes when the dilated small bowel loops are almost completely fluid-filled) and is virtually diagnostic of small bowel obstruction (Fig. 2c).
- On an AXR it is important to differentiate small bowel and large bowel dilatation.

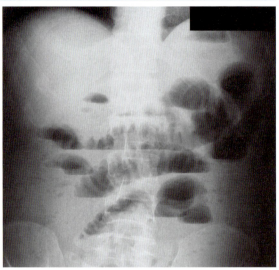

Fig.2b *Erect abdominal radiograph of the same patient as in Fig. 2a showing multiple air-fluid levels within the dilated small bowel loops. Again note the valvulae conniventes.*

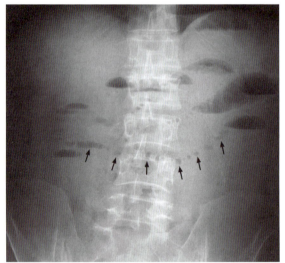

Fig.2c *Erect abdominal radiograph of another patient showing the "string of beads" sign (arrows) virtually diagnostic of small bowel obstruction.*

Discussion Case 2
Small bowel obstruction

- Several radiological features help to differentiate small bowel and large bowel dilatation (see table).
- A contrast follow through (Fig. 2d and e) may be indicated in case of equivocal radiographic findings.

	Small bowel	Large bowel
Valvulae conniventes	Present	Absent
Haustra	Absent	Present
Number of loops	Many	Few
Distribution of loops	Central	Peripheral
Radius of curvature of loop	Small	Large
Diameter of loop	30-50 mm	>50 mm
Solid faeces	Absent	May be present

Haustra - thicker incomplete bands across colonic lumen
Valvulae conniventes - closely-packed complete rings across small bowel lumen
N.B. valvulae conniventes are more prominent in the jejunum than in the ileum

- CT (Fig. 2f-i) is useful in providing more definitive information regarding the site and level of obstruction, the cause of the obstruction (e.g. malignancy) and potential complications (e.g. strangulating obstruction resulting in bowel ischaemia, infarct and perforation).

Role of imaging in the evaluation of bowel obstruction:
- To confirm the diagnosis of bowel obstruction
- To localize the site/level of obstruction
- To detect obstructing lesions like adhesions, tumours, volvulus, hernia, etc.
- To detect possible complications such as strangulation and bowel ischaemia/ infarct

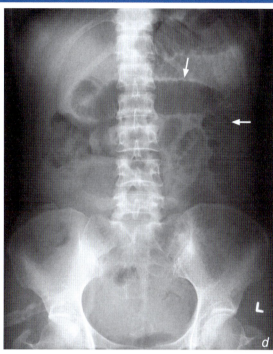

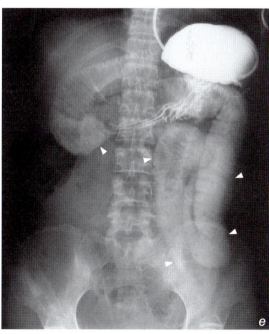

Fig. 2d, e *Supine abdominal radiograph of another patient shows dilated loops of bowel in the upper and left sided abdomen (arrows). Contrast follow through at 4 hours shows the hold up of contrast in the dilated jejunum (arrowheads) at the left side of the abdomen. Features are suggestive of small bowel obstruction.*

Discussion Case 2
Small bowel obstruction

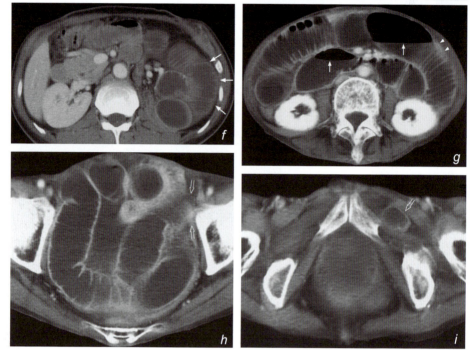

Fig. 2f *Contrast enhanced axial CT of another patient shows small bowel obstruction at the upper level with dilatation of jejunum with prominent valvulae conniventes (arrows).*

Fig. 2g-i *Contrast enhanced axial CT images of another patient shows dilated ileum with multiple air fluid levels (arrows) in the ileum where the valvulae conniventes (arrowheads) are less closely packed compared to the jejunum. There is a loop of bowel (open arrows) extending along the inguinal canal suggestive of inguinal hernia. Overall appearances raise the suspicion of strangulated hernia causing small bowel obstruction. This was later proven by surgery.*

Note:
(1) The temporal pace of development of the radiographic signs of mechanical small bowel obstruction depends on the completeness of the obstruction.
(2) Imaging studies are useful in determining the site/level of obstruction, the cause of the obstruction and in the detection of potential complications.

Discussion Case 3
Mechanical large bowel obstruction

Mechanical distal large bowel obstruction (Fig. 3a)

Discussion:
Dilatation of large bowel >5.5 cm is the hallmark of large bowel obstruction. Once this is diagnosed, the cause and its location requires further investigation.

Colonoscopy and barium enema are relatively contra-indicated in acute obstruction for fear of bowel perforation. A water soluble contrast enema or CT abdomen are safe alternatives.

A water soluble contrast enema (Fig. 3b) was performed in this patient (same patient as Fig. 3a) which demonstrated an 'apple-core' stricture of the large bowel. This appearance is due to a combination of signs:
- Concentric mucosal thickening (due to a carcinoma)
- Shouldering proximal and distal edges
- Irregularly (lobulated) thickened mucosa and/or ulcers between the edges of the lesion.

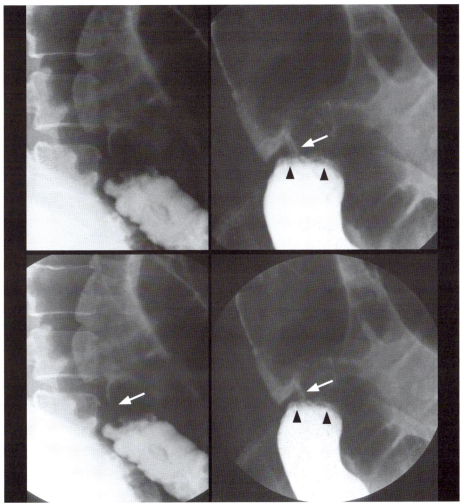

Fig.3b *Coned down view of water soluble contrast enema series of the same patient (as in Fig. 3a) demonstrating a malignant colonic stricture appearing as a typical 'apple-core' lesion (arrows), with shouldered edges (arrowheads).*

Discussion Case 3
Mechanical large bowel obstruction

In some cases of large bowel obstruction, the small bowel may also be dilated (in the presence of incompetent ileocaecal valve). The radiological appearances may be identical to paralytic ileus. In these cases, clinical finding of hyperactive bowel sounds would favour mechanical large bowel obstruction.

There are many causes of large bowel obstruction and a simple way to classify them is by location:
1. Intra-luminal: e.g. faecal impaction, gallstone, intussusception
2. Mural: e.g. neoplasm, infection (parasites), inflammatory bowel disease
3. Extrinsic: e.g. adjacent neoplasm (by compression or invasion), adjacent abscess, endometriosis

In an elderly patient the most common cause is colonic carcinoma.
N.B. large bowel obstruction is rarely caused by post-operative adhesion (as opposed to small bowel obstruction).
N.B. For more information on CA colon, please refer to case 8.

> **Note:**
> (1) Dilatation of large bowel proximal to the site of obstruction with absent rectal gas are typical AXR findings of large bowel obstruction.
> (2) Further evaluation with water soluble contrast enema or CT abdomen helps to identify the underlying cause.

Discussion Case 4
Sigmoid volvulus

Sigmoid volvulus (Fig. 4a)

Discussion:
- Sigmoid volvulus is caused by twisting of a loop of sigmoid colon (sigmoid colon has a mesentery which allows it such mobility, especially when the sigmoid colon elongates with age).
  1. The two ends of this twisted loop are kinked and become closed off (thus termed a closed-loop intestinal obstruction).
  2. This closed off loop contains gas producing bacteria and thus becomes distended with gas, forming an inverted U.
  3. The two limbs of this inverted U are attached to the rest of the sigmoid and thus rest in the left lower quadrant.
  4. Proximal to the site of the volvulus, the large bowel (working from descending colon backwards) is also obstructed and dilates.
- Once the diagnosis is established on clinical and radiographic grounds, urgent treatment by rectal tube insertion in an attempt to 'untwist' the volvulus is indicated (to prevent/minimize bowel ischaemia/infarction/necrosis)
- If the diagnosis is not certain on plain abdominal radiograph, water soluble contrast enema helps. The typical finding is smooth tapered end of contrast column: hook-like in appearance - 'bird of prey sign' (Fig. 4b-c) (where the tapered blind end is seen as a hook)

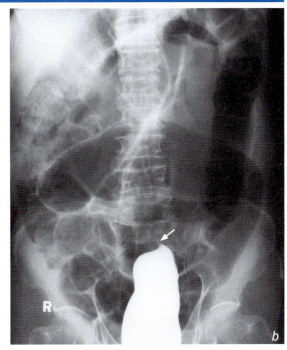

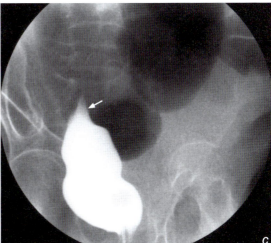

Figs. 4b, c The 'bird of prey' sign (arrow) of sigmoid volvulus as shown on a water soluble contrast enema (Image courtesy of Dr Mabel Tong, Department of Diagnostic Radiology and Organ Imaging, The Chinese University of Hong Kong).

Discussion Case 4
Sigmoid volvulus

- Volvulus may occur in many parts of the intestinal tract, these are in descending frequency: sigmoid > caecum > small bowel > stomach (Fig. 4d) > transverse colon.
- Sigmoid volvulus tends to occur in older patients while caecal volvulus tends to occur in younger (20-40 years old) patients.

Note:
(1) Abdominal radiograph is the initial investigation for suspected sigmoid volvulus.
(2) Distended loop of bowel with inverted U-shaped configuration and coffee bean appearance are characteristic radiological features of sigmoid volvulus.
(3) Immediate treatment with rectal tube insertion is indicated to untwist the volvulus to prevent further bowel ischaemia/ necrosis.

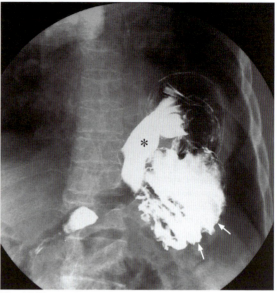

Fig. 4d *Water soluble contrast examination showing the stomach has twisted on itself - gastric volvulus. Note the fundus (arrow) is in a lower position compared to pylorus (asterisk). (Image courtesy of Dr Grace Au, Department of Diagnostic Radiology and Organ Imaging, The Chinese University of Hong Kong).*

Gallstone ileus

Gallstone ileus (Fig. 5a)

Discussion:

The findings in Fig. 5a demonstrate 'Rigler's Triad' (not to be mistaken as Rigler's sign of pneumoperitoneum):

1. Aerobilia (air in the biliary tree) suggests reflux of air from the gastrointestinal tract into the biliary tree. This in turn suggests an abnormal communication (fistula) between the gastrointestinal tract and biliary tree or gallbladder.
2. Abnormal location of a gallstone, as a laminated radio-opacity in the left lower quadrant.
3. The proximal bowel distention and paucity of distal bowel gas indicates some form of mechanical obstruction. The transition point coincides with the site of gallstone, hence the diagnosis of gallstone ileus can be made.

A water-soluble contrast follow through in the same patient (Fig. 5b, c) showed:

- Reflux of contrast from the proximal small bowel into the biliary tree
- The transition point from dilated and contrast filled (obstructed) bowel to non-dilated (distal to obstruction) bowel coincides with the site of the laminated (concentrically calcified) radiopacity.

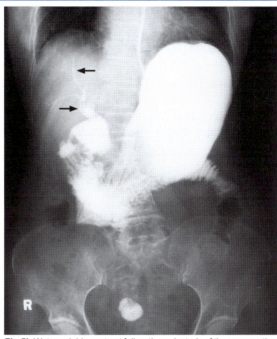

Fig.5b *Water soluble contrast follow through study of the same patient demonstrating reflux of oral contrast from the small bowel into the biliary tree (arrows) indicating abnormal gastro-biliary communication.*

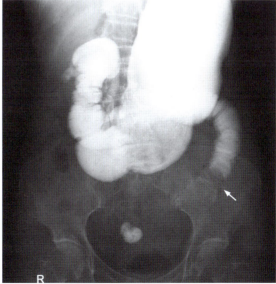

Fig.5c *A more delayed radiograph of the same patient confirms that the laminated concentric calcification to be a gallstone that has eroded into the small bowel and got impacted at the upper jejunum (arrow) to cause the small bowel obstruction – gallstone ileus.*

Discussion Case 5
Gallstone ileus

Gallstone ileus is caused by passage of a large gallstone into the small bowel (by eroding through the bowel wall), and eventually impacting itself within a narrow part of the bowel causing obstruction (partial or complete). Gallstone ileus is a rare cause (<1%) of mechanical small bowel obstruction.

A stone needs to be 25 mm or larger to cause such obstruction. The sites of obstruction in descending order of frequency are: Ileocaecal valve or other parts of small bowel >> duodenum >> sigmoid colon.

Note:

(1) The presence of bowel dilatation, aerobilia and a radio-opaque gallstone in the abdomen should raise the suspicion of gallstone ileus.

Acute appendicitis

Acute appendicitis (Fig. 6a, b)

Discussion:

Appendicitis is caused by obstruction of the appendiceal lumen (by lymphoid hyperplasia, faecolith, appendicolith, parasites, etc.) which leads to superimposed infection and ischaemia, and possibly eventual perforation. Straightforward cases with typical clinical findings may proceed directly to surgery. However, some cases of appendicitis may present with non-specific or atypical symptoms and signs. This is particularly true in patients at the extremes of the age spectrum, and in young female patients where confusion with gynaecological problems may arise.

Imaging helps in suspected cases of acute appendicitis aiming to:

1. Confirm the diagnosis - to prevent delay in treatment and decrease complications, such as perforation, and to avoid a negative laparotomy
2. Exclude/provide alternative diagnosis for the cause of the patient's symptoms
3. Detect complications (e.g. perforation, abscess or fistula formation)

AXR is often non-contributory but may sometimes demonstrate an appendicolith (Fig. 6c) in the right lower quadrant. Ultrasound is often used as an initial imaging modality to identify the inflamed appendix, associated inflammatory changes and possible complications, such as perforation.

USG findings of appendicitis include:

1. Blind-ended, distended tubular structure (longitudinal profile of inflamed appendix) (Fig. 6d)
2. Thickened hypoechoic wall (Fig. 6d)

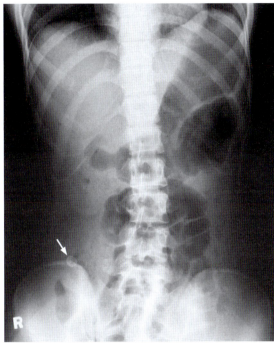

Fig.6c *Supine abdominal radiograph showing an appendicolith (arrow), in the right lower quadrant.*

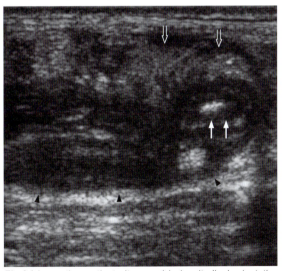

Fig.6d *In another patient ultrasound in longitudinal orientation shows a swollen appendix as a typical tubular blind-end structure (arrowheads). An appendicolith is present at the tip (arrows). The thickened hyperechoic omentum (open arrows) wraps around the inflamed appendix.*

06 GASTROINTESTINAL SYSTEM

285

Acute appendicitis

3. Concentric appearance (due to the thickened mural layers) on cross section (total diameter >6 mm on compression) (Fig. 6e)
4. Appendicolith present (Fig. 6f)
5. Surrounding free fluid.

Findings of acute appendicitis on CT include:

1. Appendicolith (homogeneous or ring-like calcifications) seen in 25-40% of cases (Fig. 6g)

Fig.6e *Same patient as Fig. 6d. Axial orientation ultrasound shows the swollen appendix (arrows) wrapped around by the thickened hyperechoic omentum (open arrows).*

Fig.6f *Longitudinal ultrasound image shows a very well-defined appendicolith (arrow) at the tip of the appendix (arrowheads).*

Fig.6g *Non-contrast axial CT image shows a small round appendicolith at the caecal end of the appendix (arrow).*

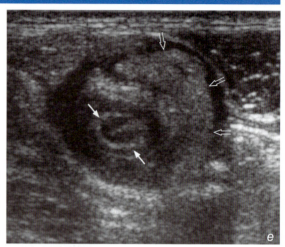

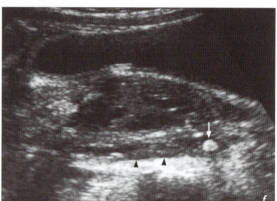

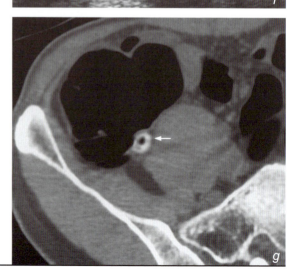

Acute appendicitis

2. The inflamed appendix which is distended and thickened (Fig. 6h, i)
3. Peri-appendiceal inflammatory fat streakiness and bowel thickening (Fig. 6h, i)

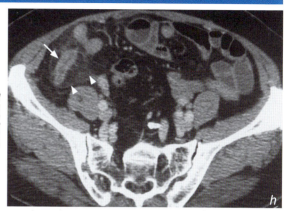

Fig.6h, i Contrast enhanced axial and sagittal CT images of a different patient show a swollen appendix (arrow) arising from the caecum associated with increased density of the peri-appendiceal fat (arrowheads) suggestive of inflammatory change. No abscess formation evident.

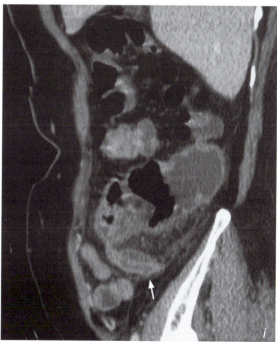

Acute appendicitis

4. Where there is perforation there will be surrounding fluid collection/ abscess formation (Fig. 6j, k) and possibly intraperitoneal free gas.

Note:

(1) In appendicitis imaging can help to confirm/ exclude the diagnosis, speed up treatment to avoid complications, prevent unnecessary laparotomy, and provide alternative diagnosis.

(2) Ultrasound or CT is the radiological investigation of choice.

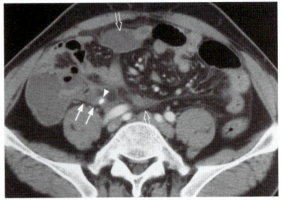

Fig.6j *Contrast enhanced axial CT image of a different patient shows an inflamed appendix (arrows) with a small appendicolith (arrowheads) at its tip. Inflammatory change is noted in the peri-appendiceal fat. There are several small collections (open arrows) in the abdomen.*

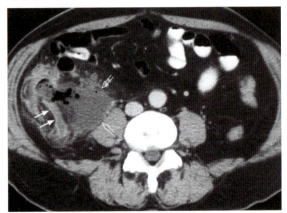

Fig.6k *Contrast enhanced axial CT shows a thickened inflamed appendix (arrows) with adjacent gas-containing abscess (open arrows).*

Acute mesenteric infarction

Acute mesenteric infarction (Fig. 7a)
- The imaging findings indicate small bowel infarction and in view of the clinical information the diagnosis is acute mesenteric infarction.

Discussion:
- Acute mesenteric infarction can be due to thrombosis or embolism (the latter commonly from a cardiac source) of the superior mesenteric artery
- The radiological findings of acute mesenteric infarction include:
  1. Small bowel dilatation – indicating an ileus (non-specific)
  2. Bowel wall thickening +/- mucosal/submucosal density increase - indicating mucosal oedema +/- submucosal haemorrhage. N.B. This bowel thickness actually represents the summation of two bowel walls (two adjacent gas-filled bowel loops in contact for this to be visible)
  3. Pneumatosis intestinalis linearis (i.e. intramural gas) - streaks of gas lucency within bowel wall suggests gangrene of involved bowel wall
  4. Portal venous gas - linear branching lucencies within the periphery of liver (due to hepato-petal flow away from the porta hepatis towards the periphery)
  5. 'Thumbprinting' of small bowel mucosal folds - reflecting oedematous mucosal folds
  6. Pneumoperitoneum - as a result of bowel perforation
- CECT abdomen findings of acute mesenteric infarction include
  1. Bowel wall thickening (Fig. 7b)
  2. Pneumatosis intestinalis linearis - intramural gas (Fig. 7c)
  3. Portal venous gas (Fig. 7d, e)
  4. Filling defects in superior mesenteric artery (represents the obstructing clot/thrombus)

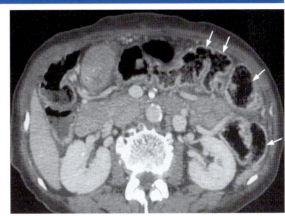

Fig. 7b CECT of a different patient shows bowel wall thickening in the colon with mucosal/submucosal high density due to oedema and haemorrhage (arrows).

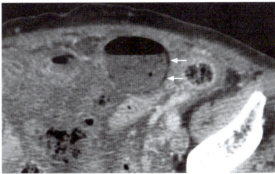

Fig.7c CECT of a different patient demonstrating pneumatosis intestinalis (arrows), i.e. gas within bowel wall indicating gangrene of bowel wall.

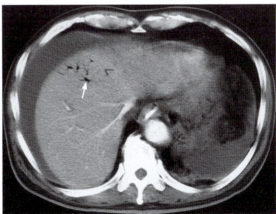

Fig.7d CECT of the abdomen of a different patient showing portal venous gas (arrow) towards the periphery of the liver, often seen in patients with mesenteric infarction.

Discussion Case 7
Acute mesenteric infarction

5. Non-enhancement of the bowel wall (Fig. 7f)
6. Fluid-filled dilated loops of small bowel (Fig. 7f)

- CECT abdomen is more informative than radiographs and allows a definitive diagnosis.
- Early diagnosis is important as mortality is high in advanced cases and urgent treatment with trans-arterial thrombolysis may potentially restore normal mesenteric circulation.

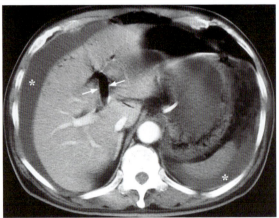

Fig.7e *Contrast enhanced CT at a lower level than Fig.7d confirms that the left main portal vein is filled with gas (arrows). Ascites is present in the right perihepatic region and left perisplenic region (asterisks).*

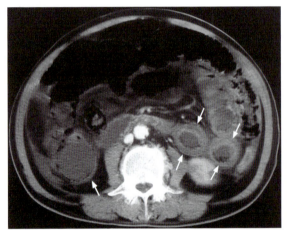

Fig. 7f *Contrast enhanced CT abdomen at the lower level of the abdomen of the same patient showing severe thickening of the small bowel (arrows) filled with fluid. The bowel wall does not show contrast enhancement and is compatible with mesenteric infarct (same patient as in Fig.7d,e).*

Acute mesenteric infarction

- In an embolic situation, other abdominal organs may be affected (Fig. 7g, h)

Note:
(1) Dilated small bowel with signs of bowel ischaemia and gangrene of involved segment are radiological features of acute mesenteric infarction.
(2) Contrast enhanced CT provides more supporting evidence for definitive diagnosis.

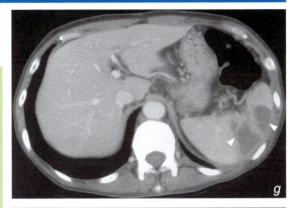

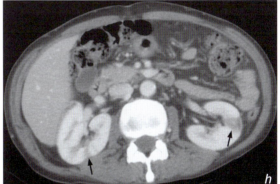

Fig. 7g, h *Abdominal CECT of a different patient with emboli originating from the heart. These images show wedge-shaped non-enhancing areas in the spleen (arrowheads) and both kidneys (arrows).*

Discussion Case 8
Carcinoma of the colon

Carcinoma of the colon (Fig. 8a)

Discussion:

- Carcinoma of the colon carries a lifetime risk of 4% in the general population and is a common cause of rectal bleeding, especially in elderly patients
- The location of colonic carcinoma, in descending order of frequency, is: rectum > sigmoid > transverse > ascending > caecum
- The two most common radiological appearances are:
  - Apple-core (ulcerating annular lesion) (Fig. 8b)
  - Fungating (multilobular protruding lesion) (Fig. 8c)

Fig.8b Double contrast enema demonstrates a severe stricture with typical apple core lesion (arrows) in the colon (Image courtesy of Dr Yolanda Lee, Department of Diagnostic Radiology and Organ Imaging, The Chinese University of Hong Kong).

Fig.8c In another patient double contrast enema shows the typical fungating mass (arrows) with mildly irregular surface arising from the posterior wall of the rectum.

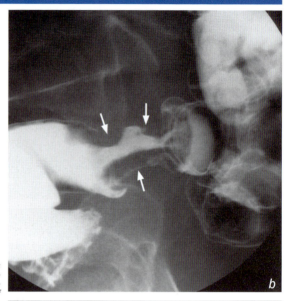

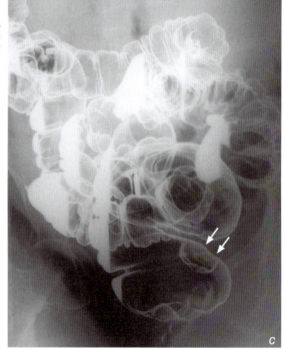

Discussion Case 8
Carcinoma of the colon

- Currently the diagnosis of colonic carcinoma is established mainly by colonoscopy and biopsy.
- The main disadvantage of colonoscopy is its invasiveness and inherent complications (e.g. bowel perforation). In difficult cases, or when colonoscopy is not possible, double contrast enema, and CT colonoscopy (Fig. 8d) are suitable alternative investigations.
- Once the diagnosis is confirmed by biopsy, the patient is usually staged with CT.

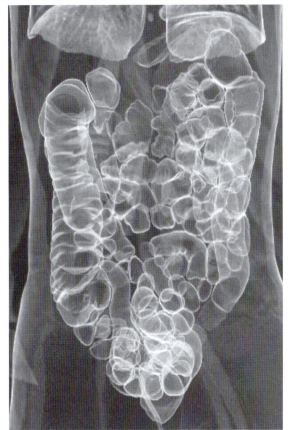

Fig.8d *CT colonoscopy (air enema projection) shows the air outlining the small bowel and large bowel which is used for screening of CA colon with low radiation.*

Discussion Case 8
Carcinoma of the colon

Imaging in patients with suspected carcinoma of colon:

1. Barium enema to detect suspicious colonic lesion in a tortuous and redundant colon (Fig. 8e, f) (difficult colonoscopy) and synchronous tumour in proximal colon in severe distal stricture (incomplete colonoscopy)

Fig.8e *Contrast enema of another patient shows a moderate sized stricture (arrows) in the distal transverse colon partially obscured by the descending colon.*

Fig.8f *Contrast enema (same patient as Fig. 8e) shows the malignant stricture in the distal transverse colon with irregular and ulcerative wall (arrows).*

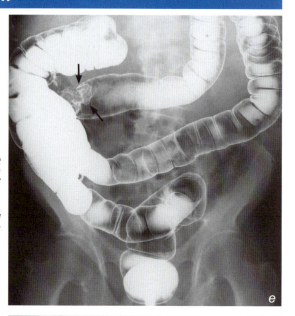

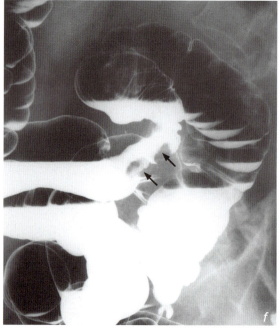

Carcinoma of the colon

2. High resolution ultrasound is useful to look for any bowel wall thickening suspicious of carcinoma (Fig. 8g)
3. Further investigations for assessment of local tumour extent, regional lymph node involvement (e.g. abdominal ultrasound/CT) (Fig. 8h, i) and systemic metastases (e.g. CXR/bone scintigraphy) and follow-up after treatment
4. Transrectal ultrasound is used for assessment of local tumour invasion for rectal carcinoma
5. MRI is sometimes used for detection and staging of carcinoma of the colon (Fig. 8j to l)

Fig.8g *Transverse sonogram of a different patient shows a Ca colon (arrows) seen as significantly thickened hypoechoic wall in the ascending colon with echogenic gas present within the narrowed lumen. This is sometimes referred to as the 'target sign'.*

Fig.8h *Contrast enhanced CT image of different patient shows the tumour mass (arrow) involving the left eccentric wall of the descending colon. There is increased adjacent mesenteric density (open arrows) which is suggestive of invasion.*

Fig.8i *Contrast enhanced CT image at a lower level than Fig. 8h shows the tumour becomes more circumferential and involves descending colon. There is associated fluid collection surrounded by a rim of the contrast enhancement (arrowheads) and extraluminal gas locule (arrow) suggesting perforation.*

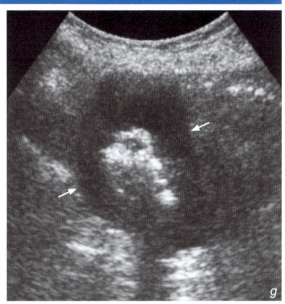
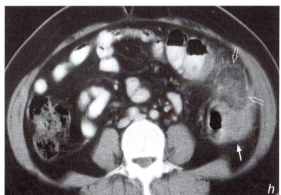
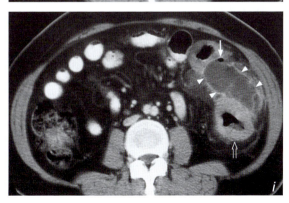

06 GASTROINTESTINAL SYSTEM

Discussion Case 8
Carcinoma of the colon

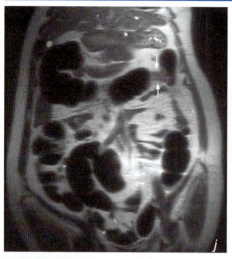 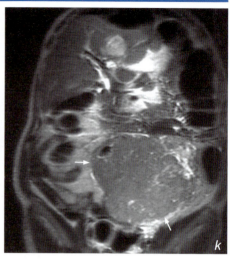

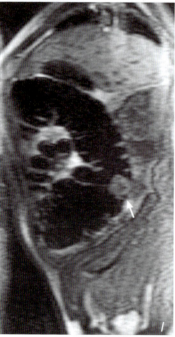

Fig.8k-n *MRI images show different appearances of CA colon. (j) Malignant stricture close to the splenic flexure (arrows). (k) A huge tumour mass occupying the left sided pelvis and lower abdomen (arrows) associated with liver metastasis (open arrows). (l) Sagittal view shows another polypoid tumour protruding into the lumen of the large bowel (Images courtesy of Prof. Wynnie Lam, Department of Diagnostic Radiology and Organ Imaging, The Chinese University of Hong Kong).*

Note:
(1) Carcinoma of the colon must be excluded in elderly patients presenting with rectal bleeding.
(2) Colonoscopy or double contrast barium enema is the investigation of choice.
(3) 'Apple-core' stricture with mucosal irregularities and ulceration are characteristic features of carcinoma of the colon on barium examination.

Discussion Case 9
Colonic diverticulosis

Colonic diverticulosis (Fig. 9a, b)

Discussion:

- Colonic diverticulosis is defined as mucosal and muscularis mucosae herniation through defects in the muscularis propria. This is thought to be mainly due to increased intra-luminal pressure, possibly as a result of a low fibre diet.
- Colonic diverticulosis most commonly affects elderly patients.
- Left-sided colon is predominantly involved in Caucasians and right-sided in Asians.
- In patients with acute diverticulitis, colonoscopy or barium enema is contra-indicated in view of risk of perforation. In this instance, CT scan helps to support the diagnosis (Fig. 9c, d) and helps to detect any complication of acute diverticulitis, e.g. collection (Fig. 9e). CT colonoscopy is now helpful in detection of a diverticulum (Fig. 9f).

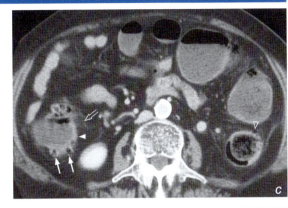

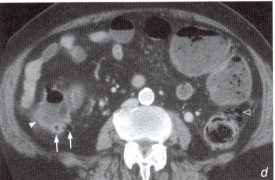

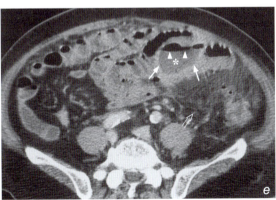

Fig.9c, d Contrast enhanced axial CT images of a different patient show that there are several small gas-filled outpouchings (arrows) from the colonic wall suggestive of diverticuli present around the fluid-filled ascending colon. Mild wall thickening (arrowheads) in the ascending colon with increased fat streakiness (open arrow) suggests acute diverticulitis. There are also several small diverticuli (open arrowhead) with no inflammatory change in the descending colon.

Fig.9e Contrast enhanced axial CT of the abdomen of another patient shows that there are several small diverticuli present in the descending colon with inflammatory change of the surrounding fat mesentery (open arrow). There is complication of acute diverticulitis with abscess (asterisk) formation in the abdomen. The abscess in the left-sided anterior abdomen shows typical appearance of the air fluid level (arrowheads) and rim of the contrast enhancement (arrows) compressing the adjacent loops of the small bowel.

Colonic diverticulosis

Note:

(1) Colonic diverticulosis should be considered in elderly patients with recurrent lower abdominal pain.

(2) Multiple smooth outpouchings from colonic wall predominantly affecting left-sided colon are the radiological findings.

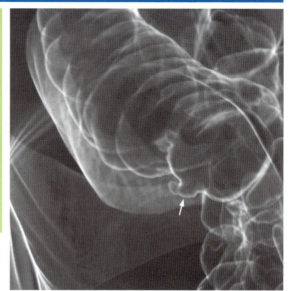

Fig. 9f *CT colonoscopy of another patient shows a diverticulum in the right ascending colon demonstrating a typical appearance of air-containing outpouching (arrow) from the colonic wall.*

Carcinoma of oesophagus

Carcinoma of oesophagus (Fig.10a) with probable liver metastases (in view of hepatomegaly with irregular outline)

Discussion:
- Causes of oesophageal stricture (narrowing > 10 mm length) include: neoplasm, infection and scarring (e.g. caustic ingestion).
  Radiological manifestations of oesophageal carcinoma on barium swallow include
  1. Stricture (i.e. circumferential or eccentric mass)
  2. Mucosal irregularities (i.e. ulcerated surface)
  3. Polyploid mass with irregular outline protruding into lumen
  4. Tracheo-oesophageal fistula – due to tumour invasion anteriorly into trachea
- Upper GI endoscopy is now more commonly employed as an initial investigation for a patient with dysphagia
- Barium swallow and upper GI endoscopy have their own advantages and disadvantages:
  1. Advantages of barium swallow - non-invasive, allows evaluation of any motility disorder
  2. Disadvantage of barium swallow - cannot provide tissue diagnosis
  3. Advantages of upper GI endoscopy - direct visualization of mucosal lesion, allows biopsy for histological diagnosis
  4. Disadvantages of upper GI endoscopy - more invasive, relatively more complications (although rare)
- Once oesophageal carcinoma is diagnosed, staging of the disease is required and this involves a CT of the thorax +/- neck USG.

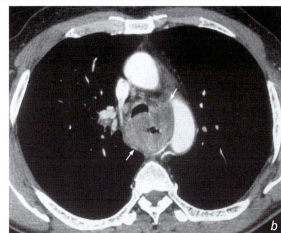

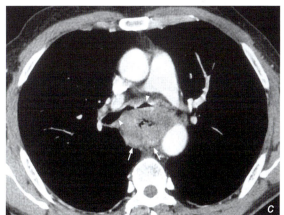

Fig.10b, c *Contrast enhanced axial CT images show a large circumferential tumour in the oesophagus (arrows) with narrowing of the lumen at the aortopulmonary (b) and subcarinal (c) level. The tumour compresses on the posterior aspect of the trachea and carina with narrowing of the right and left main bronchi (arrowheads, Fig. 10c).*

Discussion Case 10
Carcinoma of oesophagus

- Current role of imaging in patients with carcinoma of oesophagus include CT thorax (Fig. 10b to e), endoscopic ultrasound, ultrasound abdomen and radionuclide bone scintigraphy.
  1. Staging of disease – local tumour extent (T-staging by endoscopic ultrasound/CT thorax), nodal involvement (N-staging by CT thorax/USG neck) and distant metastases (M-staging by CT thorax/USG abdomen/radionuclide bone scintigraphy)
  2. Monitor response to chemotherapy or radiotherapy

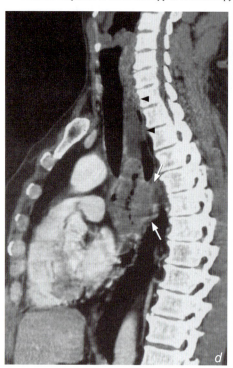
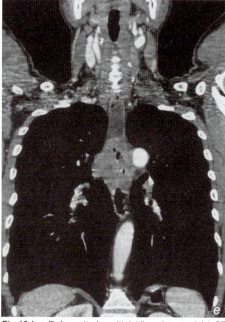

Fig.10d, e Reformatted sagittal (d) and coronal (e) CT images better demonstrate the position and extent of the large tumour of the oesophagus in the posterior mediastinum (arrows). There is evidence of fluid hold- up in the upper oesophagus (arrowheads). Same patient as in Fig. 10b, c.

Note:
(1) Carcinoma of oesophagus is a common cause of painless progressive dysphagia in an elderly patient.
(2) Upper GI endoscopy is the initial investigation of choice for diagnosis.
(3) The presence of stricture with irregular contour and mucosal irregularities are radiological features on barium swallow.
(4) Role of imaging is mainly for tumour staging and to monitor response to treatment.

Crohn's disease

Crohn's disease (Fig. 11a, b)

Discussion:

- Crohn's disease is a disease of unknown aetiology with asymmetric involvement of entire GI tract.
- Patient usually presents with recurrent episodes of diarrhoea, abdominal pain, weight loss and anaemia. Sometimes complications such as fistula-in-ano and malabsorption result.
- Fluoroscopic features of Crohn's disease (Fig. 11a-b):
  1. Cobblestone appearance: serpiginous longitudinal and transverse ulcers separated by areas of the oedema
  2. Skip lesions in the small bowel
  3. Thickened small bowel folds
  4. Separation and displacement of the small bowel loops due to lymphoedematous wall thickening/ increase in mesenteric fat and enlarged mesenteric lymph nodes
  5. Larger filling defects present in the terminal ileum suggestive of pseudopolyps which are due to islands of hyperplasic mucosa between denuded mucosa.
  6. Pseudodiverticula represents bulging area of normal wall opposite to the affected scarred wall on the antimesenteric side.

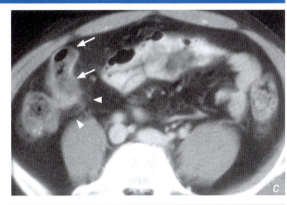

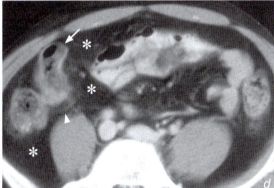

Fig. 11c, d *Axial contrast CT image of the same case as Fig. 11a, b shows abnormal dilatation of the terminal ileum (arrows). However, the details of the mucosal abnormality cannot be well delineated by routine CT scan. There is increased mesenteric density suggestive of inflammation (arrowheads). Massive proliferation of mesenteric fat (asterisks) with displacement of the small bowel to the left side is noted.*

Discussion Case 11
Crohn's disease

- CT features of Crohn's disease (Fig. 11c-f)
1. Asymmetric bowel wall thickening
2. Luminal narrowing
3. Proliferation of the mesenteric fat (creeping fat)
4. Skip areas of asymmetric bowel wall thickening

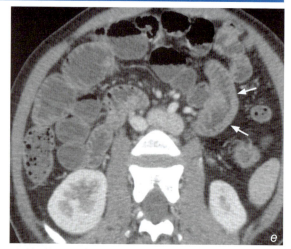

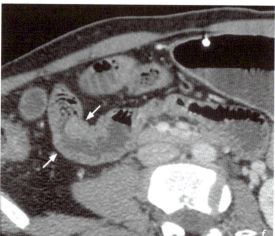

Fig. 11e, f *CT enteroclysis images show a short segment of asymmetrical bowel wall thickening (arrows) at the proximal jejunum with loss of normal valvulae conniventes. Although the rest of the small bowel is well-distended by fluid, the lumen in this short segment is narrow, suggestive of fibrotic changes. Overall features are suggestive of chronic stage of Crohn's disease (Images courtesy of Dr Simon Le, Department of Diagnostic Radiology and Organ Imaging, The Chinese University of Hong Kong).*

Remarks:
CT enteroclysis is an examination using fine cut CT images to delineate the small bowel, particularly the mucosal pathology. Before the scan, the small bowel is infused with methylcellulose via naso-duodenal tube placed at the duodeno-jejunal junction.

Discussion Case 11
Crohn's disease

- Complications of Crohn's disease include
  1. Fistula-in-ano (Fig. 11g, h)
  2. Abscess
  3. Perforation (Fig. 11i)
  4. Toxic megacolon
  5. Malignancy of the bowel (adenocarcinoma or lymphoma)
- There are other causes for focal bowel wall thickening which include infection (Fig. 11j, k) and neoplasm.

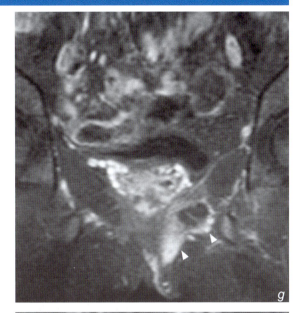

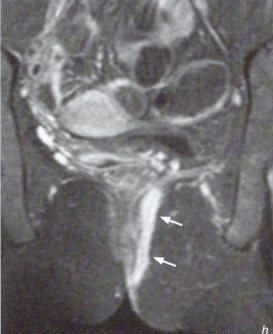

Fig. 11g, h *Coronal T2W fat saturated sequence shows a fistulous tract extending from the left lateral wall just beyond the anus and ascends in the medial left ischio-rectal fossa (arrows). No supra-levator extension. There is abscess formation in the more anterior aspect of the fistula in the left ischio-rectal fossa (arrowheads).*

Crohn's disease

Fig. 11i *Contrast axial CT of the abdomen showing an abnormal thickened loop of small bowel (arrows) in a patient with Crohn's disease. Note the ascites (asterisk) and air fluid levels (arrowheads) suggestive of a perforation (Images courtesy of Dr Simon Le, Department of Diagnostic Radiology and Organ Imaging, The Chinese University of Hong Kong).*

Fig. 11j *Axial contrast CT image shows diffuse thickening of the distal ileum (arrows). Small amount of ascites is present in the pelvis (asterisks). The patient was later confirmed to have TB ileitis with malabsorption syndrome.*

Fig. 11k *Coronal contrast reformatted CT image shows a rigid contracted cone-shaped caecum with wall thickening (arrow). There is also irregular wall thickening of the terminal ileum (arrowheads) mimicking the diagnosis of Crohn's disease. The tubular structure inferior to the caecum is fluid-filled appendix (open arrow). Biopsy confirmed TB infection of the caecum and terminal ileum.*

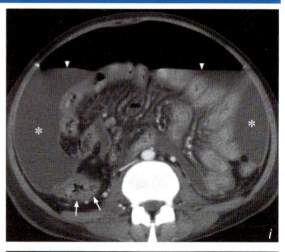

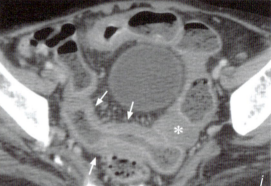

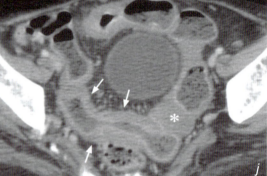

> **Note:**
>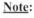
> (1) Crohn's disease is characterized by focal segment(s) of bowel wall inflammation.
> (2) Imaging helps with diagnosis and can be used for monitoring progress.

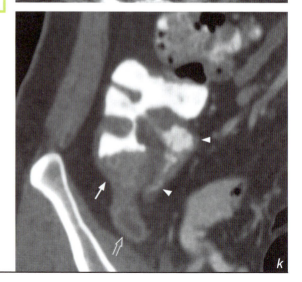

GENITOURINARY SYSTEM

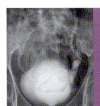

Contributors:

K.K. Shing, K.T. Wong, Gregory E. Antonio, Shlok J. Lolge, Anil T. Ahuja

Questions

Case 1 - 12	306 - 317

Discussion

Renal calculus	318 - 322
Ureteric stone	323 - 327
Non-calculus ureteric obstruction	328 - 331
Renal cell carcinoma	332 - 337
Renal laceration	338 - 339
Carcinoma of the bladder	340 - 342
Bladder calculus	343 - 345
Uterine fibroid	346 - 348
Adrenal mass	349 - 352
Testicular torsion	353
Testicular tumour	354 - 355
Ovarian tumour	356 - 358

Chapter 07

Case 1

A 52-year-old woman presented with gross haematuria associated with right loin pain for 3 days. On physical examination, she was tender over the right loin region but was afebrile. Blood tests were essentially normal. Based on these findings, a renal calculus was suspected. A KUB was performed as an initial investigation (Fig. 1a) followed by an IVU a few days later (Fig. 1b).

Questions

(1) What radiological abnormality can you see ?
- KUB : Calcified opacities projected over left renal shadow
- IVU : Filling defect in upper pole calyx and renal pelvis of the left kidney – corresponding to opacity on the KUB
  Clubbing of adjacent renal calyces - due to focal calyceal obstruction by the stones
(2) What is the diagnosis ?

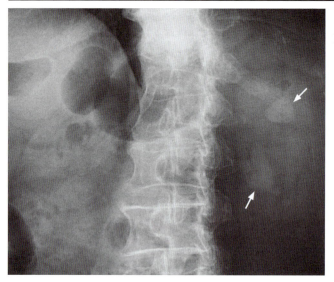

Fig.1a *Coned KUB shows radio-opacities (arrows) over the left renal area which may represent renal stones.*

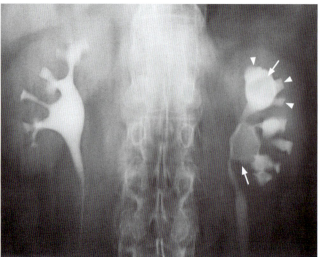

Fig.1b *A tomogram obtained during an IVU shows filling defects (arrows) in the left upper pole calyx and left renal pelvis corresponding to the opacities seen on the KUB in Fig.1a. This supports the diagnosis of left renal calculi. Note that the stones appear radiolucent against a background of contrast. Also note the clubbing of the adjacent minor renal calyces (arrowheads).*

Case 2

A 45-year-old man, with a known history of left renal calculus, complained of severe left loin pain for one day. The pain was colicky and sharp in nature and radiated to the left groin. Physical examination was essentially normal. Urine examination was positive for RBC and negative for WBC. Blood tests were unremarkable. A clinical diagnosis of ureteric colic was suspected. A KUB (Fig.2a) followed by an IVU (Fig.2b) a few days later was performed.

Questions

(1) What radiological abnormality can you see ?

   KUB - Well defined radio-opacity on the left side of L4. It is vertically aligned and along the course of the left ureter.

   IVU - The radio-opacity seen on the KUB is in the left ureter, causing hydronephrosis and proximal hydroureter

(2) What is the diagnosis ?

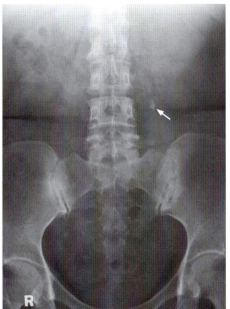

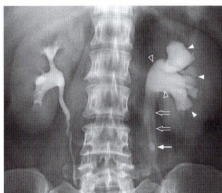

Fig.2b *A tomogram obtained during IVU examination shows left hydronephrosis (dilated renal calyces (arrowheads) and pelvis (open arrowheads)), and proximal hydroureter (open arrows). The ureteric stone (arrow) is situated at the lower end of the dilated left ureter.*

Fig.2a *KUB shows a radio-opacity (arrow) in the left paravertebral region at the level of L4, along the course of the left ureter. This was confirmed to be a ureteric calculus.*

Case 3

A 49-year-old woman was recently diagnosed with carcinoma of the cervix. She presented with bilateral loin pain and fever for 3 days. Physical examination showed ballotable kidneys with local tenderness. There was no haematuria. Laboratory investigations revealed elevated serum creatinine and white cell count. KUB showed no definite radio-opaque urinary calculus. She was suspected to have a urinary tract obstruction. An urgent ultrasound of the abdomen was performed (Fig. 3a).

Questions

(1) What radiological abnormality can you see on this longitudinal sonogram of the kidney ?
   - Enlarged left kidney.
   - Hydronephrosis with dilatation of renal pelvis.
(2) What is the diagnosis ?

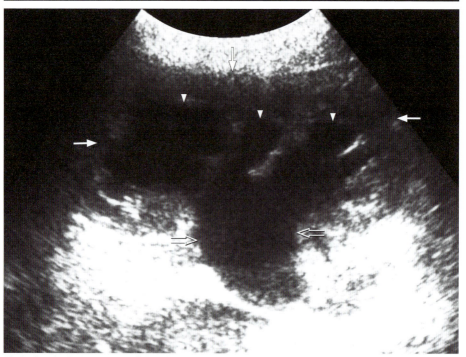

Fig.3a *Longitudinal sonogram of the left kidney (arrows) shows dilated calyces (arrowheads) and renal pelvis (open arrows) indicating hydronephrosis.*

Case 4

A 67-year-old man with no history of urinary tract calculus, complained of painless whole stream haematuria for 2 months, loss of weight and loss of appetite. Physical examination revealed a ballotable right kidney. Laboratory investigations were essentially normal. As a right renal mass was suspected, an ultrasound scan of the kidney was performed (Fig. 4a). This was followed by a contrast enhanced CT scan (Fig. 4b, c).

Questions

(1) What radiological abnormality can you see on the longitudinal sonogram ?
   - A hypoechoic mass in the lower pole of the kidney.
(2) What radiological abnormality can you see on the axial contrast enhanced CT ?
   - Large heterogeneous irregular soft tissue mass in the right kidney.
   - Thrombus in the right renal vein and IVC.
   - Enlarged retro-caval lymph node.
   - Increased streakiness in perinephric fat on the right.
   - Unremarkable left kidney.
(3) What is the diagnosis ?

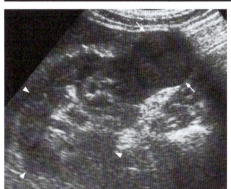

Fig.4a *Longitudinal sonogram of kidney (arrowheads) shows a hypoechoic mass in the lower pole of the right kidney which was confirmed to be a renal cell carcinoma (RCC) (arrows). On ultrasound, RCC may have a mixed echogenicity with a heterogeneous echo pattern due to areas of necrosis, liquefaction and haemorrhage.*

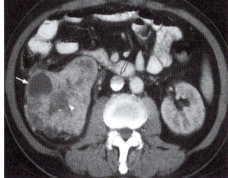

Fig.4b *Axial contrast enhanced CT (CECT) of the abdomen of the same patient shows a large irregular heterogeneous mass in the right kidney with a fluid density area (arrow) suggesting a renal cell carcinoma (RCC). The central hypodense area appears ill-defined and is suggestive of necrosis (arrowhead). Note the filling defect in the IVC which represents a tumour thrombus in the IVC (open arrow).*

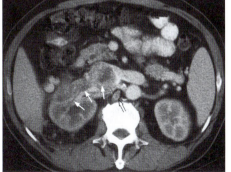

Fig.4c *More superior CECT scan shows that the mass has extended into the right renal vein (arrows). An enlarged retro-caval lymph node is present (open arrow).*

Case 5

A 16-year-old man presented with back pain and frank haematuria following a fall earlier in the day. On admission his vital signs were stable. Localized tenderness and skin bruise was noted over the right loin. The rest of the abdominal examination was unremarkable. Laboratory investigations showed normal haemoglobin level and renal function. Renal injury was suspected and a contrast enhanced CT (CECT) was performed (Fig. 5a, b).

Questions

(1) What radiological abnormality do you see on this axial CECT ?
   - Linear fissures within the parenchyma of the right kidney - representing renal laceration
   - Fluid around the right kidney - indicates haematoma or leakage of urine in the perinephric space
   - Normal contrast enhancement of fragments - signifies that major vessels within the renal pedicle are intact

(2) What is the diagnosis ?

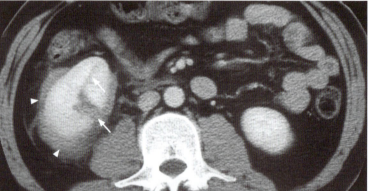

Fig.5a *Axial CECT of the abdomen shows right renal laceration (arrows) and perinephric haematoma (arrowheads). The lower pole of the left kidney is just visible on this slice. There is no difference in the degree of contrast enhancement between the two kidneys indicating that the different parts of the right kidney are normally perfused.*

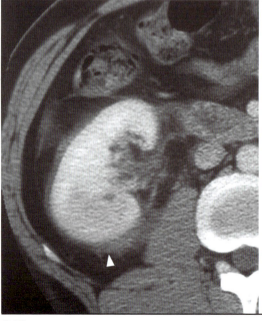

Fig.5b *Axial CECT scan of the abdomen of the same patient in Fig.5a shows fluid around the right kidney indicating a haematoma or extravasated urine (arrowhead).*

Case 6

A 74-year-old man, a chronic smoker for 50 years, presented with on and off painless gross haematuria for 2 months. Physical examination showed a vague hard mass in the suprapubic area arising from the pelvis. The prostate was not enlarged on rectal examination. Plain abdominal radiograph did not reveal any radio-opaque calculus. Urine cytology revealed malignant cells. Carcinoma of the urinary bladder was suspected and a CECT was performed (Fig. 6a-c).

Questions

(1) What abnormality do you see on the CECT ?
- Soft tissue mass with nodular thickening of bladder wall - represents the primary bladder wall tumour
- Bilateral hydronephrosis suggesting ureteric obstruction by the bladder tumour.
- Increased density in perivesical fat - indicates local tumour infiltration around the bladder

(2) What is the diagnosis ?

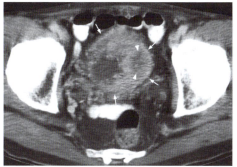 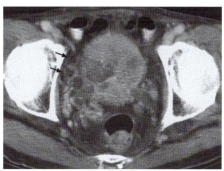

Fig.6a *Axial CECT of pelvis shows irregular nodular thickening in the bladder wall (arrows) which represents a bladder tumour. In its thickest portion, there is evidence of necrosis (arrowheads).*

Fig.6b *Axial CECT of the pelvis at a more inferior level shows gross bladder wall thickening and increased density in the perivesical fat (arrows) which indicates local tumour invasion.*

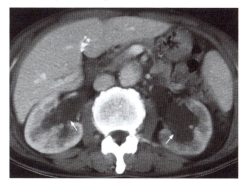

Fig.6c *Axial CECT of the abdomen shows bilateral hydronephrosis (arrows) caused by ureteric obstruction by the bladder tumour.*

Case 7

A 72-year-old man with a known history of benign prostatic hypertrophy, presented with on and off haematuria for 3 months which was associated with mild suprapubic pain, dysuria and urinary frequency. There was no fever or loin pain. Physical examination showed mild local tenderness over the suprapubic region. No abdominal or pelvic mass was detected. Laboratory investigations revealed normal white cell count. Urine cytology and culture were negative. A KUB was performed as an initial investigation (Fig. 7a).

Questions
(1) What radiological abnormality do you see on this coned down KUB ?
 - Several well-defined radio-opacities are noted in the bladder region, slightly to the left
(2) What is the most likely diagnosis ?

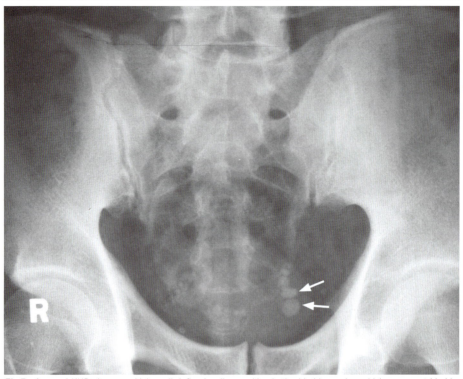

Fig.7a *A coned KUB shows multiple well-defined radio-opacities in the bladder region which represent bladder stones (arrows).*

Case 8

A 43-year-old woman presented with mild pelvic discomfort, menorrhagia and irregular menstruation for recent 6 months. Physical examination found a firm, non-tender lower abdominal mass arising from the pelvis. Laboratory investigations were unremarkable. Cervical smear did not reveal any malignant cells or atypia. A KUB was performed as an initial investigation (Fig. 8a).

Questions
(1) What radiological abnormality do you see on this coned down KUB ?
- A large amorphous, well-defined, ovoid, calcified mass in the pelvis - commonly seen in degenerated fibroids.
(2) What is the diagnosis ?

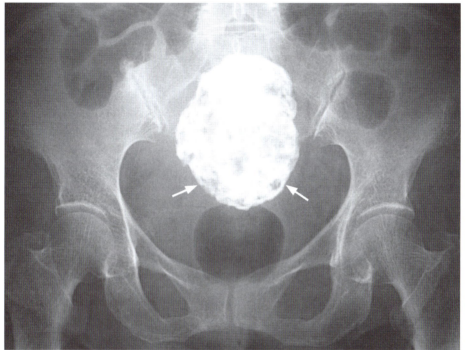

Fig.8a *A coned down KUB shows a large calcified mass in the pelvis (arrows), which is typical for a large calcified fibroid.*

Case 9

A 40-year-old woman presented with a 6-month history of hypertension and intermittent generalized muscle weakness. Physical examination showed elevated blood pressure and hypertensive retinopathy. The rest of the examination was unremarkable. Laboratory investigations revealed metabolic alkalosis. Plasma aldosterone level was raised while serum renin level was below normal limit. Biochemical parameters were suggestive of hyperaldosteronism (Conn's syndrome) and NECT of abdomen was performed (Fig. 9a-c).

Questions

(1) What radiological abnormality can be identified on the NECT ?
- Round lesion with well-defined margins in left adrenal gland
- The lesion is of low attenuation (<0 HU) - due to high lipid content
- No invasion of adjacent structures or evidence of metastases – consistent with a benign lesion rather than a malignancy
- Normal right adrenal gland

(2) What is the diagnosis ?

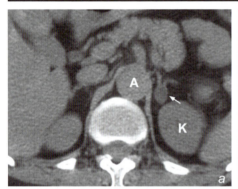

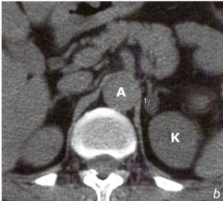

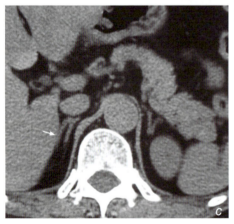

Fig.9a *Non-contrast axial CT of abdomen shows a well-defined low density nodule (arrow) in the left adrenal gland which is suggestive of an adenoma (K = left kidney, A = aorta).*

Fig.9b *Measurement of the CT number of the left adrenal nodule shows a negative value which is due to high lipid (cholesterol) content within the functional adenoma (K = left kidney, A = aorta).*

Fig.9c *Non-contrast axial CT of abdomen at a higher level shows a normal right adrenal gland (arrow).*

Case 10

A 9-year-old boy presented with acute onset of severe left sided scrotal pain for 6 hours. He was afebrile with no urinary symptoms and urine examination was negative for WCC. On physical examination the scrotum was mildly swollen and markedly tender on the left. The mother of the child claims that there have been similar episodes before which resolved spontaneously but it was more severe and persistent this time. An ultrasound of the scrotum was performed for further evaluation (Fig. 10a-d).

Questions

(1) What abnormality is demonstrated on ultrasound (grey scale and colour Doppler) ?
- The left testis is enlarged compared to the right and shows a diffuse, heterogeneous, hypoechoic echopattern. Note the paucity of vascularity within the left testis.
- Normal testicular echopattern and vascularity on the right.

(2) <u>What is the diagnosis ?</u>

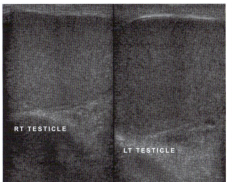

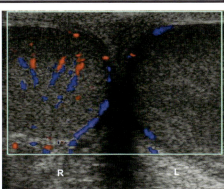

Fig.10a Sonogram of the testes showing:
- Normal right testis with a diffusely homogeneous fine, bright echopattern.
- The left testis is enlarged compared with the right and shows a diffuse, hypoechoic (dark) echopattern compared to the right.
(Image courtesy of Department of Radiology, K.E.M. Hospital, Mumbai, India)

Fig.10b Color Doppler of the testis showing normal testicular vascularity on the right. Note the paucity of vascularity in the left testis which is enlarged with a hypoechoic echopattern. Features are consistent with left testicular torsion (Image courtesy of Department of Radiology, K.E.M. Hospital, Mumbai, India).

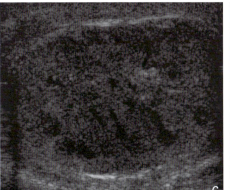

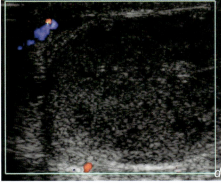

Fig.10c, d Grey scale and Doppler sonogram of the torsioned left testis showing an enlarged, hypoechoic testis with a diffusely heterogeneous echopattern and absence of testicular vascularity (Image courtesy of Department of Radiology, K.E.M. Hospital, Mumbai, India).

Case 11

A 20-year-old otherwise healthy man presented with a painless swelling of the right testis for 2 months. There was no history of haematospermia, haematuria or other genitourinary symptoms. On physical examination there was a non-tender firm enlargement of the right testis. Serum alpha fetal protein (AFP) and beta human chorionic gonadotropin (HCG) levels were not elevated. A scrotal ultrasound was performed for further evaluation (Fig. 11a,b).

Questions

(1) What abnormality is demonstrated on the ultrasound ?
   - There is a 2.5 cm well-defined hypoechoic homogeneous mass with prominent increased vascularity in the right testis.
   - No evidence of calcification.
   - Normal overlying subcutaneous tissues.
   - The left testis was normal.

(2) <u>What is the diagnosis ?</u>

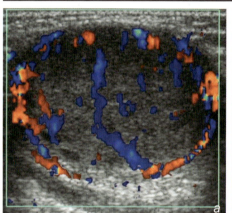 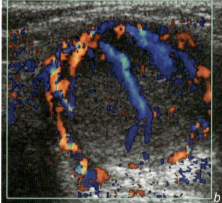

Fig.7a, b *Ultrasound shows a well-defined hypoechoic hypervascular lesion in the right testis which is highly suspicious of malignancy. Note there is no calcification and the overlying tissues are normal (Images courtesy of Department of Radiology, K.E.M. Hospital, Mumbai, India).*

Case 12

A 38-year-old woman complained of abdominal distension that has been getting worse over the last 12 months. Physical examination revealed a vague mass in the left lower quadrant. Her menstrual history and bowel habit have been unremarkable. In view of the clinical findings, a USG (Fig. 12a, b) was performed.

Questions

(1) What abnormalities can you identify on these transvaginal USG images of the left adnexal region ?
   - Loculated cystic mass in the left adnexal region.
   - Thick septum separating cysts.
   - Debris within cyst falling to the dependent region.
(2) <u>What is the most likely diagnosis ?</u>

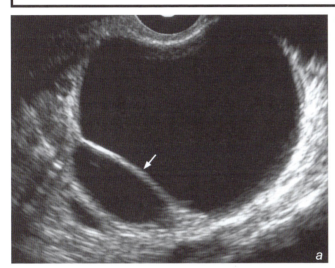

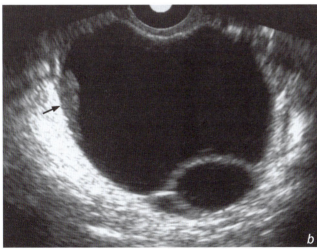

Fig.12a,b Transvaginal grey scale ultrasound images showing a large left adnexal cystic mass with multiple loculations. Note the thick septum (white arrow in Fig. 12a) and the internal debris at the dependent portion (black arrow in Fig. 12b) within this cystic lesion. No solid mural nodule was identified.

Discussion Case 1
Renal calculus

Left renal calculus with calyceal obstruction (Fig. 1a, b)

Discussion:

Renal calculus is a common cause of haematuria, particularly in the presence of loin pain.

Renal calculi are composed of crystals and/or aggregated with proteins. The crystal may contain calcium or magnesium oxalate/phosphate (which are radio-opaque and found in the majority of stones) or uric acid/ xanthine (which are not radio-opaque). As a result of this variable composition, the majority (~90%) of renal stones are radio-opaque, hence a KUB is useful as the initial investigation in a patient with suspected urinary calculus (Fig. 1c-e).

IVU is the key imaging modality for the diagnosis of
(1) Suspected urinary tract calculus
(2) Radio-lucent calculus which is not visualized on KUB
(3) Ureteric calculus which may not be demonstrated by ultrasound.

Information on IVU which is helpful in management of patients with renal stone include:
1. Size of renal stones - stones <5 mm in size are usually passed spontaneously on conservative treatment
2. Coexisting ureteric obstruction - extracorporeal shock wave lithotripsy (ESWL) may not be possible since stone fragments cannot pass down the ureter
3. Associated renal cortical scarring

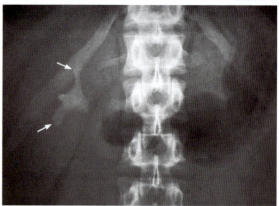

Fig.1c *Coned KUB of another patient shows a staghorn calculus (arrows) in the right renal region.*

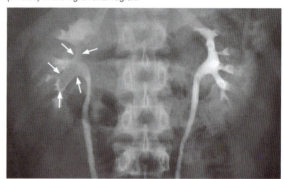

Fig.1d *IVU of the same patient in Fig.1c shows the staghorn stone as a filling defect within the contrast-filled renal pelvis(arrows).*

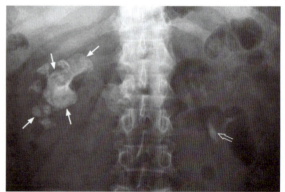

Fig.1e *Coned KUB of another patient shows a right staghorn stone (arrows). Another radio-opacity is also noted on the left side (open arrow), which is more inferior to the left renal shadow and may represent a proximal left ureteric stone (confirmed later).*

Discussion Case 1
Renal calculus

If a patient is allergic to intravenous contrast medium, ultrasound is a good alternative imaging modality for diagnosis. It evaluates the renal cortical thickness and the presence of scarring/cortical loss at the same time (Fig. 1f). A higher percentage of stones are detectable using non-contrast CT scan due to its higher spatial resolution (i.e. no overlapping of structures) and higher contrast resolution (i.e. differentiates the subtle higher density of non-radio-opaque stones from fluid and soft tissue) compared to radiographs. It can

- clearly evaluate the kidney (Fig. 1g-j), ureter and bladder
- confirm the location of the calculus
- evaluate the degree of obstruction
- evaluate other causes of renal calcifications.

However, it is relatively expensive and may not be readily available. It also involves the use of ionizing radiation and should be carefully used, particularly in children.

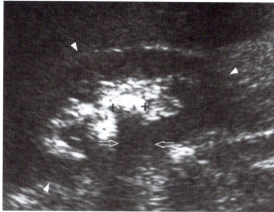

Fig.1f *Right renal USG of another patient (longitudinal axis) shows a calculus which is seen as an echogenic focus (between crosses) with posterior shadowing (open arrow) in the right kidney (arrowheads). Note ultrasound also evaluates the renal cortex and pelvi-calyceal system at the same time.*

Fig.1g *Axial NECT of the kidney shows a staghorn stone (arrow) in the right renal pelvis (same patient as in Fig.1e). Also note the dilated left renal pelvis (arrowhead).*

Fig.1h *Axial NECT of the abdomen, of the same patient as in Fig.1e, shows the radio-opacity on the left side is in the left ureter and is a proximal left ureteric stone (arrow). Note the wall thickening of the ureter (arrowheads) which represents ureteric wall oedema and is termed the 'ureteric rim sign'.*

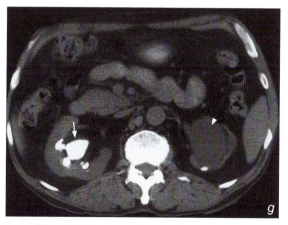

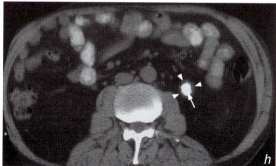

Discussion Case 1
Renal calculus

Fig.1i *Coronal reformatted NECT images show the right staghorn stone (arrow) - same patient as in Fig.1e. Note the renal scar as cortical indentation (arrowhead) and right ureter (open arrow).*

Fig.1j *Coronal reformatted NECT images show left ureteric stone (arrow) - same patient as in Fig.1e. Also note the dilated renal pelvis (arrowheads) and thin renal cortex (open arrows).*

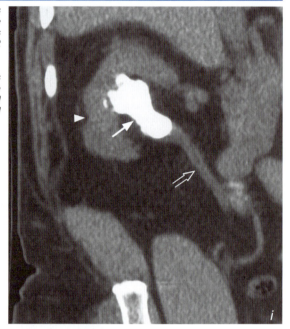

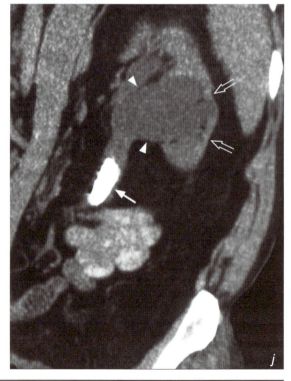

Discussion Case 1
Renal calculus

There are other conditions that will give rise to renal calcification apart from renal calculus

1) Renal tuberculosis - only one kidney affected in 75% of cases. The affected kidney becomes calcified, shrunken and non-functioning, aptly termed autonephrectomy (Fig. 1k). In patients with renal TB, 5-10% will also have pulmonary TB. A chest X-ray is a valuable further investigation.

2) Nephrocalcinosis - deposition of calcium salts in the renal parenchyma. This can be divided into two types : (i) medullary in 95% of cases (Fig. 1l, m) and cortical in 5% of cases.
   - Conditions that give rise to medullary nephrocalcinosis include hyperparathyroidism, medullary sponge kidney, renal tubular acidosis and hypercalcaemia.
   - Conditions that give rise to cortical nephrocalcinosis include acute cortical necrosis and chronic glomerulonephritis

3) Calcified renal tumour - Wilms' tumour (10%), renal cell carcinoma (15-20%)

4) Post-traumatic - healed renal injury may calcify.

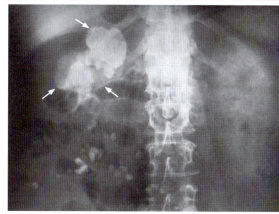

Fig.1k. *Coned KUB shows extensive calcification in the right kidney (arrows). This represents autonephrectomy in TB kidney (non-functioning kidney).*

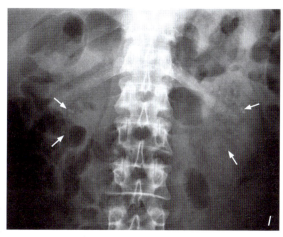

Fig.1l *Coned KUB shows multiple tiny calcifications over both renal areas (arrows). Differential diagnosis includes multiple tiny renal calculi or medullary nephrocalcinosis.*

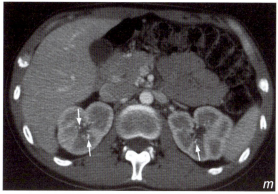

Fig.1m *Corresponding contrast enhanced axial CT though the kidneys of the same patient as in Fig.1l shows multiple tiny calcifications in the renal medulla (arrows). This is consistent with nephrocalcinosis.*

Discussion Case 1
Renal calculus

Note:

(1) Renal calculus is a common cause of haematuria.

(2) Majority of renal calculi are radio-opaque and are detectable by plain radiographs.

(3) IVU is the key imaging modality for diagnosis and treatment planning.

(4) Other established imaging modalities of choice include ultrasound and non-contrast CT scan.

(5) Other differential diagnoses of renal calcifications should be kept in mind.

Discussion Case 2
Ureteric stone

Left ureteric stone with obstruction (Fig. 2a, b)

Discussion:

Ureteric stones are renal stones which have passed down the pelvicalyceal system and become lodged within the ureter. The majority of them are therefore radio-opaque. IVU (Fig. 2c, d) is usually the second investigation after a KUB. The role of an IVU is to confirm the clinical diagnosis, determine the level and severity of obstruction and detect any complications (such as rupture of pelvicalyceal system), as all these are important for treatment planning.

Fig.2c KUB shows a radio-opacity in the left hemipelvis (arrow) along the course of the left ureter.

Fig.2d IVU of the patient in Fig.2c confirms the location of the ureteric stone (arrow) and shows hydroureter and hydronephrosis (arrowheads) proximal to it.

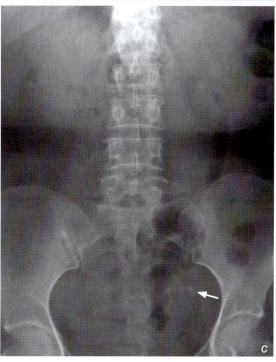

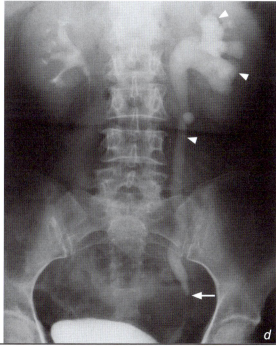

Discussion Case 2
Ureteric stone

If the patient is allergic to contrast, USG (Fig. 2e) or NECT scan (Fig. 2f, g) are alternative modalities for investigation. Although ultrasound can readily evaluate renal calculi, ureteric calculi may be missed if obscured by overlying gas in the bowel. However, a ureteric stone may be suspected if there is hydroureter and hydronephrosis seen on USG.

A non-contrast CT scan can clearly evaluate the kidneys, ureters and bladder, as well as demonstrate any associated pelvicalyceal distension. It gives better spatial and contrast resolution. Its limitation is the relative cost and hazard of ionizing radiation.

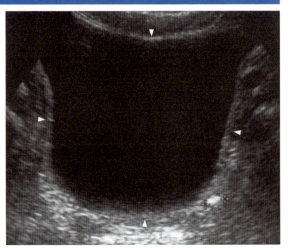

Fig.2e Transverse sonogram of the urinary bladder (arrowheads) of another patient shows an echogenic focus which corresponds to a stone (echogenic focus between the calipers) in the left vesico-ureteric junction.

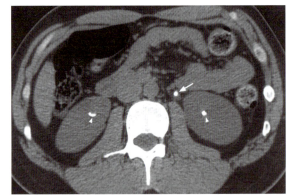

Fig.2f Axial NECT scan through the kidneys of another patient shows radio-opacities in both kidneys (arrowheads) and left ureter (arrow) representing bilateral renal stones and left ureteric stone respectively.

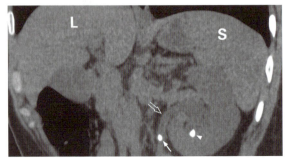

Fig.2g Coronal reformatted CT image of the patient in Fig. 2g shows the relationship of the left ureteric stone (arrow) and the dilated left ureter (open arrow). Also note the left renal stone in the lower pole of the left kidney (arrow head). (L = liver, S = spleen).

Ureteric stone

With the advanced development of MRI, the collecting system can thus be demonstrated. An MR urogram (Fig. 2h) can demonstrate obstruction along the urinary tract. Its potential is still being evaluated and is not used routinely. Apart from a ureteric stone, there are other causes of ureteric obstruction:

(1) Intraluminal
- Benign stricture: post-inflammatory, post-infective
- Malignant stricture : Transition cell carcinoma of ureter (Fig. 2i-l)
- Blood clot: any cause of haematuria
- Ureterocele: congenital condition (prevalence 1 : 5000 to 1 : 12000 children) where there is obstruction and prolapse of terminal portion of the ureter into the bladder (Fig. 2m)

(2) Extraluminal
- Pelvic tumour: by direct compression or invasion of the ureter
- Surrounding soft tissue fibrosis: can cause distortion or displacement of the ureter

In evaluating a KUB, other calcifications may mimic ureteric calculi, e.g. phlebolith. Phleboliths are venous calcifications which are typically roundish, well-defined with central lucency (compared with the usually angular, uniformly dense renal/ureteric calculus). If there is doubt on the identity of a density, it should be further assessed by IVU, ultrasound or non-contrast CT scan to determine the exact nature.

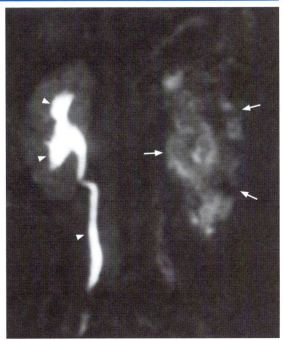

Fig.2h *MR urogram of another patient shows a normal right collecting system (arrowheads) and a hydronephrotic left kidney (arrows) as dilated renal pelvis and calyces with poor contrast enhancement and excretion (i.e. poor function due to back pressure).*

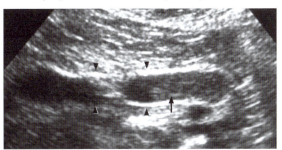

Fig.2i *Longitudinal sonogram of the ureter of another patient shows a soft tissue mass in the ureter (arrow) with obstruction and dilatation of the proximal ureter (arrowheads) representing transitional cell carcinoma of the ureter. This tumour may also be seen clearly on an IVU or CT scan.*

07 GENITOURINARY SYSTEM

Discussion Case 2
Ureteric stone

Fig.2j-l Axial CECT of another patient shows circumferential thickening of the right ureter (Fig. 2j, arrow) which was confirmed to be a transitional cell carcinoma. Also note the dilated right ureter (Fig. 2k, arrowhead) and dilated right renal pelvis (Fig. 2l, open arrow).

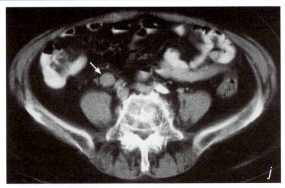

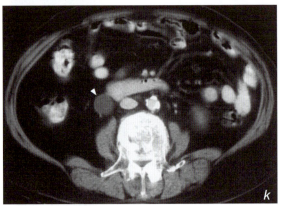

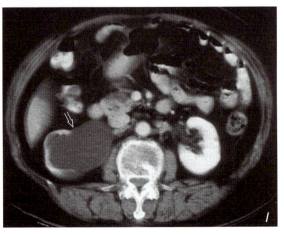

Ureteric stone

Note:

(1) Acute ureteric colic due to a ureteric stone is usually suspected based on clinical history and KUB findings.

(2) IVU, sonography and CT are the imaging modalities of choice for diagnosis.

(3) Phleboliths are common pelvic calcifications which may mimic ureteric/ bladder stone.

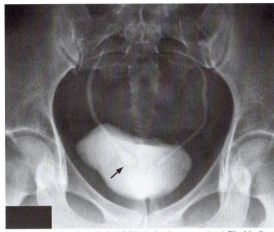

Fig.2m *Bladder view during IVU study shows contrast-filled bulbous dilated terminal right ureter with radiolucent halo (arrow) - the cobra head sign of a ureterocele. The radiolucent halo is due to the oedematous ureteric wall and bladder urothelium.*

Discussion Case 3
Non-calculus ureteric obstruction

Carcinoma of cervix with invasion/ compression of both ureters causing complete obstruction (Fig. 3a).

An urgent percutaneous nephrostomy was performed to relieve the obstruction. Antegrade pyelogram was then performed a few days later when the patient was stable and aseptic (Fig. 3b-c). The antegrade pyelogram shows bilateral hydronephrosis and hydroureter. Abrupt tapering is noted at both distal ureters with complete obstruction.

Discussion:
Urinary tract calculus and invasion/ extrinsic compression by a pelvic tumour are the two most common causes for hydronephrosis. A plain abdominal radiograph is useful to exclude a urinary tract calculus. An IVU or antegrade pyelogram helps to delineate the level and cause of obstruction in most cases.

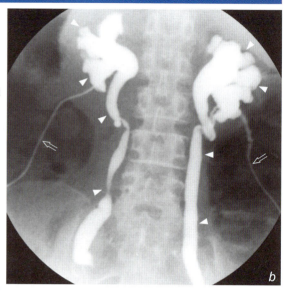

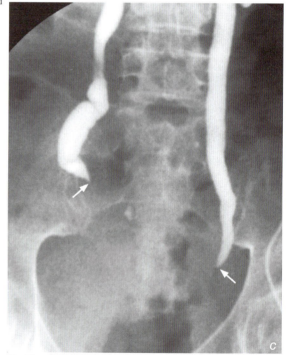

Fig.3b,c *Antegrade pyelogram, performed by injecting contrast through percutaneous nephrostomy catheters (open arrows), shows bilateral hydronephrosis and hydroureters (arrowheads). Persistent narrowing with tapered ends are present at the level of obstruction (arrows). Note there is no contrast filling into the bladder due to the bilateral obstruction.*

Discussion Case 3
Non-calculus ureteric obstruction

In cases of suspected pyelonephritis, an urgent ultrasound of kidney is useful for assessing or ruling out urinary tract obstruction (Fig. 3d, e). Early intervention may be needed to relieve the obstruction and help control the sepsis.

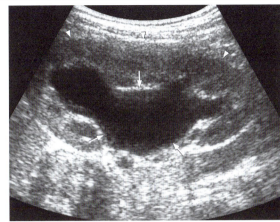

Fig.3d *Longitudinal sonogram of kidney shows hydronephrosis (arrows). There is preservation of renal cortical thickness (arrowheads) which indicates acute hydronephrosis.*

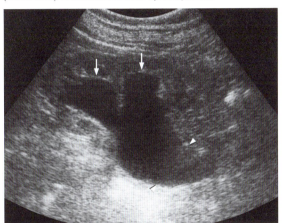

Fig.3e *Longitudinal sonogram of kidney shows hydronephrosis (arrows) and hydroureter (arrowheads) which indicates obstruction more distally. Same patient as in Fig. 3d.*

Discussion Case 3
Non-calculus ureteric obstruction

For a suspected pelvic tumour causing urinary tract obstruction, cross-sectional imaging such as ultrasound (Fig. 3f) or CT (Fig. 3g) may provide more information about the nature and extent of tumour.

Cervical cancer is the sixth most common cause of death from cancer in middle aged women. Most of them are squamous cell carcinoma and about 5% are adenocarcinoma. It is usually diagnosed by direct gynaecological examination with Pap smear or biopsy. CT is useful in staging the disease.

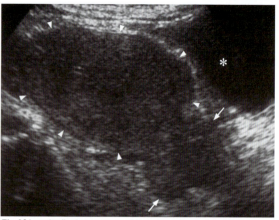

Fig.3f *Longitudinal sonogram of the uterus (arrowheads) shows an irregular mass in the cervix (arrows) which corresponds to carcinoma of the cervix. The asterisk identifies the urine-filled bladder.*

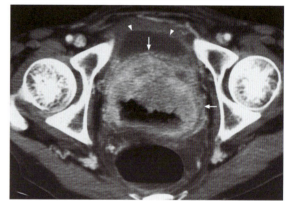

Fig.3g *Contrast axial CT scan shows a large pelvis soft tissue mass (arrows) posterior to the urinary bladder (arrowheads) which causes bilateral ureteric obstruction. The urinary bladder wall is of normal thickness.*

330

Non-calculus ureteric obstruction

MRI is another useful imaging modality (Fig. 3h, i) to assess the cervical carcinoma, although it may not be routinely used in many centres. Apart from cervical tumour, other pelvic tumours may also cause ureteric obstruction :

(1) Bladder tumour (Fig. 3j)
(2) Other gynaecological tumours, e.g. carcinoma of uterine corpus, carcinoma of ovary
(3) Extensive pelvic deposits, e.g. carcinoma of colon, peritoneal metastases
(4) Lymphoma with enlarged pelvic lymph nodes

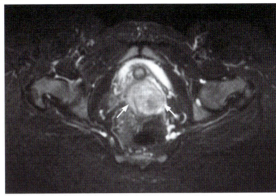

Fig.3h *Axial T2W fat-saturated MR image of the pelvis shows a soft tissue mass in the cervix which represents a cervical carcinoma (arrows).*

Fig.3i *Sagittal MR image of the pelvis of the patient in Fig. 3h shows the cervical carcinoma (arrow).*

Fig.3j *Contrast enhanced axial CT of pelvis shows gross thickening of the urinary bladder (arrows), later confirmed to be bladder carcinoma. The cervix is normal (arrowhead). Note the difference between this case and thickening of cervix in cervical carcinoma.*

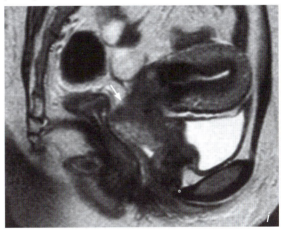

Note:

(1) Hydronephrosis is suspected in a patient with loin pain and deteriorating renal function.

(2) Obstructing urinary tract calculus and extrinsic compression by pelvic tumour are the most common causes of urinary tract obstruction.

(3) Contrast study (IVU/ antegrade pyelogram), sonography, CT and MR are the imaging modalities of choice to delineate the level, severity and cause of obstruction.

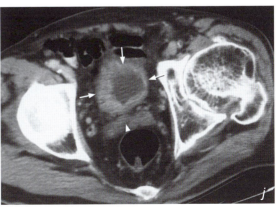

Discussion Case 4
Renal cell carcinoma

Renal neoplasm such as ***renal cell carcinoma*** (Fig. 4a-c).

Discussion:

Renal cell carcinoma (RCC) is the commonest primary malignant renal tumour in adult. Most of them are clear cell type. Other less common types are papillary, chromophobe and sacromatoid, which account for the remaining 20%.

On plain radiographs, the renal shadow may be enlarged, but it could be normal if the tumour is small. The tumour may be hypo/isoechoic on ultrasound scan (Fig.4a, d).

Contrast enhanced CT (Fig. 4e-g) features of renal cell carcinoma (RCC) include :
- Heterogeneous renal mass - hypodense components suggest areas of necrosis or cyst formation
- Inhomogeneous contrast enhancement - indicate hypervascular nature of tumour
- Soft tissue within right renal vein and IVC - due to venous tumour invasion which is more common in RCC than other malignant renal tumours (Fig. 4b, c)
- Intralesional calcification (15-20%)
- Streaky perinephric fat suggestive of tumour extension to perinephric space
- Thickening of Gerota's fascia due to tumour invasion or sympathetic inflammation
- Enlarged lymph nodes in renal hilum

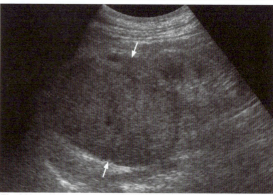

Fig.4d *Longitudinal sonogram of the kidney shows an isoechoic mass (arrows) in the upper pole of the kidney which represents an RCC.*

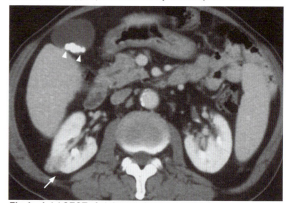

Fig.4e *Axial CECT of abdomen shows a small heterogeneous mass (arrow) in the mid-pole of the right kidney which represents a small RCC. Incidental findings of multiple small radio-opaque gallstones are noted (arrowheads).*

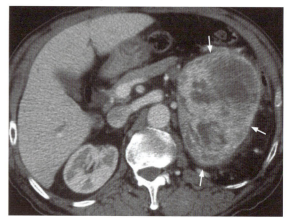

Fig.4f *Axial CECT of abdomen shows a heterogeneous enhancing mass (arrows) in the left kidney which represents an RCC.*

Discussion Case 4
Renal cell carcinoma

Approximately 1-3% of RCC are bilateral (Fig. 4h), especially in Von Hippel Lindau syndrome (uncommon autosomal dominant disease with multiple tumours involving CNS, kidney, adrenal, pancreas and liver). Transitional cell carcinoma (TCC) is a less common primary malignant tumour occurring in the kidney. Features which help to differentiate TCC from RCC include:

- More central location (because of urothelial in origin)
- Less likely to have calcification (1-5%)
- Vascular invasion is rare
- No cystic component

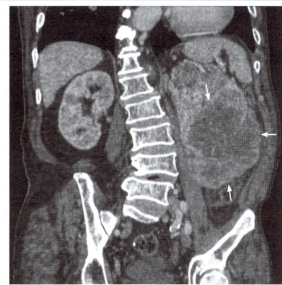

Fig.4g *Coronal reformatted CT image of the patient in Fig. 4f better demonstrates the vertical extent of the RCC (arrows).*

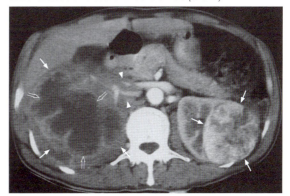

Fig.4h *Axial CECT of abdomen shows bilateral RCC (arrows). The tumour on the right side shows local invasion to the surrounding soft tissue and encasement of vascular pedicle (arrowheads). It is also causing hydronephrosis (open arrows). The tumour on the left side is smaller with no definite surrounding soft tissue invasion or hydronephrosis. Bilateral renal cell carcinoma occurs in about 1-3% of cases, especially associated with Von Hippel-Lindau syndrome.*

Discussion Case 4
Renal cell carcinoma

For staging the disease, CT is superior to ultrasound in assessing the local tumour extent, nodal metastases and vascular invasion. Further staging by CXR and bone scintigraphy is necessary before planning surgical treatment.

Apart from RCC and TCC, there are other common conditions that may mimic carcinoma, they include:
(1) Renal cyst (Fig. 4i-n) - appear as well-defined, thin walled, fluid density lesions.

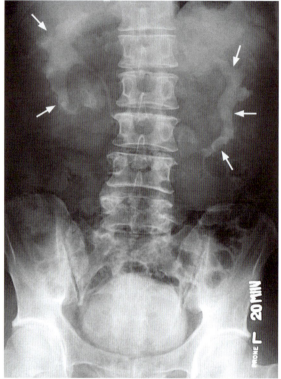

Fig.4i *Pyelogram of IVU study in a patient with multiple renal cysts shows elongated, distorted and attenuated collecting system (arrows). This is due to compression of the collecting system by multiple space occupying renal cysts.*

Renal cell carcinoma

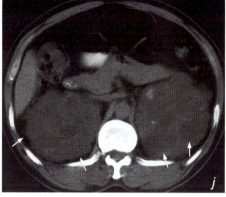
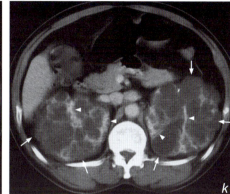
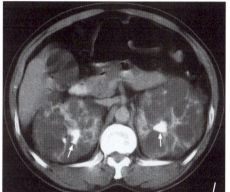
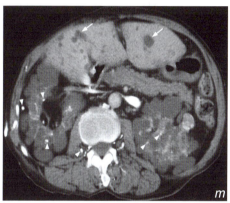
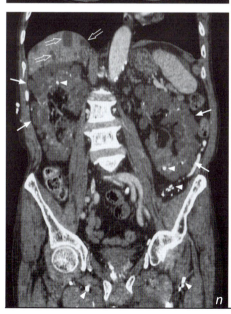

Fig.4j - l *Axial CT of the abdomen shows multiple well-defined cysts in both kidneys in pre-contrast phase (Fig. 4j). Both kidneys are enlarged with multiple slightly hypodense lesions (arrows). They represent the renal cysts in a patient with adult type polycystic kidney disease. In the porto-venous phase (Fig. 4k), the hypodense cysts (arrows) show no enhancement. Contrast enhancing functioning renal parenchyma is present in between cysts (arrowheads). In the delay phase (Fig. 4l) excreted contrast shows the collecting system (arrows) distorted by the cysts.*

Fig.4m *Axial CECT of the abdomen shows multiple cysts in both kidneys. In this patient, the renal function is impaired and there is hyperparathyroidism. As a result, multiple calcifications (arrowheads) are noted in the soft tissue and kidneys. Hyperparathyroidism is one of the causes of nephrocalcinosis. Hepatic cysts (arrows) are also noted in 25-50% of cases.*

Fig.4n *Reformatted CT image of the patient in Fig. 4m shows polycystic kidneys in coronal plane. Note multiple renal cysts (arrows), soft tissue calcifications (arrowheads) and hepatic cysts (open arrows).*

Discussion Case 4

Renal cell carcinoma

(2) Angiomyolipoma (AMC, Fig. 4o-q) - which may appear as a fat-containing mass in the kidney

(3) Xanthogranulomatous pyelonephritis (Fig. 4r) - seen as a heterogeneous mass replacing the renal parenchyma. There is often an associated calculus and evidence of extension of inflammatory change in the peri/para-renal spaces. This may easily be mistaken for RCC.

(4) Renal abscess (Fig. 4s) - which is usually a complication of renal inflammation. It is often low in attenuation and may have a rim contrast enhancement and show evidence of peri/para-renal inflammation. The diagnosis is based on a combination of clinical parameters and imaging appearance. Small abscesses may be difficult to differentiate from a primary tumour.

(5) Lymphoma (Fig. 4t) - Non-Hodgkin/Hodgkin's lymphoma of the kidney is frequently due to haematogenous dissemination or contiguous spread of adjacent disease. Primary lymphoma of the kidney is rare. Its CT appearance may be non-specific and appears as a low attenuation ill-defined lesion in the renal parenchyma. They may appear as multiple masses or diffusely infiltrative with renal enlargement. The renal function may be compromised.

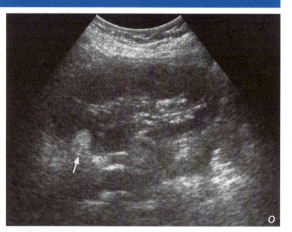

o

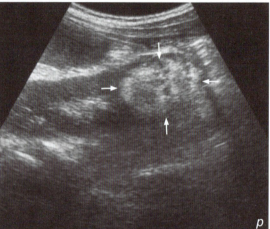

p

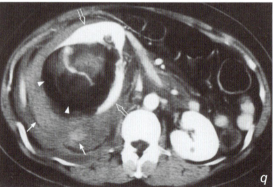

q

Fig.4o - p Longitudinal sonograms show well-defined hyperechoic lesions (arrows) of different sizes in different kidneys. They are typical for renal angiomyolipoma (AML).

Fig.4q Axial CECT of the abdomen shows a fat-containing lesion (AML) which was complicated by rupture. The fatty component is indicated by the hypodense dark area (arrowheads). The perinephric collection represent haematoma (arrows). The contrast-containing (very hyperdense) renal pelvis is displaced and distorted (open arrows). Compare it to the normal left kidney.

Renal cell carcinoma

Fig.4r Contrast enhanced axial CT scan of abdomen shows a complex mass in the right kidney. Multiple thick walled cysts are suggestive of infection with abscess formation (arrow head). Note the associated hyperdense renal stones (arrows). This combination of features suggests xanthogranulomatous pyelonephritis which may mimic RCC on imaging.

Fig.4s Contrast enhanced axial CT scan of abdomen of a different patient shows multiple hypodense lesions in both kidneys (arrows) and spleen (arrowheads). They represent renal and splenic abscesses due to TB infection in this case. However, one must note that for such small lesions, the diagnosis may depend on a combination of clinical and imaging findings.

Fig.4t Contrast enhanced axial CT scan of the abdomen of a different patient shows a solitary hypodense lesion (arrow) in the right kidney. It was found to be renal lymphoma on biopsy. Note the non-specific appearance of the lesion.

Note:
(1) The most common primary renal tumour is renal cell carcinoma.
(2) Contrast enhanced CT is the imaging modality of choice.
(3) Heterogeneous hypervascular renal mass +/- venous tumour extension are characteristic CT features of renal cell carcinoma.
(4) Other causes of renal mass should be investigated by ultrasound or CT.

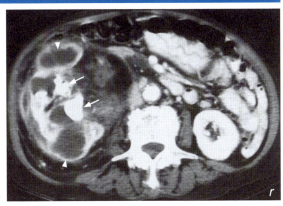

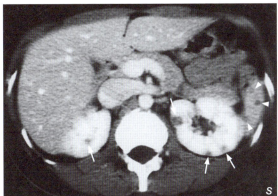

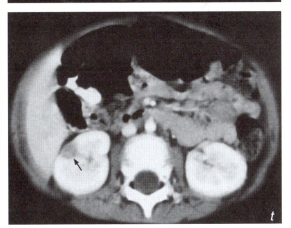

07 GENITOURINARY SYSTEM

Discussion Case 5
Renal laceration

Renal laceration (Fig. 5a, b)

Discussion:
Renal trauma is a common injury presenting to the emergency department. The indications for imaging include :
(1) Penetrating injury with haematuria
(2) Blunt trauma with haematuria and hypotension
(3) Microscopic haematuria with positive peritoneal lavage
(4) Blunt trauma with known association of renal injury (contusion/haematoma of flank, fractured lower rib, fractured transverse process and fractured thoracolumbar spine)

Renal injuries are classified into 4 categories according to the severity:
- Category 1 - contusion/laceration not involving the renal collecting system
- Category 2 - laceration which communicates with renal collecting system with resultant extravasation
- Category 3 - major renal laceration/ damage to vascular pedicle
- Category 4 - ureteropelvic junction avulsion/renal pelvis laceration

In suspected renal injury, an immediate contrast enhanced CT scan of the abdomen in different phases is useful to assess the degree of renal injury, integrity of the renal vascular pedicles and integrity of the collecting system.

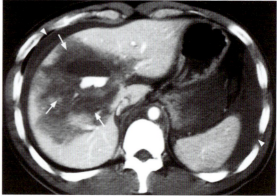

Fig.5c *Contrast enhanced axial CT scan of abdomen shows large hypodense area in the liver indicating liver contusion/ laceration (arrows). Note the trace fluid around the liver and spleen (arrowheads).*

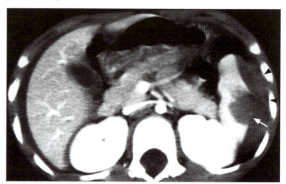

Fig.5d *Contrast enhanced axial CT scan of abdomen shows a splenic laceration (arrow) with surrounding haemorrhage (arrowheads).*

Fig.5e *Sagittal reformatted non-contrast enhanced CT shows an intraperitoneal rupture of bladder. The bladder (asterisk) is filled with contrast using a Foley catheter (arrowheads). Note the extravasation of contrast (arrows) into the peritoneal cavity outlining air-containing bowel (cross) (Image courtesy of Dr Deyond Siu, Department of Diagnostic Radiology and Organ Imaging, The Chinese University of Hong Kong).*

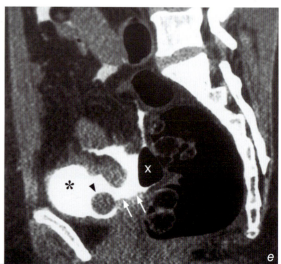

338

Discussion Case 5
Renal laceration

Possible CT findings of renal injury include :
- Wedge-shaped non-perfused renal parenchyma - represents renal infarction due to occlusion of segmental arteries
- Contrast extravasation in early phase - suggests active bleeding
- Contrast extravasation in delayed phase - indicates laceration involving the pelvi-calyceal system

Apart from delineating the extent of renal injury, contrast enhanced CT also assesses the contralateral kidney, detects injury of other intra-abdominal organs, e.g. liver and spleen (Fig. 5c, d), and evaluates the pelvis (Fig. 5e) all at the same time.

Note that in a patient with pyelonephritis (Fig. 5f, g), areas of low attenuation may also be seen in the kidney on CECT. These mimic renal laceration and the diagnosis is based on a combination of clinical parameters, history and imaging appearance.

> **Note:**
> (1) Renal injury has to be excluded in a patient with abdominal trauma presenting with haematuria and localized pain/tenderness in the loin area.
> (2) Contrast enhanced CT is the imaging modality of choice.

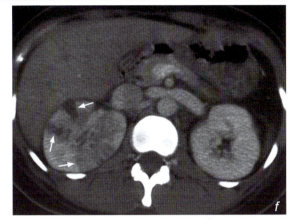

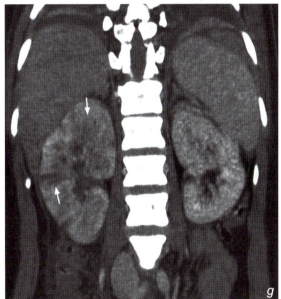

Fig.5f,g *Axial and coronal reformatted images of a CECT show multiple low attenuation areas within the right kidney (arrows) in a patient with pyelonephritis (mimicking a renal laceration). This patient has a clinical picture of pyelonephritis with no history of abdominal trauma.*

Carcinoma of the bladder

Carcinoma of the bladder (Fig. 6a-c)

Discussion:
Carcinoma of the bladder is the most common tumour in the urinary tract. Transitional cell carcinoma is the commonest histological type of malignant bladder tumour, others are squamous cell carcinoma and adenocarcinoma. The diagnosis is usually made on cystoscopy and biopsy.

CT helps in the assessment of the primary tumour, its local and regional extent, nodal involvement and presence of distant metastasis.

There are 3 main pathological appearances of bladder carcinoma:
(1) Exophytic papillary lesion
- frond-like outgrowth from the bladder wall (Fig. 6d - f)

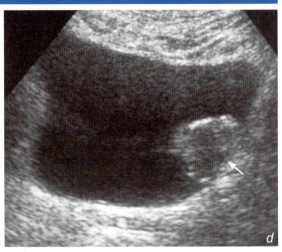

Fig.6d Transverse sonogram through the bladder shows a soft tissue nodule (arrow) in the left postero-lateral wall of the bladder indicating a bladder tumour.

Fig.6e Axial CECT of the pelvis shows a soft tissue density mucosal outgrowth (arrows) from the left lateral and posterior wall of the bladder, indicating bladder tumours.

Fig.6f Delayed phase of contrast enhanced axial CT of the pelvis shows filling defects (arrow) in the right lateral aspect of the contrast filled bladder which represent a bladder tumour.

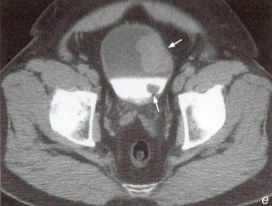

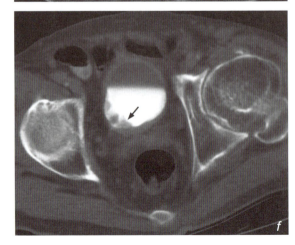

Carcinoma of the bladder

(2) Infiltrative type with diffuse
    bladder wall thickening (Fig. 6g)
(3) Carcinoma-in-situ
The first two can be demonstrated with
imaging.

Intravenous urography (Fig. 6h) and CT
(Fig. 6i, j) are useful for detection of
synchronous tumours arising from the
urothelium of the upper urinary tract
(e.g. kidney/ureter). The bladder tumour
itself can also be visualized on contrast
filled bladder views during IVU
examination (Fig. 6h) and as a soft tissue
mass on an ultrasound scan (Fig. 6d).

There may be other CT findings of
carcinoma of the bladder :
- Calcification
- Invasion of adjacent structures (e.g.
  seminal vesicle, small bowel loops,
  etc.)

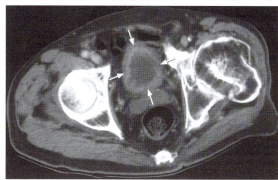

Fig.6g *Axial CECT of the pelvis shows diffuse circumferential thickening of the bladder wall (arrows) which is in keeping with infiltrative type of TCC bladder.*

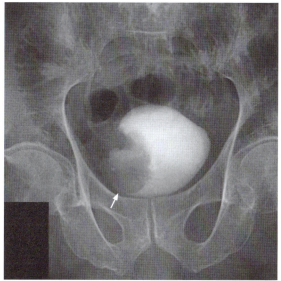

Fig.6h *Bladder view of an IVU study shows a large filling defect (arrow) in the right lateral aspect of a contrast filled bladder, indicating a bladder tumour.*

07 GENITOURINARY SYSTEM

341

Carcinoma of the bladder

Note:

(1) Carcinoma of the urinary bladder has to be excluded by cystoscopy in elderly patients with painless haematuria, especially if there is no evidence of urinary tract calculus.

(2) Contrast enhanced CT of the abdomen and pelvis is the imaging of choice for assessment of local tumour involvement and detection of metastases.

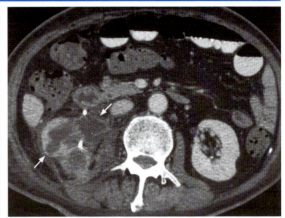

Fig.6i *Contrast enhanced axial CT of the abdomen (in a patient with bladder TCC) shows a large right renal TCC with invasion of surrounding soft tissue.*

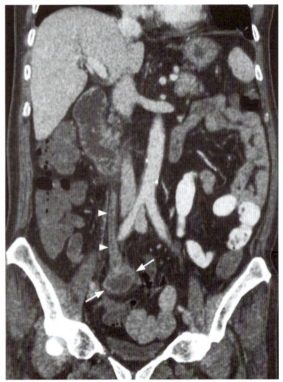

Fig.6j *Coronal reformatted image of a CECT (in a patient with bladder TCC), same patient as in Fig. 6i also shows a right ureteric TCC (arrow) with proximal dilatation of the ureter (arrowheads).*

Bladder calculus

Bladder stone (Fig. 7a)

Discussion:
The majority of bladder calculi are of high calcium content and hence are radio-opaque.
There are several types of bladder calculi

(1) Stasis calculi (70%) - in bladder outflow tract obstruction (in patient with prostatic hypertrophy causing bladder outflow tract obstruction (Fig. 7b).

(2) Migrant calculi - renal calculi passing into the bladder

(3) Foreign body nidus calculi - stent, catheter, suture or intestinal mucosa in bladder augmentation, ileal conduit

(4) Idiopathic

In patients with suspected bladder calculus, a KUB is usually the first modality of investigation, as most of the bladder stones are radio-opaque (Fig. 7c). An IVU is useful in assessing the bladder and the upper tract. The bladder calculus appears as a filling defect in the contrast filled bladder (Fig. 7d)

Fig.7b *Longitudinal sonogram of the pelvis shows enlarged prostate (arrows) which is a common cause of outflow tract obstruction and haematuria in elderly (B = bladder).*

Fig.7c *Plain radiograph shows a bladder stone (arrow).*

Fig.7d *Oblique bladder view, during IVU of the patient in Fig. 7c shows filling defect (arrow) in contrast filled bladder which represents a bladder stone.*

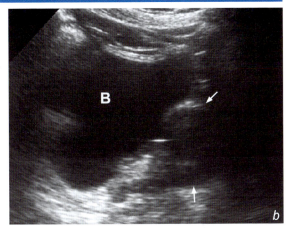

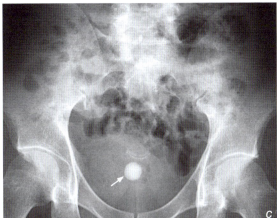

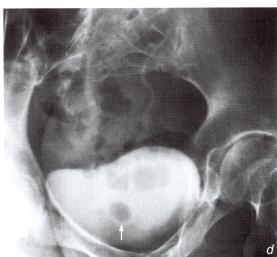

07 GENITOURINARY SYSTEM

Bladder calculus

Ultrasound is another good modality to assess and confirm the presence of a bladder stone especially radio-lucent stones (Fig. 7e). These can also be demonstrated on unenhanced CT scan (Fig. 7f).

Other causes of pelvic calcification that can mimic bladder stones
  (1) phleboliths (Fig. 7g) - very commonly seen calcification in the pelvis. They are typically roundish with radiolucent centre. Further investigation such as IVU, ultrasound or non-contrast CT scan may be needed to differentiate less typical appearing lesions.

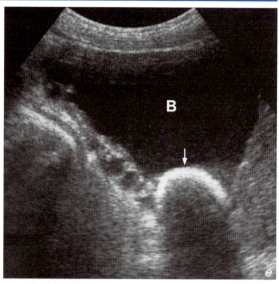

Fig.7e Transverse sonogram of the pelvis shows bladder stone (arrows) causing posterior shadowing (B = bladder).

Fig.7f Non-contrast CT of the pelvis shows a large calculus (arrow) in the bladder. The bladder wall is hypertrophied (arrowheads) due to outflow obstruction (which caused urinary stasis).

Fig.7g Pelvic radiograph shows well-defined roundish radio-opacities with lucent centre outside the bladder shadow representing phleboliths (arrows), which are common calcifications in the pelvis. They are concretions in the veins and are easily mistaken for urinary tract calculi.

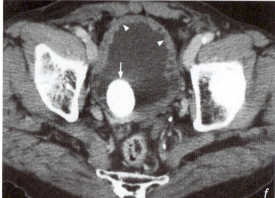

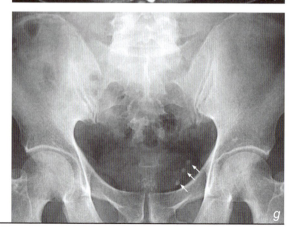

Discussion Case 7
Bladder calculus

(2) Prostatic calcifications in male patient (Fig. 7h) - commonly seen in prostate with increasing age. They are usually clusters of tiny and irregular calcifications in the midline of lower pelvis.

(3) Gynaecological calcifications in female patient - several conditions will give rise to calcifications in the pelvis, such as calcified fibroid (Fig. 8b, c) and dermoid cyst (Fig.7i). Typically, calcifications in the fibroid are amorphous and popcorn like. For those in dermoid, they may be tooth-like and associated with a fatty component.

(4) Bladder wall calcification -
   a) Inflammation -
      TB Schistosomiasis
      Post-RT/chemocystitis
   b) Neoplasm (uncommon) -
      Transitional cell carcinoma
      Squamous cell carcinoma

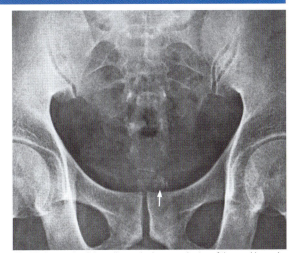

Fig.7h *A coned pelvic radiograph shows a cluster of tiny and irregular calcifications in the lower pelvis which are prostatic calcifications.*

Note:

(1) The presence of lower urinary tract symptoms in patients with chronic bladder outflow tract obstruction raises the possibility of urinary bladder calculus.

(2) Large rounded calcified opacity in pelvis is the typical finding on plain radiograph.

(3) IVU, ultrasound or non-contrast CT will confirm the diagnosis and assess the upper tract.

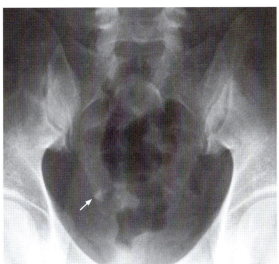

Fig.7i *Plain abdominal radiograph of pelvis shows tooth-like calcification (arrow) in the pelvis which was found to be a dermoid.*

Uterine fibroid

Calcified uterine fibroid (Fig. 8a)

Discussion:

Uterine leiomyoma, also known as uterine fibroid, is benign and the most common gynaecological neoplasm. When they are symptomatic, their usual presentations include: suprapubic mass, pain or menorrhagia.

A leiomyoma may undergo calcification as it degenerates, and become visible on plain radiograph (~5%) (Fig. 8b, c). The diagnosis is usually made on ultrasound (Fig. 8d, e). On USG, it appears as a well-defined hypoechoic mass in the myometrium of the uterus.

CT scan is not a routine investigation for assessing the fibroid, but it is often seen as incidental CT finding as enlarged uterus with or without calcifications (Fig. 8f).

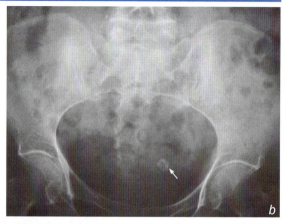

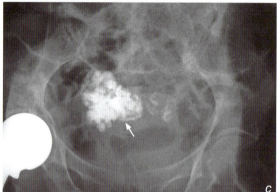

Fig.8b,c *Plain X-rays of the abdomen show amorphous calcifications (arrows) in the pelvis of different patients representing calcified uterine fibroids.*

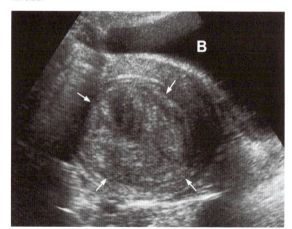

Fig.8d *Transverse sonogram of the pelvis shows a heterogeneous hypoechoic mass in the uterus (arrows) which represents a uterine fibroid (B = bladder).*

Discussion Case 8
Uterine fibroid

Malignant change is very rare (~0.2%) in a uterine fibroid.

Other differentials of pelvic calcification in a female include dermoid (Fig. 8g-i), bladder stones (Fig. 7a, c) and phleboliths (Fig. 7g).

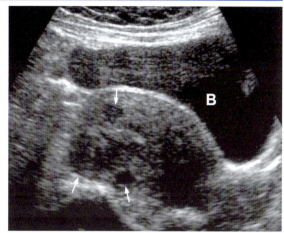

Fig.8e *Longitudinal sonogram of the pelvis shows several small hypoechoic masses in the uterus (arrows) representing small uterine fibroids (B = bladder).*

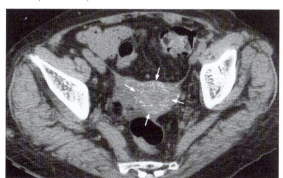

Fig.8f *Non-contrast axial CT through the pelvis shows multiple tiny calcifications in the uterus representing a calcified uterine fibroid (arrows).*

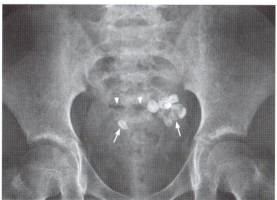

Fig.8g *Plain X-ray of the pelvis shows multiple faceted 'tooth-like' calcific densities (arrows) and fat densities (arrowheads). Features are typical for a dermoid (ovarian teratoma).*

Discussion Case 8
Uterine fibroid

Note:

(1) Uterine fibroid should be suspected if there are gynaecological symptoms and a palpable pelvic mass.

(2) Ultrasound of pelvis is the imaging modality of choice.

(3) Plain radiograph may show characteristic amorphous calcification in a degenerated fibroid.

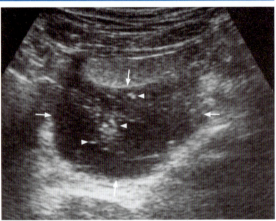

Fig.8h *Transverse sonogram of the patient in Fig. 8g shows a complex mass with echogenic content suggestive of a dermoid cyst.*

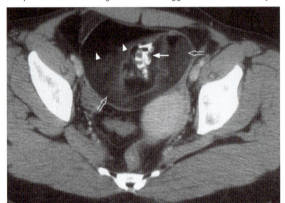

Fig.8i *Contrast enhanced axial CT through the pelvis shows a dermoid. Note the calcifications (arrow), fat (arrowhead) and solid component (open arrows).*

Discussion Case 9
Adrenal mass

Conn's syndrome (Fig. 9a-c) caused by left adrenal adenoma. The diagnosis is based on clinical, biochemical findings and imaging is used mainly to identify the underlying cause.

Discussion:

Conn's syndrome, also known as primary hyperaldosteronism, is a disease of autonomous excess secretion of mineralocorticoid with hypertension and hypokalaemia. It is caused by:

(1) Adrenal adenoma (80%) - solitary in ~70% and multiple in ~10% (Fig. 9d-f)

Fig.9d, e Non-contrast axial CT of abdomen shows well-defined nodules (arrows) in both right (Fig. 9d) and left (Fig. 9e) adrenal glands in keeping with bilateral adrenal adenomas.

Fig.9f Contrast enhanced axial CT of abdomen in another patient shows large adenomas (arrows) in both adrenal glands.

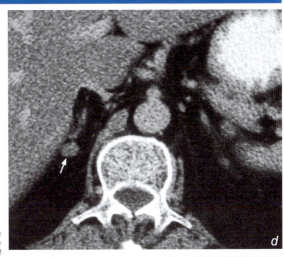

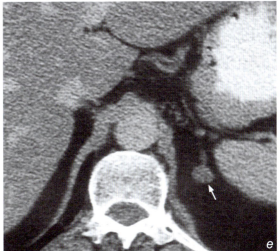

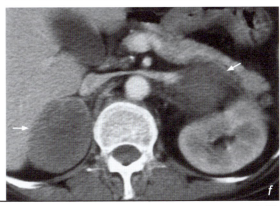

Discussion Case 9
Adrenal mass

(2) Bilateral adrenal hyperplasia in ~20% (Fig. 9g)

(3) Adrenocortical carcinoma in less than 1% (Fig. 9h)

It can be investigated by NECT scan (N.B. intravenous contrast may precipitate a hypertensive crisis. If contrast is still needed, the patient should be premedicated with a beta-blocker, e.g. propranolol). A nodular lesion with a slight negative CT number, indicating the presence of fat content, is diagnostic for an adenoma.

Radioactive iodocholesterol scintigraphy (nuclear medicine) can be used for assessing the function of the adrenal nodule (Fig. 9i, j).

Fig.9g *Contrast enhanced axial CT scan of the adrenal glands shows enlargement of both adrenal glands (arrows). No focal nodule or mass can be identified. Features are suggestive of adrenal hyperplasia.*

Fig.9h *Contrast enhanced axial CT scan of the abdomen shows a large irregular soft tissue mass in the left suprarenal region, which represents a carcinoma in the left adrenal gland (arrows) with invasion into the left kidney (arrowheads). Note the incidental gallstones.*

Fig.9i *Tc-99m Iodocholesterol scintigraphy shows unilateral increased radioactive tracer uptake in the right adrenal region (arrow). This is suggestive of a functional adenoma (L = liver).*

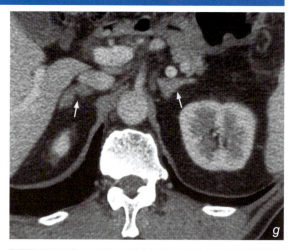

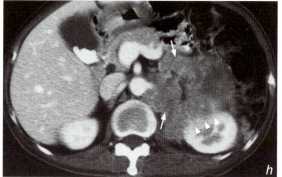

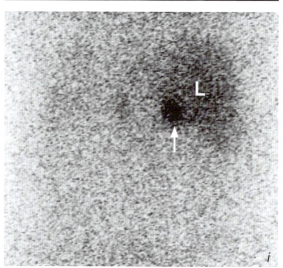

Discussion Case 9
Adrenal mass

If the CT number of the adrenal mass is not negative, the nature of that adrenal mass is indeterminate. Other differentials of adrenal mass should be considered, and these include:

(1) Adrenal cortex -
 (a) Adenoma can cause Conn's syndrome (mineralocorticoid) or Cushing's syndrome (glucocorticoid)
 (b) Hyperplasia
 (c) Carcinoma
(2) Adrenal medulla -
 (a) Phaeochromocytoma (Fig. 9k, l) - a rare catecholamine-secreting tumour of chromaffin tissue causing hypertension

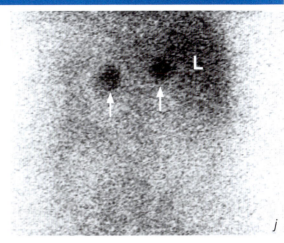

j

Fig.9j Tc-99m Iodocholesterol scintigraphy shows increased radioactive tracer uptake in both adrenal regions (arrows). Features are more suggestive of adrenal hyperplasia. The other possible differential is bilateral adrenal adenoma (L = liver).

Fig.9k Non-contrast axial CT scan of the adrenals shows solid mass in the left adrenal (arrow) which was confirmed to be a phaeochromocytoma.

Fig.9l Another case of large phaeochromocytoma (arrows) in the left adrenal seen as a heterogeneous mass in the suprarenal region. 10% of cases will have calcification. 10% are bilateral, 10% are extrarenal and 10% of cases are familial. It is also known as '10% tumour'.

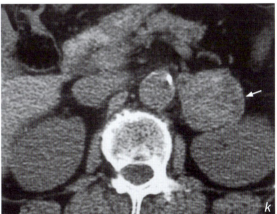

k

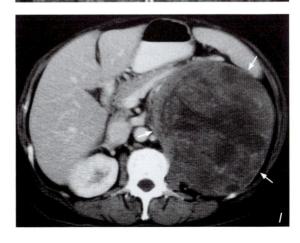

l

Adrenal mass

(b) Neuroblastoma (Fig. 9m) - most common solid abdominal tumour in infant. It is of neural crest cell origin

(c) Myelolipoma (Fig. 9n)

(3) Adrenal metastases (Fig. 9o) - commonly from lung (40%), breast (20%), thyroid, colon

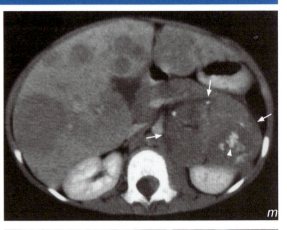

Fig.9m *Contrast enhanced axial CT of abdomen of a child shows a large suprarenal tumour (arrows) with calcifications (arrow head) representing a neuroblastoma.*

Fig.9n *Axial CECT of the abdomen demonstrates a mass lesion (asterisk) of fat density, splaying the two limbs (arrows) of the left adrenal gland and indenting the medial aspect of the spleen (arrowheads). The fat density makes this an adrenal myelolipoma.*

Fig.9o *Contrast enhanced coronal reformatted CT of abdomen shows bilateral adrenal masses (arrows) in a patient with lung tumour. This is highly suspicious of adrenal metastases which occurs in about 20% of cases.*

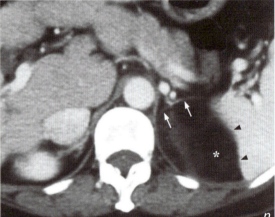

Note:

(1) Diagnosis of Conn's syndrome is based on characteristic biochemical findings.

(2) CT abdomen is the imaging modality of choice to identify the underlying cause.

(3) Low-density adrenal lesion with well-defined margins are typical features of adenoma on CT.

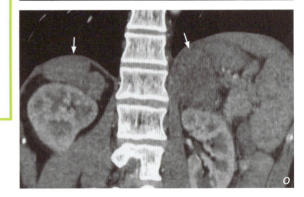

Testicular torsion

Acute left testicular torsion (Fig. 10a-d)

Discussion:

- Testicular torsion is a surgical emergency, and it typically affects young males especially those with abnormally lying testes such as horizontal or inverted (bell and clapper configuration) testes.

- Undescended testes have a 10-fold increased risk of developing torsion.

- Majority of testes can be salvaged if surgical intervention is carried out within 6 hours after the onset of symptoms.

- Only 10-20% of testes can be salvaged if surgical intervention is carried out beyond 12 hours after the onset of symptoms.

- On ultrasound in the acute phase the torsioned testis is enlarged with diffuse hypoechogenicity, and may appear abnormal in position. The epididymis may show similar changes of enlargement and decreased echogenicity. There may also be reactive hydrocele and scrotal oedematous thickening. The cardinal feature is absence of testicular and epididymal flow on Doppler examination.

- In the subacute phase the testis becomes heterogeneous in echotexture due to haemorrhagic infarction, and in the chronic phase the testis is atrophic and homogeneously hypoechoic.

- A torsioned testis that spontaneously untwists may appear normal on ultrasound but its viability may still be jeopardized.

- If ultrasound is not available or inconclusive, scintigraphy is also highly accurate in evaluating testicular torsion.

> **Note:**
> (1) The cardinal sonographic feature of testicular torsion is absence of testicular and epididymal flow on Doppler in an enlarged, oedematous testis.
> (2) Torsion-detorsion sequence may result in false negative sonographic findings.

Testicular tumour

The sonographic appearance and history are suggestive of a testicular neoplasm, probably primary germ cell tumour especially a *seminoma* (Fig. 11a, b).

Discussion:
- Testicular carcinomas are the most common malignancy affecting male patients in the 15-30 age group, and typically present as painless testicular enlargement.
- Risk factors include cryptorchidism (Fig. 11c, d), family history of testicular cancer, maternal diethylstilboestrol use and testicular atrophy.
- An undescended testis has a 30-fold increased risk for developing malignancy. The further away it is from the scrotum, the higher is the risk.
- Testicular malignancies can be classified into germ cell tumours (95%), non-germ cell/stromal tumours, and metastases.
- Germ cell tumours include seminoma (40%), mixed tumours (40%, teratocarcinoma being most common), and non-seminomatous germ cell tumours which include teratoma (10%), embryonal cell carcinoma (10%), choriocarcinoma, and yolk sac carcinoma.
- Serum alpha fetal protein (AFP) level is elevated in mixed tumours, embryonal cell carcinoma and yolk sac carcinoma.

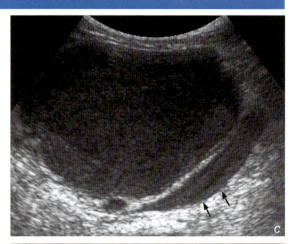

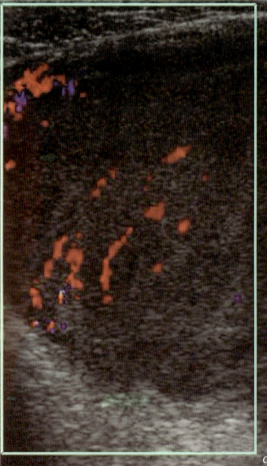

Fig.11c, d This 40-year-old patient presented with a single testis in the scrotum and a large abdominal mass. Fig. 11c Longitudinal grey scale sonogram showing a large, hypoechoic, heterogeneous abnormal mass compressing the iliac veins (arrows) (Image courtesy of Department of Radiology, K.E.M. Hospital, Mumbai, India).
Fig.11d Doppler examination of the mass (with a high resolution transducer) shows large vessels within the tumour which is hypoechoic and heterogeneous in echopattern (Image courtesy of Department of Radiology, K.E.M. Hospital, Mumbai, India).

Testicular tumour

- Beta human chorionic gonadotrophin (HCG) level is elevated in pure seminoma (10%), embryonal cell carcinoma and choriocarcinoma.
- Non-germ cell tumors include the Leydig cell tumour and the Sertoli cell tumour, which may be endocrinologically active and produce symptoms such as precocious virilization, feminization and gynaecomastia.
- The most common primary tumours that metastasize to the testis include malignancies from the prostate, kidney, and lymphoma/leukaemia.

On Ultrasound (1) Seminoma typically appears as a focal hypoechoic lesion but occasionally may show diffuse infiltration. It is usually well circumscribed with a sharp tumour-parenchymal interface, and may cause architectural distortion and bulging of the tunica albuginea.

(2) Mixed tumours and non-seminomatous germ cell tumours (especially embryonal cell carcinoma) usually appear more ill-defined and heterogeneous with cystic components and calcifications.

(3) Larger testicular tumours tend to be hypervascular on Doppler ultrasound while smaller tumours tend to be hypovascular. In general the cell type does not correlate with the flow pattern.

- The precise histological diagnosis can only be made on biopsy/surgical specimen.

- The aim of ultrasound is to demonstrate whether the pathology is intratesticular or extratesticular, single or multiple, unilateral or bilateral.

At times it may be difficult to differentiate a testicular neoplasm from testicular inflammation, in which case it is useful to search for other evidence of inflammation such as enlargement of the epididymis and scrotal wall thickening. It should, however, be noted that hydrocele may be present in both conditions.

Note:
(1) Testicular carcinomas typically present as painless testicular enlargement.
(2) Solitary intratesticular lesions are more likely to be neoplastic, while extratesticular lesions, especially when multiple and bilateral, tend to be benign.

Discussion Case 12
Ovarian tumour

Ovarian mass, confirmed to be a mucinous cystadenoma at surgery (Fig. 12a, b). A trans-vaginal USG reveals more information due to its higher resolution (USG probe closer to the adnexal region) compared to a trans-abdominal examination.

Discussion:
a: Mucinous cystadenoma
- Around 90% of ovarian neoplasms in premenopausal women are benign compared to only 50% being benign for those in post-menopausal women.
- Ovarian cystadenomas are benign tumours of epithelial origin (rather than germ cell or stromal cell) and may be mucinous or serous (latter more common).
- In mucinous cystadenomas, the epithelium produces a glycoprotein resembling mucin. Mucinous cystadenomas are usually unilateral (95%) and multi-locular (compared to the usually unilocular serous cystadenoma). These may grow to a large size (up to 30 cm) and may rupture (resulting in pseudomyxomatous peritonei, seeding of epithelial cells onto peritoneum).
- On USG the typical features are:
- Multiple cysts.
- Cysts separated by thick septae (compared to the thin septae in serous cystadenomas).
- Cysts may contain debris or diffuse low-level (mucin) echogenicity.
- N.B. The presence of an intra-cystic solid component is a feature of malignancy (cystadenocarcinoma).
- CT and MRI show features similar to the sonographic findings (Fig. 12c-e).

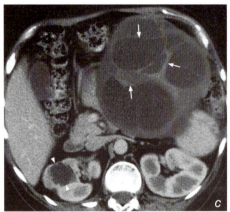
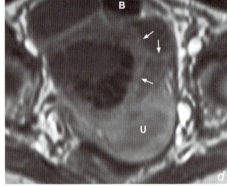
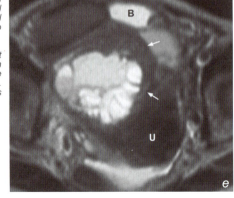

Fig.12c Axial NECT image shows a large multiloculated cystic lesion with numerous thick and thin internal septations (arrows). No calcification or solid mural nodules present. Note the attenuation is comparable to a cyst (arrowhead) in the right kidney.

Fig.12d, e Axial MRI T1W and T2W images of a different patient show a large multiloculated cystic lesion with numerous septations present within the cyst. Note the thick septations (arrows) within the complex cyst. This was found to be a mucinous cystadenoma. Uterus (U) and urinary bladder (B).

Ovarian tumour

b: Ovarian mucinous cystadenocarcinoma (Fig. 12f, g)

- This is a malignant ovarian epithelial neoplasm which produces a mucin-like substance. Other common malignant ovarian neoplasms include serous cystadenocarcinoma, endometrioid tumour and clear cell adenocarcinoma and metastasis (Krukenberg tumour (Fig. 12h)).
- Ovarian mucinous cystadenocarcinoma occur mostly in the fourth and fifth decades.
- Approximately 20% of these lesions are bilateral.
- The typical imaging features reflect the pathology and include:
  - Cystic lesion with solid component.
  - Cysts may contain debris or diffuse low-level (mucin) echogenicity.
  - Solid component containing cysts and/or demonstrating vascularity.
  - Abnormal blood flow within solid component (low resistance vessels, which suggests that the vessels are themselves abnormal).
  - Ascites with/without peritoneal metastasis (pseudomyxomatous peritonei).
- CT and MRI are useful at providing a global assessment of the extent and relationships of the tumour (Fig. 12i-k).

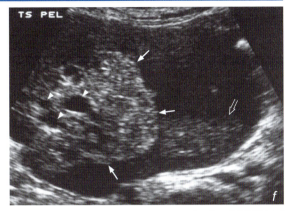

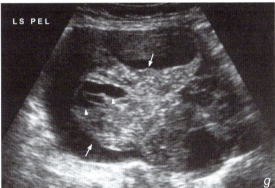

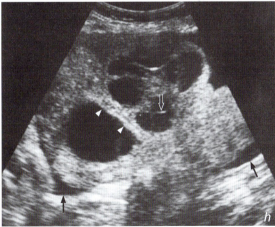

Fig.12f, g *Transverse (a) and longitudinal (b) transabdominal ultrasound images of the pelvis showing a large complex mixed solid and cystic lesion. Note the irregular contour (arrows) and multiple small cystic areas (arrowheads) within the solid component of the lesion. There is echogenic debris within the major cystic component (open arrow).*

Fig.12h *Longitudinal transabdominal ultrasound image shows a markedly enlarged ovary which is outlined by the free fluid in the pelvis (arrow). There are solid and cystic components within the lesion. Internal septations (arrowheads) and debris (open arrow) are also seen within the tumour mass. Patient had history of CA stomach. Surgery showed this to be ovarian metastasis (Krukenberg tumour).*

Discussion Case 12
Ovarian tumour

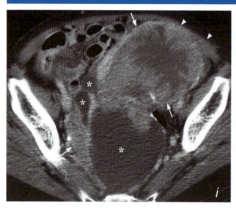

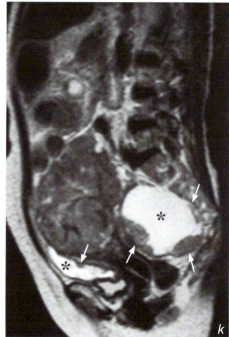

Fig.12i *Axial CECT shows a huge tumour mass in the pelvis with solid (arrows) and cystic (asterisks) components. The tumour shows heterogeneous contrast enhancement with low attenuation centre suggestive of early central necrosis. Note the normal fat plane between the tumour mass and the left anterior abdominal wall is lost (arrowheads), raising the suspicion of local invasion.*

Fig. 12j, k *Axial (j) and sagittal (k) T2W MRI images of a different patient show a huge cystadenocarcinoma occupying almost the whole pelvis. The tumour mass shows mixed cystic (asterisks) and solid component. Mural nodules are present within the cystic component (arrows). Large solid component is present in the anterior and superior aspect of the lesion. Malignant free fluid is present on the right side of the lesion (arrowheads).*

<u>**Note:**</u>
(1) A unilateral multilocular cystic adnexal lesion with thick septae should be considered a mucinous adenoma until proven otherwise.
(2) A cystic adnexal lesion with a solid component should be considered malignant unless proven otherwise.

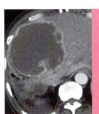

HEPATOBILIARY SYSTEM

Contributors:

David P.N. Chan, Alex W.H. Ng, K.T. Wong, Gregory E. Antonio, Edmund H.Y. Yuen, Anil T. Ahuja

Questions

Case 1 - 11	360 - 370

Discussion

Cholelithiasis	371 - 372
Acute cholecystitis	373 - 374
Acute cholangitis	375 - 376
Hepatic haemangioma	377 - 378
Hepatocellular carcinoma	379 - 381
Pyogenic liver abscess	382 - 383
Liver metastases	384 - 385
Splenic rupture	386 - 387
Acute pancreatitis	388 - 390
Chronic pancreatitis	391 - 392
Carcinoma of pancreas	393 - 394

Chapter 08

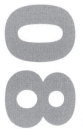

Case 1

A 47-year-old obese woman presented with on and off epigastric pain for 4 months. The pain was dull in nature and aggravated by fatty meals. Physical examination was essentially normal. Laboratory investigations showed normal liver function and white cell count. The clinical diagnosis of gallstone was suggested and an abdominal x-ray (AXR) (Fig.1a) was performed as a routine initial investigation.

Questions

(1) What abnormalities can you identify on the AXR ?
 - Calcification projected over right upper quadrant
 - Faceted outline of the calcification (the calcification is outside the right renal shadow ruling out the possibility of being radio-opaque renal stone)
 - Note the degenerative lumbar spine

(2) <u>What is the diagnosis ?</u>

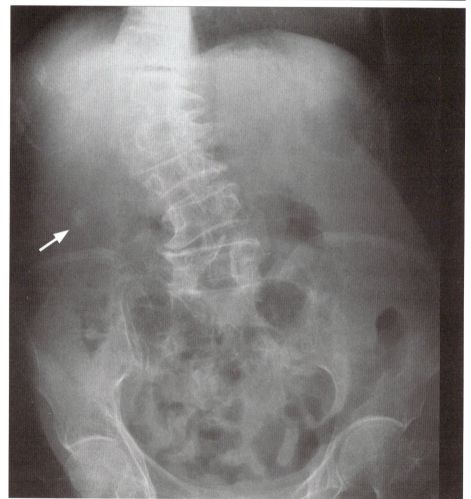

Fig.1a *Abdominal radiograph showing faceted calcification in the right upper quadrant suggestive of gallstone (arrow).*

Case 2

A 72-year-old woman, with a known history of gallstones, complained of right upper quadrant pain and fever for 2 days. On abdominal examination, there was localized tenderness, guarding and rebound tenderness over the right upper quadrant. Laboratory investigations revealed a raised white cell count. Bilirubin and alkaline phosphatase levels were within normal limits. The clinical diagnosis of acute cholecystitis was suggested and a CT abdomen was performed (Fig. 2a-c).

Questions

(1) What abnormalities can you detect on this CT ?
- Distended gallbladder - cystic duct obstruction leading to accumulation of inflammatory exudate
- Gallstones - majority of cases of acute cholecystitis are calculus-related
- Gallbladder wall thickening (>3 mm in a fasting state) - mucosal oedema due to acute inflammation
- Peri-cholecystitic fluid (soft tissue streakiness) - exudate around GB in the presence of inflammation

(2) What is the diagnosis ?

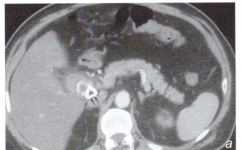
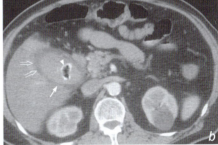
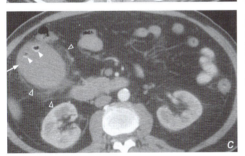

Fig.2a,b and c *Contrast enhanced axial computed tomography at three levels showing multiple gallstones (arrowheads) within a distended gallbladder (arrows) showing wall thickening (open arrows), pericholecystic fluid and streakiness of fat (open arrowheads). These are signs of inflammation indicating acute cholecystitis. Note the impacted large calculus (double arrows), and gas within stones, which is a common finding.*

Case 3

A 57-year-old obese woman with a known history of gallstone disease presented with right upper quadrant pain, high fever and jaundice for 2 days. On general examination she looked ill, was tachycardic and hypotensive. Abdominal examination revealed marked local tenderness and guarding over the right upper quadrant. The gallbladder was not palpable and Murphy's sign was negative. Laboratory investigations showed leukocytosis, raised bilirubin and alkaline phosphatase. The clinical diagnosis of acute cholangitis was suggested and a USG abdomen (Fig. 3a, b) was performed.

Questions

(1) What ultrasound abnormalities do you see ?
- Echogenic foci casting posterior acoustic shadowing in distal common bile duct (CBD)
  - represent gallstones which have passed through cystic duct into CBD
- Dilatation of common bile duct – due to distal CBD obstruction
- Multiple small stones are present in the intrahepatic part of the left main bile duct

(2) <u>What is the diagnosis ?</u>

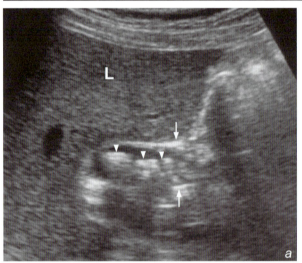

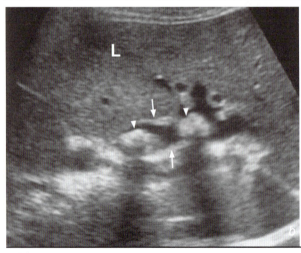

Fig. 3a,b *Longitudinal (a) and transverse sonograms at the porta hepatis (b) showing multiple echogenic ductal stones (arrowheads) causing dilatation of the common bile duct (arrows in Fig. 3a) and the left intrahepatic duct (arrows in Fig. 3b). L=liver.*

Case 4

A 42-year-old woman presented with right upper quadrant pain for 4 months. There were no associated systemic symptoms. She was afebrile and not jaundiced on general examination. Hepatomegaly with a smooth edge was detected on palpation of the abdomen. Laboratory investigations revealed normal liver function and the alpha fetal protein (AFP) level was within normal limits. Viral hepatitis serology was negative. A CT of the abdomen was performed for further evaluation (Fig. 4a-d).

Questions

(1) What abnormality is demonstrated on this four-phase dynamic contrast enhanced CT ?
- There is a well-defined, non-calcified lesion in the right lobe of the liver. It shows initial peripheral, nodular enhancement on the arterial phase, centripetal enhancement pattern with gradual 'central filling in' on the portal venous and delayed phases. On all phases the enhancing portions of the lesion show the same density as the other major arterial vascular compartments.

(2) <u>What is the most likely diagnosis ?</u>

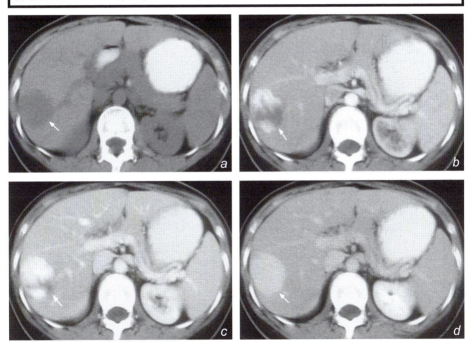

Fig.4a,b,c and d Contrast enhanced axial computed tomography showing the typical contrast enhancement pattern of a hepatic haemangioma (arrow). It is hypodense in the pre-contrast CT scan (a), with progressive centripetal enhancement on arterial phase (b), portal venous phase (c) and complete 'filling in' on the 5 minute delay phase (d).

Case 5

A 66-year-old man, a known hepatitis B carrier, complained of mild right upper quadrant pain, weight loss and generalized malaise in the recent 2 months. He was cachectic with stigmata of chronic liver disease (i.e. spider naevi, palmar erythema). Examination of the abdomen revealed hepatomegaly which was hard and non-tender. Laboratory investigations showed raised bilirubin and alkaline phosphatase. Alpha fetal protein level was markedly elevated. The clinical diagnosis was hepatocellular carcinoma and a CECT (Fig. 5a, b, c) was performed for further evaluation.

Questions

(1) What abnormalities can you see on the CECT ?
- Large heterogeneous enhancing mass in right lobe of liver
- Non-opacification of right portal vein indicates portal venous thrombosis
- Soft tissue filling defect within lumen of IVC - represents tumour thrombus
- Underlying cirrhosis: as evident by the nodular, irregular edge

(2) What is the most likely diagnosis ?

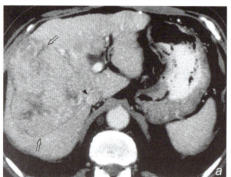
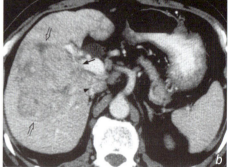
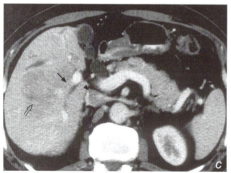

Fig.5a,b,c *Contrast enhanced axial computed tomography at three different levels showing a heterogeneously enhancing hepatocellular carcinoma (open arrows) in right lobe of liver with tumour thrombus extending into the right portal vein (arrows) and inferior vena cava (arrowheads). Note the nodular, irregular liver edge suggesting cirrhosis.*

Case 6

A 64-year-old woman, with a known history of insulin dependent diabetes mellitus, complained of right upper quadrant pain, fever, chills and rigor for 2 days. On general examination, she was febrile and looked ill. Abdominal examination showed hepatomegaly with local tenderness. Laboratory investigations revealed raised white cell count and normal bilirubin and alkaline phosphatase level. The alpha fetal protein level was within normal limits. A provisional diagnosis of liver abscess was suggested and a CECT (Fig. 6a ,b) was performed for further evaluation.

Questions

(1) What abnormalities can you see on the CECT ?
   - Well-defined hypodense hepatic lesion - due to pus/inflammatory exudate within an abscess cavity
   - Thick irregular wall - due to host response to inflammation
   - Peripheral rim enhancement (of abscess wall) - hyperaemia around periphery of abscess
   - Loculation
   - Right pleural effusion - reaction to adjacent subdiaphragmatic inflammation
   - No evidence of underlying cirrhosis
(2) <u>What is the most likely diagnosis ?</u>

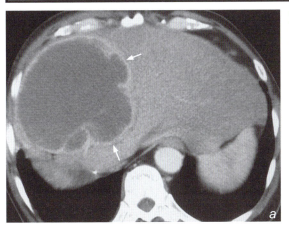

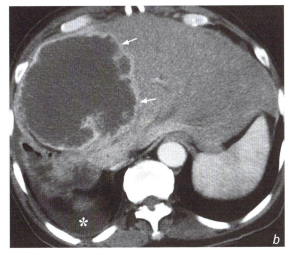

Fig.6a,b *Contrast enhanced axial computed tomography showing a large right lobe hepatic abscess (arrows) as a well-defined hypodense lesion with a thick, irregular enhancing wall. Note the presence of a small right pleural effusion (asterisk) which is a reaction to the adjacent subdiaphragmatic inflammation.*

Case 7

A 72-year-old man, with a history of colonic carcinoma operated 2 years earlier, complained of vague upper abdominal pain and weight loss for 3 months. Physical examination revealed hepatomegaly with nodular edges and which was non-tender. Laboratory investigations showed raised chorio-embryonic antigen. Alpha fetal protein level was normal. The working diagnosis of liver metastases was suggested and a CECT (Fig. 7a) was performed for further evaluation.

Questions

(1) What abnormalities can you see on the CECT ?
   - Multiple hypodense, non-enhancing lesions in both lobes of liver of various sizes
   - No evidence of a cirrhotic liver
   - Mass lesion in the left adrenal gland
(2) <u>What is the most likely diagnosis ?</u>

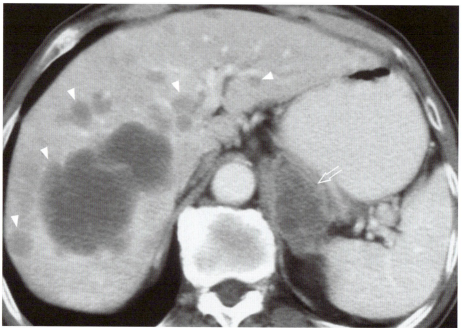

Fig.7a *Contrast enhanced axial computed tomography showing multiple hepatic metastases appearing as hypodense (poorly enhancing) lesions of various sizes (arrowheads). Note the enlarged, heterogeneous left adrenal mass (open arrow) representing adrenal metastasis.*

Case 8

A 30-year-old woman accidentally fell from a height of 10 metres and landed on her left side. She subsequently complained of severe left upper abdominal pain. On general examination she was pale and tachycardic but normotensive. Examination of abdomen revealed marked tenderness over left lower chest wall and left upper abdomen. Plain chest radiograph showed fractures of left lower ribs with evidence of a pneumothorax. Haemoglobin level remained low after transfusion of 2 units of blood and a clinical diagnosis of splenic injury was suggested. A CECT abdomen was performed for further evaluation (Fig. 8a, b).

Questions

(1) What radiological abnormalities can you see on this CECT ?
  - Shattered spleen - indicates rupture of splenic parenchyma
  - Fluid in peri-splenic space - represents haematoma from adjacent splenic rupture
  - Fluid in peritoneal space - indicates haemoperitoneum

(2) What is the diagnosis ?

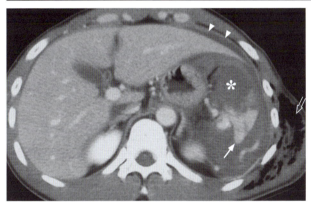

Fig.8a *Contrast enhanced computed tomography showing a ruptured spleen (arrow). Note the presence of perisplenic haematoma (asterisk) and haemoperitoneum (arrowheads) seen as a crescent of fluid around the left lobe of liver. Surgical emphysema is also present in the left chest wall (open arrow). Note the other organs can be clearly evaluated at the same time.*

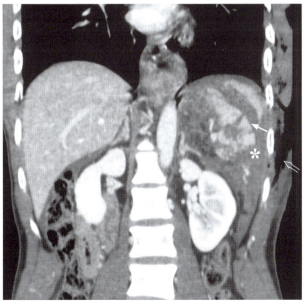

Fig.8b *Contrast enhanced computed tomography with coronal reformation showing the ruptured spleen (arrow). Note the presence of perisplenic haematoma (asterisk) and surgical emphysema (open arrow) in left chest wall.*

Case 9

A 68-year-old patient, a chronic drinker, complained of severe epigastric pain for one day. The pain was of sudden onset, radiating to the back and associated with repeated vomiting. Physical examination showed local tenderness and guarding over the epigastrium. Blood tests revealed markedly elevated serum amylase, liver function test was normal and white cell count was not elevated. The clinical diagnosis of acute pancreatitis was suggested and a CECT abdomen (Fig. 9a-c) was performed for further assessment.

Questions

(1) What abnormalities can you see on this CECT ?
   - Swollen and oedematous pancreas with ill-defined margins
   - Dilated pancreatic duct
   - Dilated common bile duct
   - Aerobilia

(2) <u>What is the diagnosis ?</u>

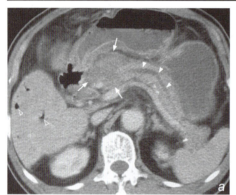
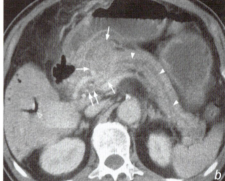
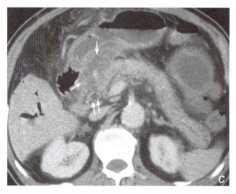

Fig.9a, b, c *Contrast enhanced axial computed tomography shows a markedly swollen and low density (oedematous) pancreatic head with ill-defined margins (arrows) in a patient with acute pancreatitis. Note the presence of pneumobilia (open arrowheads), dilated pancreatic duct (arrowheads) and common bile duct (double arrows). In contrast, the body and tail of the pancreas are well visualized and of normal size and appearance.*

Case 10

A 63-year-old man, a chronic heavy drinker for 30 years, presented with on and off epigastric pain for 3 months. He had three episodes of acute pancreatitis in the past 8 years which required hospital admission. Physical examination was essentially normal. Laboratory investigations showed elevated plasma glucose level and mildly raised amylase. Liver function test and white cell count were normal.

A CT abdomen (Fig. 10a) was performed for further assessment.

Questions

(1) What abnormalities can you detect on this CECT ?
   Pancreatic tissue replaced by:
   - Multiple coarse pancreatic calcifications
   - Dilated pancreatic duct
(2) What is the diagnosis ?

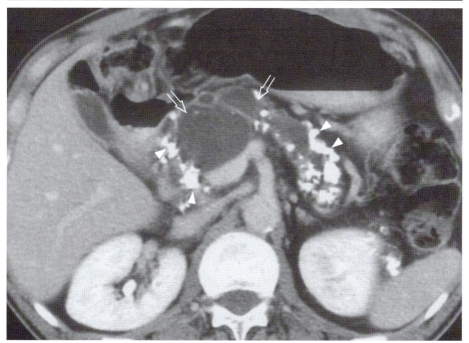

Fig.10a *Contrast enhanced axial computed tomography shows multiple coarse calcifications (arrowheads) and a dilated pancreatic duct (open arrows) in chronic pancreatitis.*

Case 11

A 75-year-old man complained of painless progressive jaundice and pale stools for 2 months, loss of weight and appetite recently. General examination showed a cachectic and jaundiced patient. A vague epigastric mass was detected on abdominal examination. Laboratory investigations revealed hyper-bilirubinaemia and a raised alkaline phosphatase level. Alanine transaminase level was within normal limits. The clinical diagnosis of obstructive jaundice was suggested and a CECT (Fig. 11a, b) was performed for further evaluation.

Questions

(1) What abnormalities can you see on this CECT ?
- Heterogeneous mass in head of pancreas
- Multiple irregular hypodense non-enhancing hepatic lesions
- Ascites

(2) What is the most likely diagnosis ?

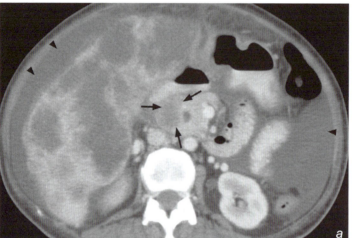

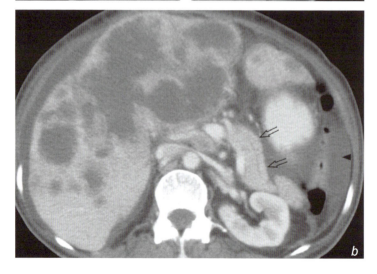

Fig.11a,b *Contrast enhanced axial computed tomography at different levels shows a poorly enhancing neoplasm in the pancreatic head (arrows) with multiple hepatic metastases and ascites (arrowheads). Note the rest of the pancreas looks normal (open arrows).*

Discussion Case 1
Cholelithiasis

Gallstone (Fig. 1a)

Discussion:
- Cholelithiasis is a common cause of epigastric/right upper quadrant pain in middle-aged obese female patients.
- Gallstones are composed of crystals of cholesterol monohydrate and variable amounts of calcium carbonate/phosphate/bilirubinate (the latter being radio-opaque)
- Only ~15-20% of gallstones are radio-opaque, hence AXR is not always helpful (compared to renal calculi)
- It may be difficult to differentiate a radio-opaque gallstone from a right renal stone, especially if the gallstone is projected over right renal shadow. A US examination easily overcomes this as it can evaluate the gallbladder and kidney separately
- Ultrasound features of gallstones within the gallbladder include (Fig. 1b, c):
  1. Echogenic foci in the dependent portion of the gallbladder
  2. Dense posterior acoustic shadowing
  3. Change in position by changing patient posture - (some) stones are mobile within gallbladder
- Ultrasound is highly accurate (~98%) in the diagnosis of gallstones, easily available and does not involve ionizing radiation.
- With CT, gallstones usually appear as rounded or faceted calcified densities within the gallbladder (Fig. 1d). However, tiny non-calcified stones may be missed by CT.
- Gallstone related complications include acute/chronic cholecystitis, biliary tract obstruction, acute cholangitis and carcinoma of gallbladder. All of these can be evaluated by ultrasound and CT.

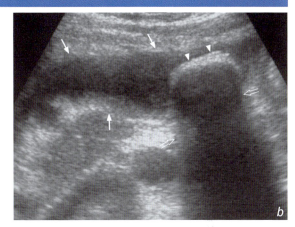

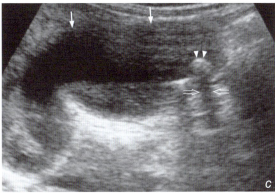

Fig.1b,c *Two examples of ultrasound of the gallbladder (arrows) showing different size gallstones (arrowheads) as echogenic foci casting dense posterior acoustic shadowing (open arrows).*

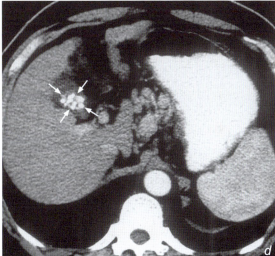

Fig.1d *Contrast enhanced axial computed tomography showing multiple gallstones (arrows) as a cluster of small calcified foci within a contracted gallbladder.*

Cholelithiasis

- An adenomyoma should not be mistaken for a gallstone. This is usually seen as an immobile, focal, smooth sessile mass in the fundus of the gallbladder, of soft tissue density (Fig. 1e).

Note:

(1) Epigastric pain associated with fat intolerance in an obese middle-aged female is likely to represent gallstone disease.

(2) Ultrasound is the initial imaging investigation of choice.

(3) Only ~15-20% of gallstones are radio-opaque and detectable by plain radiograph.

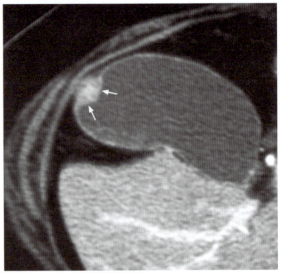

Fig.1e *Contrast enhanced CT of the gallbladder showing a focal, sessile, smooth soft tissue mass (arrows) in the wall fundus of the gallbladder. The appearances are of an adenomyoma.*

Discussion Case 2
Acute cholecystitis

Acute cholecystitis (Fig. 2a-c)

Discussion:
- Approximately nine out of ten cases of acute cholecystitis are due to cystic duct obstruction by a gallstone (calculous cholecystitis). In diabetic patients, cholecystitis may occur without a gallstone causing obstruction (acalculous cholecystitis, Fig. 2d). The static bile itself is an irritant causing acute inflammation of the gallbladder wall, which becomes oedematous and hyperaemic. In addition, there may be superimposed infection to add to the inflammation.
- Ultrasound (Fig. 2e, f) and CT (Fig. 2a-c) is commonly used to confirm the diagnosis, by showing gallbladder mural thickening, pericholecystic fluid, gallstone
- In addition to the signs of inflammation, USG has additional advantages in that:
  1. It has higher spatial resolution and can demonstrate a shaggy/irregular gallbladder wall - which is suggestive of gallbladder gangrene
  2. It is done real-time and can be used to illicit localized tenderness on probe pressure on gallbladder (sonographic Murphy's sign)

Fig.2 e,f Ultrasound showing features of acute cholecystitis with gallstone(arrowheads) in a gallbladder with thickened wall (arrows) and the presence of pericholecystic fluid (open arrows). Note the posterior acoustic shadow due to the presence of gallstones (open arrowheads). L=liver.

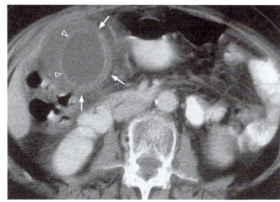

Fig.2d Contrast enhanced axial computed tomography showing acalculous cholecystitis as a distended gallbladder with wall thickening (arrow) and mucosal contrast enhancement (open arrowheads). Note the absence of a gallstone.

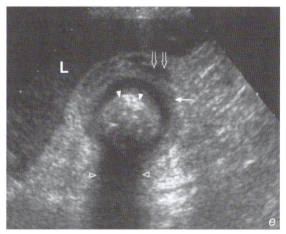

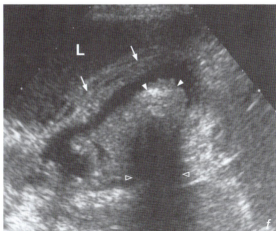

Acute cholecystitis

- On the other hand, USG may be
  equivocal in very early cholecystitis.
  In these cases cholescintigraphy
  (nuclear medicine) is more sensitive.
  The examination relies on
  demonstrating an obstructed cystic
  duct (rather than gallbladder
  inflammation) to make the diagnosis.
- Complications of acute cholecystitis
  include:
  1. Gallbladder perforation (which may
     lead to peritonitis or abscess
     formation, Fig. 2g, h)
  2. Gallbladder empyema
  3. Gallbladder gangrene
  4. Ascending infection (cholangitis)

Note:
(1) Acute cholecystitis is
    most commonly due to
    impaction of gallstone in
    the cystic duct.
(2) A distended thick-
    walled gallbladder
    with gallstones,
    peri- cholecystic fluid
    collection and localized
    tenderness are typical
    findings.

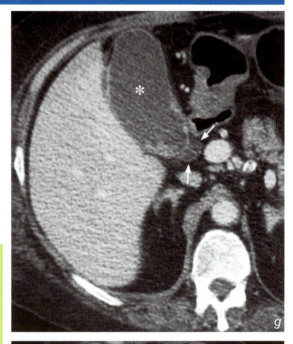

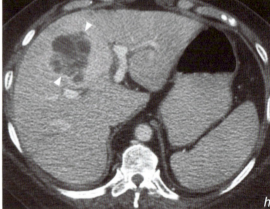

Fig.2 g,h *Contrast enhanced axial CT showing a distended gallbladder (asterisk) with perforation (arrows) and adjacent intrahepatic abscess formation (arrowheads).*

Acute cholangitis

Acute cholangitis (Fig. 3a, b)

Discussion:

- Acute cholangitis is defined as acute inflammation of the bile ducts. This usually involves obstruction to the bile duct resulting in bile stasis and accumulation. The static bile may be sterile or there may be a superimposed infection (usually from bacteria ascending via the sphincter of Oddi). Patients with the superimposed infection are usually septic
- There are many causes of biliary obstruction which include:
    1. Gallstone(s) - in approximately one third of cases
    2. Duct scarring (stricture) from previous surgery
    3. Parasitic infestation
    4. Malignant tumour - such as pancreatic carcinoma, carcinoma of the ampulla of Vater, etc.
- The aim of imaging is to demonstrate the presence of an obstructed biliary system and to elucidate the cause. Ultrasound (Fig. 3a, b) is the initial imaging investigation of choice due to its wide availability as well as being radiation-free. Aside from USG, CT can also be used to establish the diagnosis (Fig.3c, d). CT is especially useful when the obstructing cause is obscured by bowel gas (ultrasound is unable to interrogate)

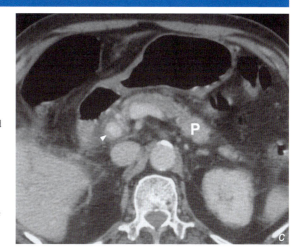

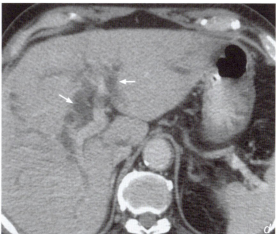

Fig.3c,d Contrast enhanced axial computed tomography showing a stone obstructing the distal end of the common bile duct (arrowheads) causing dilatation of the intrahepatic ducts (arrows) in both lobes of liver. P=pancreas.

Discussion Case 3
Acute cholangitis

- Treatment is aimed at relieving and/ or removing the biliary obstruction. Endoscopic Retrograde Cholangio-Pancreatography (ERCP) (Fig. 3e, f) is the most common method of stone extraction and biliary drainage
- In patients with contraindications to ERCP or if the cause of obstruction cannot be quickly resolved, percutaneous transhepatic biliary drainage (PTBD) under ultrasound and fluoroscopic guidance is an alternative method for biliary decompression.

Note:

(1) Ultrasound is the initial imaging modality of choice for suspected acute cholangitis.

(2) A CBD stone with dilatation of the CBD and intrahepatic ducts are classical ultrasound features of acute cholangitis.

(3) ERCP is commonly used to provide biliary decompression.

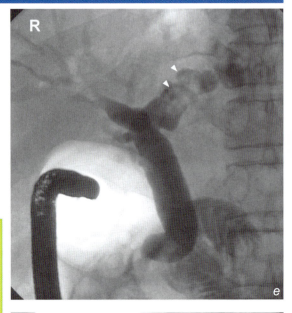

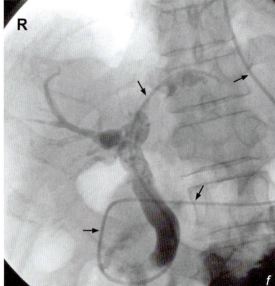

Fig.3e,f *ERCP showing multiple filling defects (arrowheads) within the left intrahepatic duct compatible with intrahepatic stones. Nasobiliary drain (arrows) was inserted for biliary drainage.*

Hepatic haemangioma

Hepatic haemangioma (Fig. 4a-d)

Discussion:

- Hepatic haemangioma is a benign tumour which consists of vascular spaces lined by endothelial cells (cavernous haemangioma)
- It is the most common benign tumour and the second most common tumour (after metastases) in the liver
- The characteristic (diagnostic) imaging feature of haemangiomas reflect the perfusion and vascularity of the lesions. The typical sequential CT contrast enhancement (Fig. 4a-d) pattern is:
  1. Early, peripheral nodular enhancement in the arterial phase
  2. Progressive centripetal enhancement in the portal venous and delayed phases
  3. Sometimes with complete 'filling in' in the delayed phase
  4. The lesion is isodense to blood vessels on all phases
- There are some exceptions to this pattern of contrast enhancement:
  - Small (<2 cm) haemangiomas may show rapid homogeneous enhancement
  - Giant (>10 cm) may not show the complete 'fill-in' due to the presence of central scarring/fibrous tissue, haemorrhage
- A technetium-99m labelled RBC scan (Fig. 4e) can also be used for diagnosing a haemangioma. This typically shows the lesion as a 'cold' lesion on the initial dynamic phase, with increasing activity on delayed images. Tc-99m labelled RBC scan showing this sequence of red blood cell accumulation in a lesion is specific for the diagnosis of a haemangioma. However, due to its inherent limited spatial resolution, the haemangioma has to be larger than 2 cm to be discernible using this modality

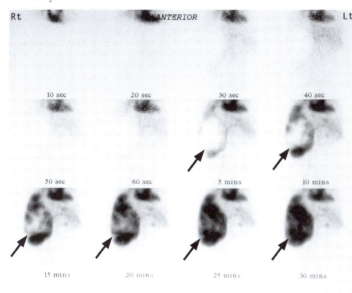

Fig.4e Sequential images from a Tc-99m labelled RBC scan of a different patient show gradual accumulation of red blood cells within a large hepatic cavernous haemangioma (arrows). This centripetal pattern of accumulation parallels that of contrast enhancement with contrast enhanced CT.

08 HEPATOBILIARY SYSTEM

Discussion Case 4
Hepatic haemangioma

- On ultrasound (Fig. 4f), small hepatic haemangiomas usually appear as well-defined homogeneous hyperechoic lesions with no mass effect. Larger haemangiomas usually appear more heterogeneous and hypoechoic. It is the modality of choice in follow up of the lesions.
- Large haemangiomas may rupture (rare) and may also sequester a significant amount of platelets to cause thrombocytopenia (Kasabach Merrit syndrome)

Note:
(1) Hepatic haemangioma is the most common benign hepatic tumour and the second most common hepatic tumour.
(2) It shows characteristic centripetal vascular enhancement pattern on dynamic CT.
(3) Diagnosis can be confirmed by RBC scan.

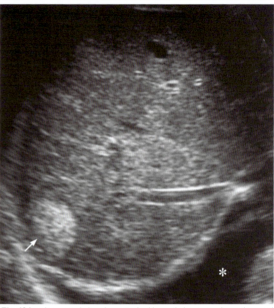

Fig.4f *An ultrasound showing a typical hepatic haemangioma (arrows) appearing as a homogeneously echogenic lesion with well-defined borders. Note the incidental pleural effusion (asterisk).*

Discussion Case 5
Hepatocellular carcinoma

Hepatocellular carcinoma (Fig. 5a-c)

- A hepatic mass could be due to many different causes including neoplasms, infection, etc. However, the presence of portal and systemic venous thrombi are much more in favour of primary hepatocellular carcinoma than metastases from other primary tumours

Discussion:

- Hepatocellular carcinoma is one of the commonest malignant neoplasms in Asians due to the high prevalence of chronic hepatitis B infection and subsequent cirrhosis. The lesion may be solitary or multifocal.
- Although ultrasound accurately evaluates a HCC, currently CECT is often used as the modality of choice in tumour staging while USG is used for screening cirrhotic patients and to follow-up HCC during/after treatment
- The typical CT findings of HCC include (Fig. 5a-g) :
  1. Single or multiple mass(es) which may be hypo- or isodense (compared to the rest of the liver)
  2. Arterial phase contrast enhancement (Fig. 5d, e)
  3. Heterogeneous portal venous phase contrast enhancement (enhancement corresponds to hypervascular areas and non-enhancement suggests tumour necrosis)
  4. Portal venous thrombosis (by tumour invasion), seen as a contrast filling defect. The tumour thrombus itself may show some arterial phase contrast enhancement
  5. Evidence of underlying cirrhosis and portal hypertension (Fig. 5f)
     - irregular liver contour, splenomegaly, ascites
  6. Intrahepatic biliary ductal dilatation (due to distal compression)

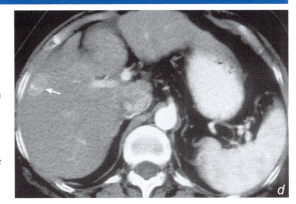

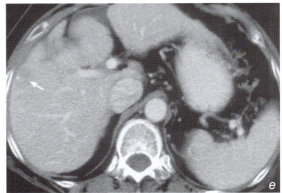

Figs.5d,e Contrast enhanced axial computed tomography shows enhancement of a small hepatocellular carcinoma (arrows). It shows increased enhancement (hypervascular) on the arterial phase and decreased enhancement (compared with the rest of the liver) on the portal venous phase.

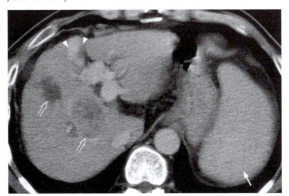

Fig.5f Contrast enhanced axial computed tomography (CT) of a different patient shows a heterogeneously enhancing hepatocellular carcinoma (open arrows) in the right lobe of the liver. This patient has portal hypertension as evident by the presence of splenomegaly (arrow) and recannulation of the umbilical vein (arrowheads).

Discussion Case 5
Hepatocellular carcinoma

- On USG, HCC usually appears as a heterogeneous mass, sometimes with mass effect (distortion or displacement of the hepatic/portal vessels) if the lesion is large (Fig. 5g)
- MRI features of HCC (Fig. 5h, i) are similar to those found on CT: heterogeneous on plain scan and hyperintense on arterial phase after gadolinium injection

Fig.5g *Ultrasound showing hepatocellular carcinoma (arrows) as a heterogeneous lesion with mass effect causing displacement of the hepatic vein (arrow-heads).*

Fig.5h,i *MRI T1-weighted sequence showing a small hepatocellular carcinoma (arrow) in right lobe of liver which is hypointense on the precontrast scan and hyperintense on arterial phase after gadolinium injection.*

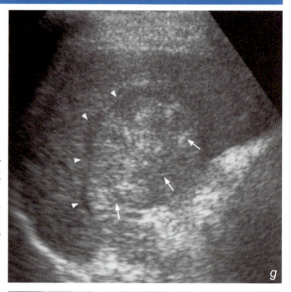

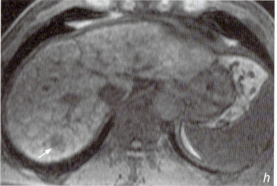

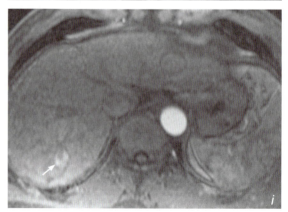

Hepatocellular carcinoma

- The major differential diagnoses of a liver neoplasm are HCC, cholangiocarcinoma (Fig. 5j, k) and metastases (see case 7). Clinical information such as hepatitis B status and raised alpha fetal protein level supports the diagnosis of HCC. If the mass is hypervascular in the arterial phase of contrast enhanced CT and if portal venous thrombosis is present, HCC is more likely than metastases.
- Apart from diagnosis and monitoring progress, imaging also plays an important therapeutic role. These include endovascular treatment (such as chemo-embolization/selective internal radiation) and local ablative therapy (e.g. microwave/alcohol injection) under ultrasound guidance.

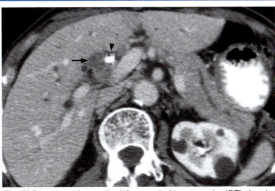

Fig. 5j *Contrast enhanced axial computed tomography (CT) showing a cholangiocarcinoma appearing as a soft tissue lesion (arrow) along the biliary ductal system at the porta hepatis. This was causing biliary obstruction and treated with a biliary stent (arrowhead).*

Note:

(1) HCC is a common malignant tumour in Asians and CECT is the imaging modality of choice.

(2) On CECT, a large, hypervascular liver mass, underlying liver cirrhosis and portal venous thrombosis are characteristic radiological features of HCC.

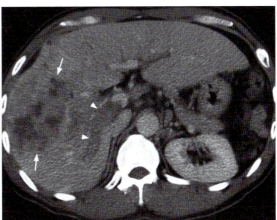

Fig. 5k *Contrast enhanced axial CT showing an ill-defined heterogeneous mass (arrow) in the right lobe of the liver. Note the associated right portal vein thrombosis (arrowheads). This was proven to be a cholangiocarcinoma mimicking an HCC. Note the absence of cirrhosis change in the liver and no evidence of portal venous hypertension.*

Discussion Case 6
Pyogenic liver abscess

Pyogenic liver abscess (Fig. 6a, b)

Discussion:

- Liver abscesses are often idiopathic and their causes include direct inoculation (trauma/surgery), ascending cholangitis, septic emboli, etc.
- E. coli is the most common organism
- Sonography is the modality of choice for screening liver abscesses (Fig. 6c, d). Once detected, a needle aspiration under USG guidance could be performed for microbiological evaluation. In addition, a CECT is often performed for evaluating the rest of the abdomen and chest aside from the liver abscess(es)
- The typical CT findings of liver abscess include (Fig. 6a, b, e):
  1. Hypodense (compared to the rest of the liver) lesion with well-defined borders
  2. Contrast enhancement of a thick and irregular wall (central non-enhancement due to pus)
  3. Ring of oedema surrounding the abscess (a zone of inflammation incited by the abscess)
  4. Gas within the abscess, may be seen if infected by a gas-producing organism
- The radiological features of a liver abscess are not entirely specific (necrotic tumour may mimic its appearances). Diagnosis relies on a combination of clinical information (i.e. fever, RUQ pain, raised WCC, septicaemia and predisposing factors e.g. DM) and radiological findings.

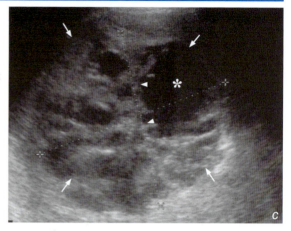

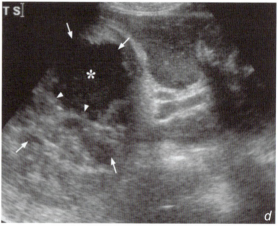

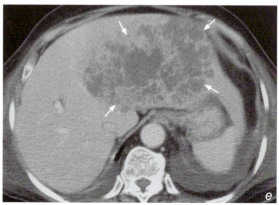

Fig.6c,d *Ultrasound shows a large liver abscess (arrows) in right lobe of liver with multiple thick septae (arrowheads) and a large cystic component containing low-level echoes (asterisk). Calipers indicate the size of abscess (14 cm x 12 cm).*

Fig.6e *Contrast enhanced axial computed tomography (CT) shows a large left lobe hepatic abscess (arrows) as a multi-loculated hypodense lesion with septations.*

Pyogenic liver abscess

- Role of imaging in patient with suspected liver abscess includes:
  1. Establish the clinical diagnosis and confirmation by image-guided aspiration
  2. Therapeutic by imaging-guided drainage (Fig. 6f), which is less invasive than surgical drainage

Note:
(1) Diagnosis of liver abscess is based on clinical information and imaging findings.
(2) Contrast enhanced CT, US abdomen are the commonly used modalities.
(3) Imaging-guided aspiration and drainage offer a less invasive mode of treatment.

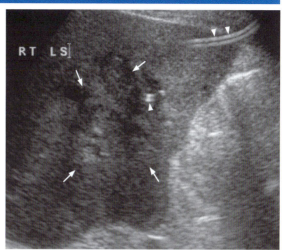

Fig.6f *Follow-up ultrasound of the patient in Fig. 6c, d after imaging-guided drainage. The draining catheter (arrowheads) is within the liver abscess and most of the cystic component of the abscess has been drained.*

Discussion Case 7
Liver metastases

Hepatic metastases from a carcinoma of colon (Fig. 7a)

Discussion:
- The liver is the most common site for metastatic involvement. Metastases are much more common than a primary malignancy of the liver.
- The CT findings of liver metastases include:
  1. Hypodense lesion(s) in the liver (Fig. 7a, b). In some cases isodense or hyperdense metastases are seen
  2. Contrast enhancement in the arterial phase may be seen (hypervascular metastases are typically from: renal cell, breast, colonic or ovarian carcinomas, carcinoid and melanoma)
  3. Portal venous phase contrast enhancement is variable
  4. Internal calcification (Fig. 7c)
     - Occurs in mucinous carcinoma of colon, osteosarcoma, neuroblastoma, squamous cell carcinoma, etc.
  5. Hypodense centre/areas without contrast enhancement (Fig. 7d)
     - Indicates area(s) of central tumour necrosis
- Sometimes it is difficult to differentiate liver metastases from hepatocellular carcinoma. Certain clues for diagnosis include:
  1. Clinical information
     - History of primary tumour, especially those with high incidence of liver metastases such as carcinoma of lung, breast and colon, would favour metastases
     - Underlying chronic hepatitis B or cirrhosis predisposes to hepatocellular carcinoma (HCC)
     - Tumour markers - in the presence of liver lesions, AFP level is raised in HCC, while a raised CEA indicates metastases from colorectal primary tumour

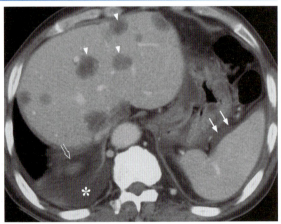

Fig.7b *Contrast enhanced axial computed tomography (CT) showing multiple hepatic metastases as hypodense, poorly enhancing lesions (arrowheads). Note the right pleural effusion (asterisk) and ascites (arrows). Mass lesion in the right adrenal gland (open arrow) represents another site of metastasis.*

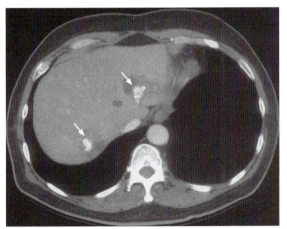

Fig.7c *Contrast enhanced axial computed tomography (CT) showing multiple calcified liver metastases (arrows) in both lobes of the liver. Patient had a history of mucinous carcinoma of colon.*

Liver metastases

2. Radiological features
   - Number of hepatic lesions
     - multiple lesions favour metastases rather than HCC
   - Vascularity of lesions
     - HCC is more hypervascular than most metastases and HCC enhances in the arterial phase of a contrast enhanced CT scan
   - Portal venous invasion
     - more common in HCC than metastases
- Sonography (Fig. 7e) is the most widely used screening modality for the detection of liver metastases. It is accurate, readily available, cost effective and is ideal for serial monitoring as it does not require contrast injection and does not use ionizing radiation. It also acts as an imaging guide for biopsy of equivocal lesions. The disadvantage is that it is often unable to accurately evaluate the primary lesion, particularly in the chest.

Note:
(1) Multiple liver lesions in a patient with known primary malignancy indicate metastases until proven otherwise.
(2) Contrast enhanced CT or ultrasound abdomen is the imaging modality of choice.
(3) Clinical information and imaging findings provide clues to differentiate between metastasis and HCC.

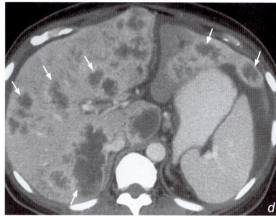

Fig.7d *Contrast enhanced axial computed tomography (CT) showing multiple necrotic liver metastases (arrows) in both lobes of liver appearing as hypodense lesions with fluid density centres and irregular enhancing walls.*

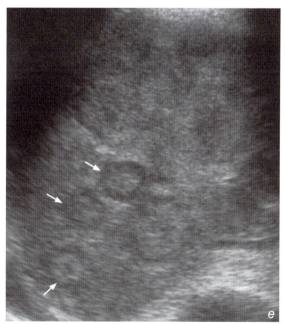

Fig.7e *Ultrasound showing multiple liver metastases (arrows) as isoechoic nodules with surrounding hypoechoic rims (halo sign).*

Discussion Case 8
Splenic rupture

Splenic rupture (Fig. 8a, b)

Discussion:

- The spleen is the most common organ involved in blunt abdominal injury
- The severity of injury ranges from subcapsular haematoma, parenchymal haematoma, splenic laceration to splenic rupture
- Typical CT findings of splenic injury reflect the possible range of abnormalities and include (Fig. 8 a-c):
  1. Subcapsular haematoma
     - indents the splenic surface but confined by the splenic capsule
  2. Contrast extravasation
     - indicates presence of active bleeding
  3. Splenic laceration
     - seen as a linear or triangular defect in the substance of the spleen extending to the surface
  4. S plenic rupture
     - seen as two or more fragments of spleen (these may still enhance with contrast, indicating that they are still receiving some blood supply)
- Splenic rupture may be delayed for a few days after the injury
- Although ultrasound is an ideal investigation for bedside evaluation of a patient with severe abdominal trauma, it does have a few limitations, including:
  1. Pain over the injured area or a wound (open or dressed) interferes with scanning (probe pressure cannot be applied). In addition lines, tubes, ECG monitors, etc. make the interrogation even more difficult
  2. A patient in pain, an unstable spine or with multiple tubes/lines inserted, cannot be moved into the optimal US scanning positions

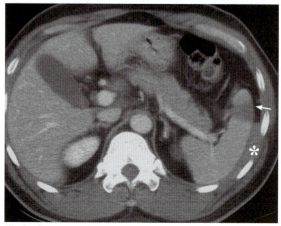

Fig.8c Contrast enhanced computer tomography (CT) showing a splenic laceration (arrow) and perisplenic heamatoma (asterisk).

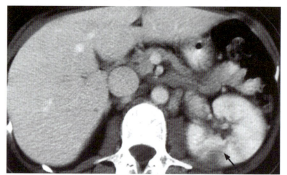

Fig.8d Contrast enhanced computer tomography (CT) with suspected splenic injury. No splenic injury is seen but there is a laceration (arrow) in the left kidney.

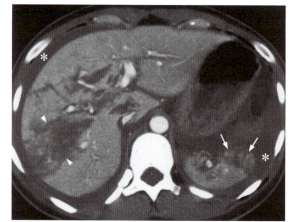

Fig. 8e Contrast enhanced CT of the abdomen in a patient with blunt abdominal trauma shows a splenic rupture (arrows), liver laceration (arrowheads) and haemoperitoneum (asterisk).

Splenic rupture

3. An initial small splenic tear or haematoma may not be seen
4. There may be an associated ileus which results in gaseous distention of bowel. This further obscures visualization of the abdomen by US
5. CT provides a quicker global overview of the entire abdomen and retroperitoneal structures (Fig. 8d-f)
6. Other parts of the patient (Fig. 8g) (thorax, spine and brain, etc.) may be injured and need some form of imaging. CT is usually requested for these regions, a CT of the abdomen can therefore be added at the same time

CECT is therefore regarded as the investigation of choice if the patient's general condition permits imaging.

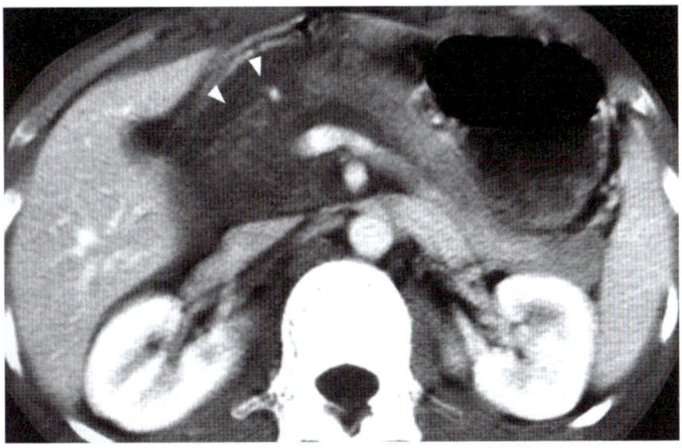

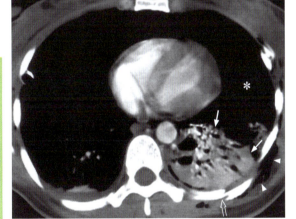

Fig. 8f *Contrast enhanced computer tomography (CT) with suspected splenic injury. No splenic injury is seen but the pancreatic head is not well defined and there is extensive haematoma (arrowheads) around the pancreas representing injury to the pancreatic head.*

Note:

(1) Spleen is the commonest organ involved in blunt abdominal injury.

(2) The presence of left lower rib fractures and localized peritoneal signs raise the possibility of splenic injury.

(3) Contrast enhanced CT is the imaging modality of choice if the patient's general condition permits imaging.

Fig. 8g *Contrast enhanced CT of the thorax in a patient with splenic injury shows rib fracture (open arrow), lung contusion (arrows), surgical emphysema (arrowheads). On lung windows a large pneumothorax was seen at the site of the asterisk. This is the advantage of CT over US as it can evaluate the thorax (which is often injured in blunt abdominal trauma) and the rest of the body at same time.*

08

HEPATOBILIARY SYSTEM

387

Discussion Case 9
Acute pancreatitis

Acute pancreatitis (Fig. 9a-c)

Discussion:
- This signifies an acute inflammation of the pancreas and may be caused by gallstones, alcoholism, infection, trauma, drugs, etc.
- The pancreatic pathology is well demonstrated by CT and findings include:
  1. Swollen and oedematous (decreased density) pancreas with ill-defined margins (signify the presence of acute inflammation within pancreatic tissue)
  2. Peripancreatic fluid collection/ abscess formation (Fig. 9d)
  3. Pseudo-cyst formation (Fig. 9e)
     - 'pseudo' meaning that this collection of fluid is not lined by epithelium (which is seen in a true cyst). This usually forms 6-8 weeks after the acute episode
  4. Lack of normal parenchymal enhancement within the pancreas after intravenous contrast administration
     - Indicates pancreatic necrosis in cases of necrotizing pancreatitis (Fig. 9f)
  5. Dilatation of adjacent bowel loops
     - So-called 'sentinel loop' sign which indicates local paralytic ileus in response to adjacent inflammation
  6. Changes of oedema/inflammation in soft tissue around the pancreas, kidney.
- Chest radiographic changes in acute pancreatitis include:
  1. Left sided pleural effusion with elevated amylase levels
  2. Elevation of the left hemidiaphragm and left lower lobe atelectasis
  3. Pericardial effusion
  4. Fistula formation between pancreas and pleura or bronchus

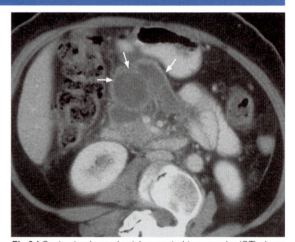

Fig.9d *Contrast enhanced axial computed tomography (CT) shows a pancreatic abscess (arrows) appearing as a multiple loculated hypodense lesion with a thick enhancing wall.*

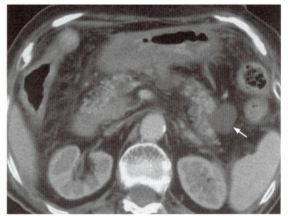

Fig.9e *Contrast enhanced axial computed tomography (CT) showing a small pancreatic pseudocyst (arrow) in pancreatic tail in a patient with recent history of pancreatitis.*

Acute pancreatitis

- Diagnosis of acute pancreatitis is usually clinical and based on presentation of acute epigastric pain with markedly elevated serum amylase
- Although USG is an ideal investigation for bedside examination in the acutely ill patient, it has some limitations in the evaluation of acute pancreatitis. These include:
  1. The associated severe abdominal pain may not allow transducer pressure to be applied
  2. Air in the dilated transverse colon and small bowel loops (associated ileus) obscures visualization of the pancreas
  3. Changes associated with acute pancreatitis may be subtle on USG (Fig. 9g)

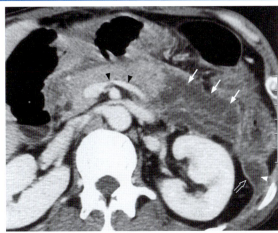

Fig.9f *Contrast enhanced axial computed tomography (CT) shows non-enhancement of the swollen pancreatic body and tail (arrows) compatible with pancreatic necrosis. The pancreatic head and neck are not enlarged and enhance normally. Note the inflammation in left paracolic gutter (arrowhead) and thickening of left Gerota's fascia (open arrow). Note the normal splenic vein (black arrowheads).*

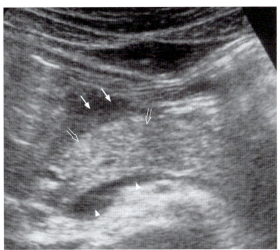

Fig.9g *Ultrasound shows pancreatitis change with peripancreatic fluid (arrows) in the region of pancreatic neck. The pancreas (open arrows) is not demonstrably swollen. Note the normal splenic vein (arrowheads) which is a useful landmark. Note the tail of the pancreas is not optimally seen as it is obscured by overlying air.*

Acute pancreatitis

- Role of imaging in acute pancreatitis includes:
  1. Exclude biliary cause of pancreatitis (i.e. gallstone-related cause) which necessitates early endoscopic intervention by ERCP
  2. Detect complications, including pancreatic necrosis (which carries a higher mortality than acute oedematous pancreatitis), abscess/pseudocyst formation, splenic artery pseudoaneurysm, splenic vein thrombosis (Fig. 9h).

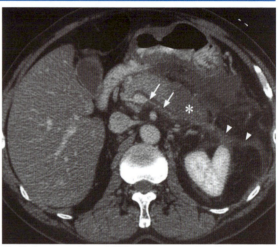

Fig.9h *Contrast enhanced CT in acute pancreatitis with oedematous pancreas (asterisk) inflammaling change in peripancreatic soft lesion, thickened Gerotia fascia (arrowheads). Note the absence of enhancement along the course of the splenic view (arrows), suggesting thrombosis. Compare it to the normally enhanced splenic vein in Fig. 9f.*

Note:

1. Imaging modality of choice for suspected acute pancreatitis is contrast-enhanced CT.
2. Swollen pancreas with inflammatory changes in adjacent structures are hallmark radiological features of acute pancreatitis.
3. Imaging helps to exclude biliary causes and detect complications.

Chronic pancreatitis

Chronic pancreatitis (Fig. 10a)

Discussion:

- Chronic pancreatitis represents on-going inflammatory pancreatic disease, characterized by irreversible damage to the pancreas.
- Alcoholism and gallstone disease are the commonest cause of chronic pancreatitis.
- The pathological changes are well-demonstrated using CT, these include:
  1. An atrophic pancreas, with irregular contours (Fig. 10b)
  2. Multiple coarse pancreatic calcifications, sometimes can be seen on AXR (Fig. 10c) or USG (Fig. 10d)
  3. Dilated pancreatic duct
  4. Inhomogeneous pancreatic parenchymal attenuation
     - indicates residual parenchymal tissue with intervening fibrosis
  5. Thickened surrounding membranes and fascia giving the organ ill-defined margins
  6. Biliary duct dilatation
- Acute attacks of pancreatitis (acute on chronic) may be marked by acute epigastric pain. In these cases, signs of acute inflammation may be present on imaging (Fig. 10e, f)

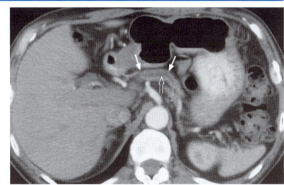

Fig.10b *Contrast enhanced axial computed tomography (CT) showing an atrophic pancreas (arrows) with dilated pancreatic duct (open arrows).*

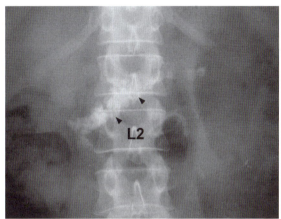

Fig.10c *Magnified AXR shows a cluster of coarse calcification (arrowheads) along the perceived location of the pancreas (L1 and L2 levels).*

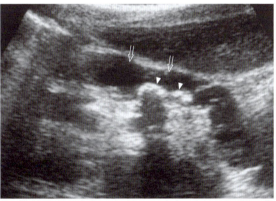

Fig.10d *Ultrasound shows evidence of chronic pancreatitis with multiple small calcifications (arrowheads) within a dilated pancreatic duct (open arrows).*

Discussion Case 10
Chronic pancreatitis

- Role of imaging in patients with suspected chronic pancreatitis:
  1. Confirm the clinical diagnosis
  2. Detect complications such as vascular thrombosis/ pseudoaneurysm and pseudocyst formation
- If contrast CT is not available, ultrasound abdomen or endoscopic retrograde cholangio-pancreatography (ERCP) would be suitable alternatives for diagnosis

Note:

(1) Chronic pancreatitis is characterized by multiple intraductal/parenchymal calcifications and pancreatic ductal dilatation.

(2) Contrast enhanced CT abdomen is the imaging modality of choice.

(3) ERCP or ultrasound is an alternative investigation if CT is not available.

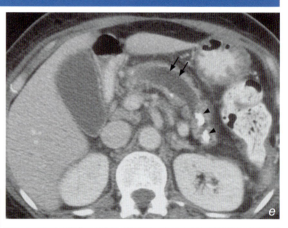

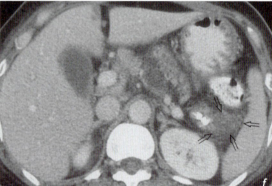

Fig.10e,f Contrast enhanced axial computed tomography (CT) showing evidence of acute on chronic pancreatitis. There is marked dilatation of the pancreatic duct (double arrow) and coarse calcification (arrowheads) indicating chronicity. There is increased peripancreatic density (open arrows) around the pancreatic tail indicating acute inflammation.

Discussion Case 11
Carcinoma of pancreas

Carcinoma of the head of the pancreas with multiple hepatic metastases (Fig. 11a, b)

Discussion:

- The pancreas is composed of exocrine (enzyme producing) and endocrine (hormone producing) tissue. Either component can develop into a neoplastic lesion, those of exocrine origin (adenomas and adenocarcinomas) are more common
- Adenocarcinoma of the pancreas is a common cause of painless obstructive jaundice in elderly patients (Fig. 11c, d)
- The head of the pancreas is the commonest site of involvement
- The imaging findings of adenocarcinoma of the pancreas include (Fig. 11a-f):
  1. Mass lesion in the pancreas (head more commonly affected than body or tail of pancreas)
  2. Tumour mass engulfing and narrowing superior mesenteric vessels
     - indicates vascular encasement
  3. Dilatation of pancreatic duct (due to obstruction by the tumour mass) and dilatation of intrahepatic and extrahepatic ducts (due to obstruction at the distal end of the common bile duct by the tumour)
  4. Peri-pancreatic and porta hepatis lymphadenopathy
     - represents regional nodal metastases
- CT is the most commonly used imaging modality for the diagnosis and staging of pancreatic neoplasms

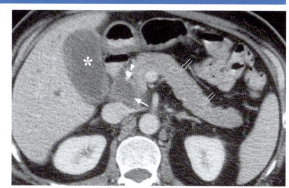

Fig. 11c *Contrast enhanced axial computed tomography (CT) shows a hypodense tumour in pancreatic head (arrow). The rest of the pancreas appears normal (open arrows). Note the presence of biliary stent (arrowhead) which was inserted to relieve common bile duct obstruction by the tumour. However, the gallbladder (asterisk) remains distended.*

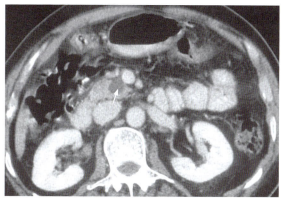

Fig. 11d *Contrast enhanced axial computed tomography (CT) of a patient who presented with weight loss. There is an incidental finding of a small cystic tumour in the pancreatic head (arrow). No mass effect or biliary obstruction is present in this case.*

Carcinoma of pancreas

- ERCP or ultrasound (Fig. 11g) abdomen are alternative modalities for investigation of patients with suspected pancreatic carcinoma
- Role of imaging in patients with obstructive jaundice:
  1. Determines the level and nature of biliary obstruction
  2. Confirms the diagnosis by imaging guided biopsy/fine needle aspiration
  3. Achieves biliary drainage by percutaneous transhepatic biliary drainage (PTBD)

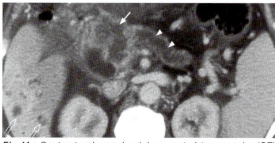

Fig.11e Contrast enhanced axial computed tomography (CT) showing a large necrotic tumour in the pancreatic head (arrow). The pancreatic duct is dilated (arrowheads). Note the presence of multiple small irregular hypodense lesions in right lobe of liver (open arrows) representing liver metastasis.

> **Note:**
> (1) Carcinoma of pancreas is a common cause of painless obstructive jaundice in elderly patients.
> (2) Contrast enhanced CT abdomen is the imaging modality of choice.
> (3) Heterogeneous mass with dilatation of pancreatic duct and biliary tree are typical radiological features of pancreatic head carcinoma.

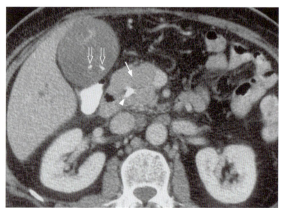

Fig.11f Contrast enhanced axial computed tomography (CT) showing a pancreatic head tumour (arrows) which appears as a bulky mass lesion with similar contrast enhancement as the surrounding normal pancreatic tissue. A biliary stent (arrowhead) was inserted to relieve common bile duct obstruction. Small gallstones (open arrows) are present in the distended gallbladder.

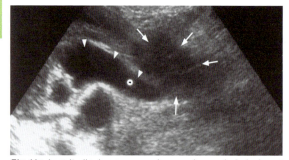

Fig.11g Longitudinal sonogram shows a hypoechoic lesion at pancreatic head (arrows). Note its mass effect with compression on the distal common bile duct causing proximal common duct dilatation (arrowheads).

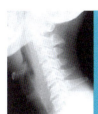

HEAD & NECK

Contributors:

K.T. Wong, Edmund H.Y. Yuen, Ann D. King, Anil T. Ahuja

Questions

Case 1 - 9   396 - 404

Discussion

Impacted foreign body	405 - 406
Acute epiglottitis	407 - 408
Retropharyngeal abscess	409 - 410
Sinusitis	411 - 412
Carotid-cavernous fistula	413 - 414
Parathyroid adenoma	415 - 417
Acoustic neuroma	418 - 420
Optic neuritis	421 - 422
Orbital fracture	423 - 424

Chapter 09

Case 1

A 64-year-old man presented with persistent foreign body sensation for 3 days. The uncomfortable feeling began after dinner and has gradually become worse. A direct laryngoscopy in the emergency department did not reveal any impacted foreign body. A plain radiograph of the neck was performed for further investigation (Fig. 1a).

Questions

(1) What abnormality is seen on the lateral neck radiograph ?
- Curvilinear calcific density impacted in the retropharyngeal soft tissues.
- Thickening of the retropharyngeal soft tissues raising the suspicion of secondary infection.
- Loss of cervical lordosis suggesting muscle spasm.

(2) What is the diagnosis ?

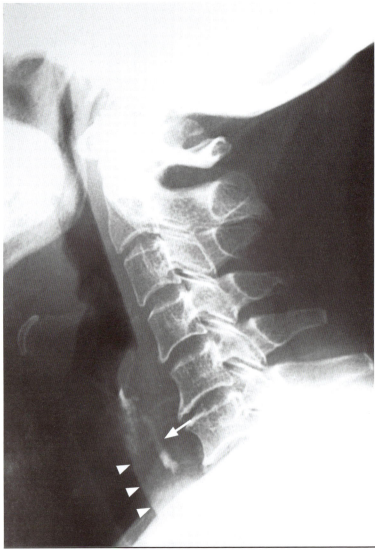

Fig.1a *Lateral radiograph of the neck shows a radio-opaque foreign body (fish bone, [arrow]) impacted at the level of pharyngo-oesophageal junction. There is associated retropharyngeal soft tissue swelling (arrowheads) causing anterior bulging of the trachea.*

Case 2

A 47-year-old man presented to the emergency department with difficulty in breathing, high fever and sore throat for 2 days. On physical examination, the patient was septic looking and dyspnoeic with an audible inspiratory stridor. He was stable otherwise with an SaO2 of 92% on room air. A lateral radiograph of the neck was performed (Fig. 2a).

Questions

(1) What abnormalities are seen on this radiograph ?
   - Markedly swollen epiglottis with 'thumb-printing' appearance
   - Thickening of aryepiglottic folds
(2) What is the diagnosis ?

HEAD & NECK

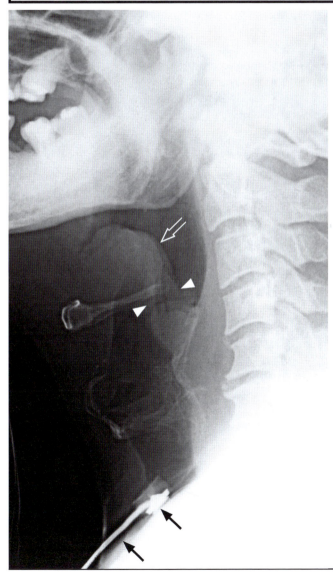

Fig.2a Lateral radiograph of the neck shows a markedly thickened epiglottis (open arrow) – 'thumb sign'. Also note the thickened aryepiglottic folds (arrowheads) due to tracking of the infection from epiglottis. Features are highly suggestive of acute epiglottitis. Note the tube in the trachea to maintain the air way (arrows).

Case 3

A 42-year-old man presented to the emergency department with severe sore throat and painful swallowing. He was running a fever of 39 °C, and physical examination revealed a rigid neck and inflammatory change of the oropharyngeal mucosa. A lateral radiograph of the neck was performed for further evaluation (Fig. 3a).

Questions

(1) What abnormalities are seen on this radiograph ?
- Widened retropharyngeal soft tissues
- A localized gas locule in the retropharyngeal space

(2) What is the diagnosis ?

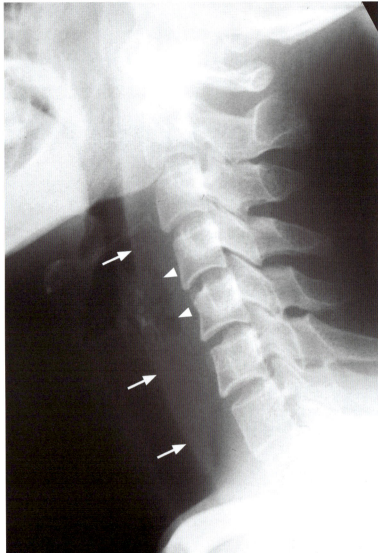

Fig.3a Lateral radiograph of the neck shows thickening of the retropharyngeal soft tissues (arrows) and localized gas lucency within (arrowheads) suggestive of a retropharyngeal abscess.

Case 4

A 23-year-old man complained of repeated episodes of intermittent nasal obstruction and purulent discharge not responding to treatment. As a part of imaging of the sinuses, plain radiographs (Fig. 4a, b, c) and CT (Fig. 4d, e) of paranasal sinuses was performed.

Questions

(1) What do you see on the plain radiographs and CT of the sinuses ?

Plain radiographs:
- Loss of normal aeration and opacification of the left maxillary and frontal sinuses
- No obvious bone destruction

CT sinuses:
- Opacification of left frontal, maxillary and anterior ethmoid sinuses
- Sclerosis of the bony sinus wall in the form of thickening and increased density

(2) <u>What is the most likely diagnosis ?</u>

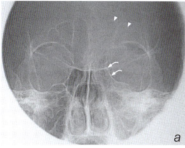

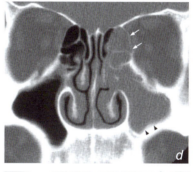

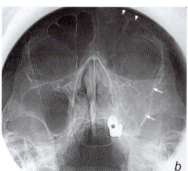

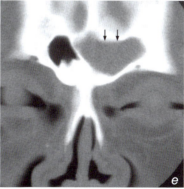

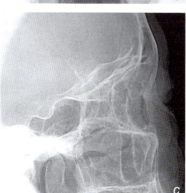

Fig.4a,b,c
Radiographs of the paranasal sinuses in (a) frontal view, (b) Water's view and (c) lateral view show opacification of the left maxillary (arrows), left frontal (arrowheads) and left ethmoid sinuses (curved arrows). Note the normal appearances of well-aerated frontal and maxillary sinuses on the right. There is no obvious associated bone destruction. Asterisk identifies metallic dental work.

Fig.4d,e Coronal non-enhanced CT of paranasal sinuses shows complete opacification of left frontal sinus (arrows in [e]), left anterior ethmoid sinus (arrows in [d]) and left maxillary sinus (arrowheads in [d]). Subtle sclerotic bone changes in the sinus walls indicate the chronicity of sinusitis.

09 HEAD & NECK

Case 5

A 65-year-old woman presented with gradual onset left eye proptosis and redness for 2 months. On examination there was increased intraocular pressure, restricted extraocular movement and a persistent orbital bruit. A carotid-cavernous fistula was suspected and an urgent CT of the orbit was performed (Fig. 5a, b).

Questions

(1) What abnormality do you see on the initial CT of the orbit ?
  - Enlargement of the left superior ophthalmic vein
  - Diffuse enlargement of extraocular muscles on the left
(2) <u>What is the diagnosis ?</u>

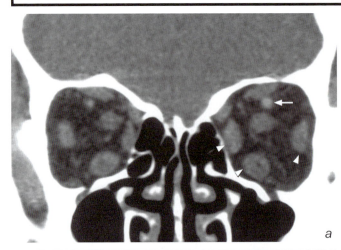
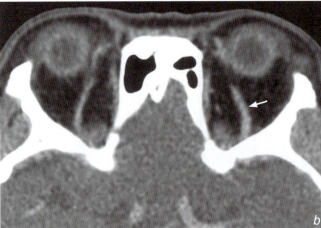

Fig.5a,b *(a) Coronal & (b) axial contrast enhanced CT orbit shows enlargement of the left superior ophthalmic vein (arrow) and diffuse enlargement of extraocular muscles in the left orbit (arrowheads) in a patient with carotid-cavernous fistula.*

Case 6

A 56-year-old woman presented with weight loss, generalized malaise and muscle weakness for 6 months. Physical examination revealed a mild degree of proximal muscle weakness in both upper and lower limbs. Routine biochemical tests showed elevated serum calcium level and parathyroid hormone level. The clinical diagnosis was primary hyperparathyroidism and an ultrasound examination of the neck was performed (Fig. 6a,b).

Questions
(1) What abnormality do you see on this ultrasound of the neck ?
   - Solitary well-defined round hypoechoic nodule posterior to the lower pole of left thyroid gland
(2) What is the diagnosis ?

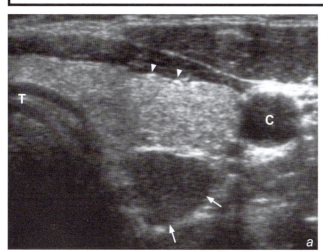

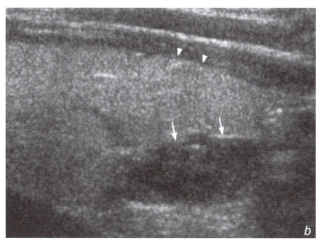

Fig.6a,b (a) *Transverse and* **(b)** *longitudinal grey scale sonograms of the neck show a well-defined homogeneous hypoechoic nodule (arrows) posterior to the lower pole of left lobe of thyroid gland (arrowheads). In a patient with biochemical evidence of primary hyperparathyroidism, it most likely represents a parathyroidadenoma. T=Trachea, C=Common carotid artery.*

Case 7

A 65-year-old man presented with gradual onset right sided hearing loss in the recent 5 months. Pure tone audiogram revealed high tone sensorineural hearing loss on the right side and an MRI examination was performed (Fig. 7a, b, c).

Questions

(1) What abnormalities do you see on this MRI ?
- Soft tissue mass centred at right cerebellopontine angle
- Homogeneous enhancement after intravenous gadolinium administration
- Intracanalicular extension of the mass into the right internal acoustic meatus

(2) What is the diagnosis ?

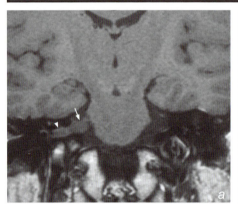
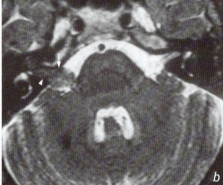
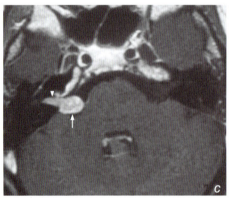

Fig.7a,b,c *(a) Coronal T1-weighted, (b) axial T2-weighted and (c) axial post-gadolinium enhanced T1-weighted MR image show a homogeneously enhancing mass centred at the right cerebellopontine angle (arrow) with extension along the 7th-8th nerve complex into the right internal acoustic meatus (arrowhead). Features are typical of an acoustic neuroma.*

Case 8

A 29-year-old woman presented with visual loss of acute onset and pain on movement of the right eye for 2 months. Examination of the fundi was unremarkable and an MRI examination of orbits and brain was performed (Fig. 8a, b, c).

Questions

(1) What is the imaging abnormality ?
- Smooth thickening of the right optic nerve
- Homogeneous enhancement following intravenous gadolinium administration

(2) What is the diagnosis ?

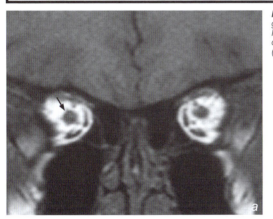

Fig.8a,b,c *(a) Coronal T1-weighted; post-gadolinium fat-suppressed (b) axial & (c) coronal MRI of orbit shows smooth thickening of the right optic nerve with homogeneous enhancement (arrows) in a patient with right optic neuritis.*

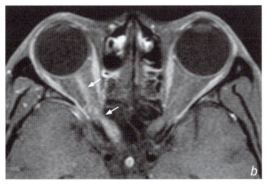

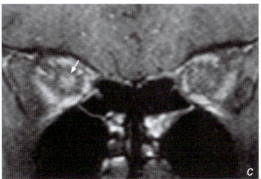

Case 9

A 28-year-old man involved in a road traffic accident sustained blunt injury to his left eye. Clinically there was left periorbital swelling and bruising and examination of the extraocular eye movement showed impaired vertical gaze with associated diplopia. A CT of the orbit and brain was performed for further evaluation (Fig. 9a, b).

Questions

(1) What abnormality do you see on this CT of the orbit ?
  - Fracture of the floor of left orbit
  - Herniation of extraconal fat and inferior rectus muscle into the roof of left maxillary sinus
  - Orbital emphysema
(2) What is the diagnosis ?

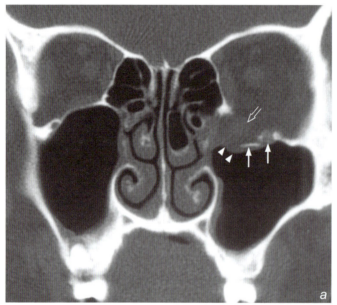

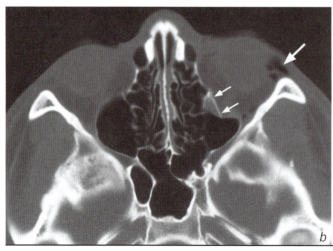

Fig.9a,b (a) Coronal and (b) axial CT orbit (bone window) show fractures of the floor of left orbit (arrows) with herniation of extraconal fat (arrowheads) and inferior rectus muscle (open arrow) into the roof of left maxillary sinus. Note orbital emphysema (large arrow), a clue to the presence of a fracture.

Discussion Case 1
Impacted foreign body

Radio-opaque foreign body, probably a piece of bone (Fig. 1a).

Discussion:

- The tonsillar fossae, tongue base, valleculae and pyriform fossae are the common sites of impaction
- Swallowed fish and chicken bones are the usual culprits
- Radiography is usually not necessary if the impacted foreign body can be detected on clinical examination and removed, especially if it is impacted at the tonsillar fossa/tongue base. Imaging is useful in patients with a high clinical index of suspicion but negative physical findings
- Small, slender foreign bodies may not appear radio-opaque on a radiograph
- Care must be taken not to confuse the ossified laryngeal cartilage (hyoid, thyroid and cricoid) as foreign bodies (Fig. 1b). Laryngeal cartilaginous ossification may appear irregular and heterogeneous but they remain confined to their anatomical location
- Widened retropharyngeal and parapharyngeal soft tissues may suggest secondary infection
- Abnormal location of gas such as surgical emphysema or pneumomediastinum is suggestive of secondary perforation (Fig. 1c, d)
- In patients with suspected perforation of a hollow viscus, one must not use barium in a 'swallow' study. Contact of barium with the mediastinum or peritoneum results in a severe inflammatory reaction and may result in potentially fatal mediastinitis/peritonitis. Iodinated water soluble contrast should be used in such cases.

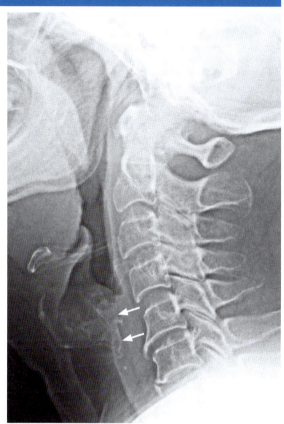

Fig.1b *Lateral radiograph of the neck shows normal ossification of the thyroid cartilage (arrows) which may be mistaken for an impacted radio-opaque foreign body. The typical coarse nodular configuration of the ossification and its location are key features to avoid misdiagnosis.*

Discussion Case 1
Impacted foreign body

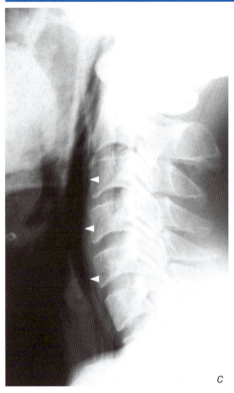

c

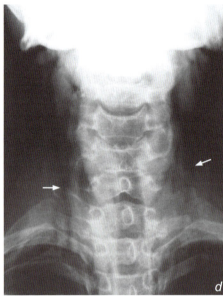

d

Fig.1c,d Lateral (c) and frontal (d) radiograph of the neck shows abnormal gas lucencies in subcutaneous soft tissues of neck (arrows) and within the retropharyngeal soft tissue (arrowheads) indicating surgical/ subcutaneous emphysema, due to a secondary perforation in a patient with impacted foreign body.

Note:
(1) Radiographs may be helpful in locating an impacted foreign body if clinical examination is negative in patients with a high index of suspicion clinically.
(2) Complications such as secondary infection/abscess formation and perforation should be carefully looked for on the radiograph.

Discussion Case 2
Acute epiglottitis

Acute epiglottitis (Fig. 2a)

Discussion:

- Acute epiglottitis is an acute, potentially fulminating infection of the upper airway and commonly occurs in children between 2 and 6 years of age (but can also occur in adults)
- The most common causative agent is Haemophilus influenzae type B
- If there is high clinical index of suspicion of acute epiglottitis, every effort should be made to minimize patient manipulation as this may exacerbate the degree of upper airway obstruction. Therefore a lateral radiograph of the neck helps to confirm the diagnosis without having to examine the epiglottis.
- Further imaging is usually not necessary as prompt treatment is instituted
- Retropharyngeal abscess and laryngotracheobronchitis (croup) share a common clinical presentation with acute epiglottitis. Plain radiograph may help to differentiate these conditions:
  (1) Retropharyngeal abscess
      - Widened retropharyngeal soft tissues (Fig. 2b)
      - Focal gas collection within the retropharyngeal soft tissues
  (2) Laryngotracheobronchitis (croup)
      - Narrowing of the subglottic airway (Steeple sign, Fig. 2c)
      - Over-distension of the hypopharynx
      - Normal epiglottis and retropharyngeal soft tissues

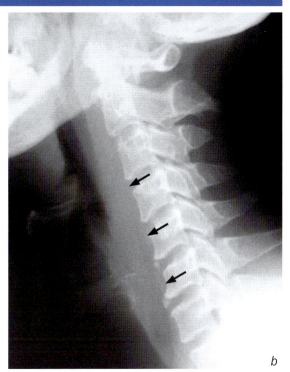

b

Fig.2b *Lateral radiograph of the neck shows thickening of the retropharyngeal soft tissues (arrows) in a patient with retropharyngeal abscess. Also note the normal appearance of epiglottis and aryepiglottic folds in this patient.*

Fig.2c *Frontal radiograph of the neck and upper thorax shows a smooth narrowing of the subglottic airway (arrows) - 'Steeple sign' - in a child with laryngotracheobronchitis (croup).*

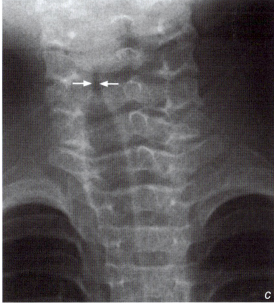

c

Discussion Case 2
Acute epiglottitis

Note:

(1) A swollen epiglottis on a lateral neck radiograph in the appropriate clinical context confirms the diagnosis of acute epiglottitis. Further imaging is usually not necessary as prompt treatment is crucial.

(2) Plain radiographs help to differentiate it from retropharyngeal abscess and laryngotracheobronchitis (croup) which may clinically mimic acute epiglottitis.

Discussion Case 3
Retropharyngeal abscess

Retropharyngeal abscess (Fig. 3a)
- A contrast enhanced CT neck was performed (Fig. 3b) which showed:
- Prominent retropharyngeal soft tissues
- Large rim-enhancing lesions with necrotic centre in retropharyngeal soft tissue consistent with an abscess

Discussion:
Retropharyngeal abscess -
- May originate from dental disease, pharyngitis, rupture of suppurative retropharyngeal lymphadenitis, penetrating trauma (+/- foreign body) and vertebral osteomyelitis.
  - Plain radiograph findings include:
    - widened retropharyngeal space (non-specific)
      - on a lateral radiograph the prevertebral soft tissues from C1 to C3/4 levels should only be a few mm thick. Below this level its thickness should not exceed ¾ of the AP diameter of the corresponding vertebra.
      - gas locules (highly suggestive of abscess formation)
- CT findings:
  - Prevertebral retropharyngeal soft tissue swelling
  - Oedematous and necrotic tissues appear hypodense
  - Ring enhancement indicates capsular formation around the abscess
  - Gas locules (specific for an abscess)
  - Fat streakiness/stranding of adjacent tissues indicate inflammatory change
  - The retropharyngeal space extends from the skull base down to the T4 level. It is therefore essential that the examination covers this entire region for adequate visualization of the abscess.
- The role of CT for suspected retropharyngeal abscess is:
  (1) Helps to confirm the diagnosis
  (2) Delineates the exact extent of abscess involvement; in particular, involvement of parapharyngeal space and mediastinum which may alter surgical management (Fig. 3c).

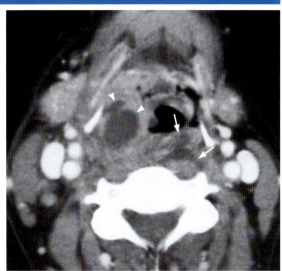

Fig.3b *Contrast enhanced axial CT of the neck shows soft tissue thickening and pus collections in retropharyngeal space (arrows) and right hypopharynx (arrowheads).*

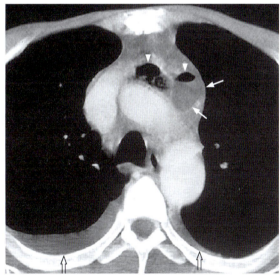

Fig.3c *Contrast enhanced axial CT of superior mediastinum shows pus tracking down from retropharyngeal space to the superior mediastinum anterior to the aortic arch (arrows). The presence of gas (arrowheads) within the collection supports the diagnosis of abscess formation in the mediastinum. Note the small pleural effusions (open arrows) bilaterally.*

Retropharyngeal abscess

(3) Exclude underlying predisposing factors such as a foreign body.

> **Note:**
> (1) Gas locules within widened retropharyngeal soft tissues on plain radiographs in the appropriate clinical setting is highly suggestive of retropharyngeal abscess.
> (2) CT is the imaging modality of choice for exact anatomical localization and extent of the abscess.

Sinusitis

Chronic sinusitis (Fig. 4a-e) involving left maxillary, frontal and ethmoid sinuses.

Discussion:

- Acute sinusitis is usually the result of bacterial superinfection of viral rhinitis and usually responds to antibiotic treatment, and further investigation (including imaging) is usually not required
- Chronic sinusitis is related to obstruction of normal mucociliary drainage pathway of paranasal sinuses. The accumulation of secretion predisposes to chronic inflammation and secondary infection (often caused by a combination of aerobic and anaerobic flora)
- Knowledge about the normal mucociliary drainage pathway is therefore necessary:
  (1) The middle meatus drains the frontal, maxillary and anterior ethmoid sinuses
  (2) The sphenoethmoidal recess drains the posterior ethmoid and sphenoid sinuses
- Standard radiographic projections for paranasal sinuses include:
  (1) Frontal view - demonstrates frontal and ethmoid sinuses
  (2) Waters' view - demonstrates maxillary and frontal sinuses
  (3) Lateral view - demonstrates sphenoid sinuses (note: maxillary, ethmoid and frontal sinuses are overlapped)
- Plain radiographs are unable to provide anatomical detail (due to overlap of structures) and delineate the entire extent of the sinus disease
- CT of the paranasal sinuses is indicated in the following circumstances:
  - when the diagnosis is uncertain
  - chronic sinusitis unresponsive to medical therapy
  - to look for complications of sinusitis

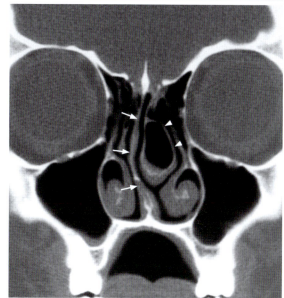

Fig.4f *Coronal non-contrast CT of paranasal sinuses shows deviation of nasal septum to the right (arrows) and a large concha bullosa on the left (arrowheads) – pneumatization of middle turbinate.*

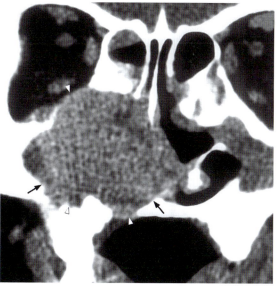

Fig.4g *Coronal contrast enhanced CT of paranasal sinuses shows an infiltrative soft tissue mass in the right maxillary sinus (arrows) causing adjacent bony destruction (involving lateral and inferior sinus walls, floor of right orbit and lateral wall of right nasal cavity, arrowheads) and tumour extension to the nasal cavity. The appearances are suggestive of a malignant tumour (biopsy proven squamous cell carcinoma).*

09 HEAD & NECK

411

- to delineate the exact location and extent of sinus disease, and to identify anatomical variations (e.g. large concha bullosa, deviated nasal septum (Fig. 4f) for surgical planning
- to provide navigation for intraoperative guidance
- when malignancy is suspected (Fig. 4g)
- The goal of Functional Endoscopic Sinus Surgery (FESS) is to establish patency of the obstructed drainage pathway with minimal anatomical distortion. It may include uncinectomy, infundibular/ostial enlargement, bullectomy, ethmoidectomy and sphenoidectomy (Fig. 4h)

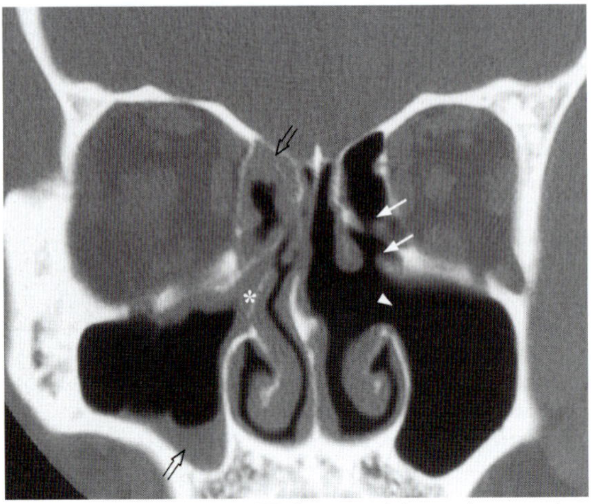

Fig.4h Coronal non-contrast CT of paranasal sinuses shows previous left ethmoidectomy (arrows) and left uncinectomy with widened left infundibulum (arrowhead) in a patient with history of functional endoscopic sinus surgery (FESS). Note the presence of chronic sinusitis in right anterior ethmoid and maxillary sinus (open arrows) and intact right uncinate process (asterisk).

Note:
(1) Uncomplicated cases of acute sinusitis are managed medically and CT is not routinely indicated.
(2) Imaging (usually coronal CT) is indicated in chronic sinusitis with atypical features, or when complications are suspected or surgical intervention is considered.

09 HEAD & NECK

Carotid-cavernous fistula

Left carotid-cavernous fistula (Fig. 5a, b)

Discussion:

- Carotid-cavernous fistula is an abnormal communication between the cavernous portion of internal carotid artery and veins of cavernous sinus
- It is most commonly post-traumatic in origin and spontaneous rupture of an aneurysm in the cavernous portion of internal carotid artery is a less common cause
- Patients usually present with pulsating exophthalmos, chemosis and conjunctival oedema
- Enlargement of the superior ophthalmic vein (due to high flow) is an important clue on CT
- An MR angiogram may allow accurate depiction of the carotid-cavernous fistula and abnormal blood flow within venous sinuses and superior ophthalmic vein (Fig. 5c, d)

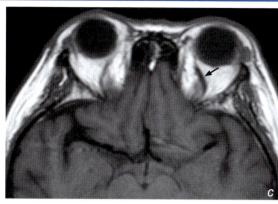

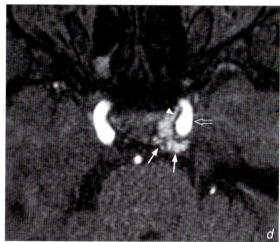

Fig.5c,d *(c) Axial T1-weighted MR of orbit shows engorgement of the left superior ophthalmic vein (arrow). (d) MR angiogram shows the presence of hyperintense flow signal in the left cavernous sinus (arrows) with a fistula (arrowhead) arising from the adjacent cavernous portion of left internal carotid artery (open arrow).*

Discussion Case 5
Carotid-cavernous fistula

- Conventional angiography is usually not necessary for diagnosis and is mainly reserved for suspected cases with equivocal findings on CT/MRI and for trans-catheter intervention (Fig. 5e, f)
- Embolization of the carotid-cavernous fistula is the treatment of choice for most cases and has a high success rate. Following a successful procedure the ocular signs resolve in a week to 10 days.

Note:

(1) Carotid-cavernous fistula should be suspected in patients with pulsating proptosis and chemosis.

(2) Enlargement of superior ophthalmic vein and enlargement of extra-ocular muscles are clues to the diagnosis on CT/ MRI.

(3) MR angiogram allows direct visualization of the fistula between internal carotid artery and cavernous sinus.

(4) Trans-catheter embolization is the initial treatment of choice for most cases.

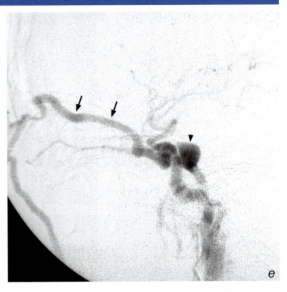

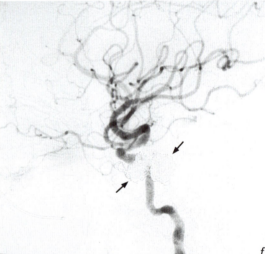

Fig. 5e,f *(e) Digital subtraction angiogram (lateral projection) of left internal carotid artery shows early contrast opacification of cavernous sinus (arrowhead) and superior ophthalmic vein (arrows). (f) The carotid-cavernous fistula is successfully treated with embolization with complete obliteration of the fistula upon deployment of embolization coils (arrows).*

Parathyroid adenoma

Parathyroid adenoma (in view of the clinical history and biochemical findings, Fig. 6a, b)

Discussion:
- The clinical symptoms of primary hyperparathyroidism may be non-specific, and the diagnosis is based on biochemical tests showing elevated serum calcium and parathyroid hormone level.
- A solitary parathyroid adenoma is the underlying cause in approximately 85%. Less common causes include multiple adenomas, parathyroid hyperplasia, parathyroid carcinoma and parathyroid cyst
- Typical ultrasound features of parathyroid adenoma include:
  1. Ovoid/round well-defined homogeneous hypoechoic nodule
  2. Posterior to and separated from thyroid gland
  3. Larger lesion may appear heterogeneous in echopattern (Fig. 6c)
  4. Calcification is rare
  5. Hypervascular on power Doppler ultrasound (Fig. 6d)

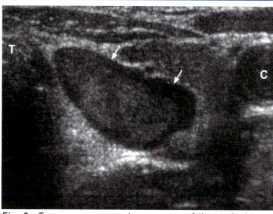

Fig. 6c *Transverse grey scale sonogram of the neck shows a heterogeneous echopattern in a large arrowhead shaped parathyroid adenoma (arrows) T=trachea, C=common carotid artery.*

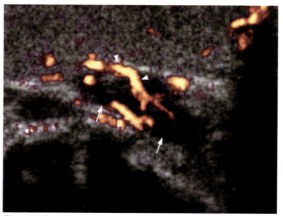

Fig. 6d *Power Doppler sonogram shows hypervascularity (arrowheads) within a parathyroid adenoma (arrows).*

09 HEAD & NECK

415

Discussion Case 6
Parathyroid adenoma

- SestaMIBI scintigraphy offers both functional and anatomical delineation of hyperactive parathyroid glands.
- Abnormal parathyroid glands show increased tracer uptake with delayed washout. If there is a solitary focus of increased tracer uptake (Fig. 6e), parathyroid adenoma is the most likely diagnosis. Alternatively if there are multiple 'hot spots' or diffuse uptake in the thyroid area, parathyroid hyperplasia should be suspected
- CT and MRI may be used for detection of parathyroid adenoma and typical features include:
CT (Fig. 6f) -
1. Soft tissue nodule posterior to/ closely related to the thyroid gland
2. Homogeneous enhancement after intravenous contrast administration
MRI (Fig. 6g) -
1. Soft tissue nodule in close proximity to thyroid gland
2. Intermediate signal on T1WI
3. Hyperintense on T2WI, especially with fat suppression technique
4. Homogeneous enhancement after i.v. gadolinium
- Which investigation is most suitable to detect parathyroid adenoma?
1. If expertise with ultrasound is available, then it is the ideal initial imaging technique as it is easily available, inexpensive and does not use ionizing radiation or intravenous contrast. If a parathyroid adenoma is clearly demonstrated then the surgeon may choose to proceed to surgery directly (as the incidence of a double adenoma is quite low, <4%) without any further imaging. However, in many centres sestaMIBI is often used as the initial imaging technique as it demonstrates multiple lesions and the presence of an adenoma at unusual sites. However, it involves radiation and may not be available in all centres.

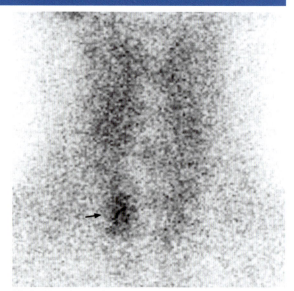

Fig.6e *Planar image of sestaMIBI scintigraphy shows a solitary focus of increased tracer activity in the right lower neck (arrow) compatible with a hyperfunctioning parathyroid adenoma (in the appropriate clinical / biochemical setting).*

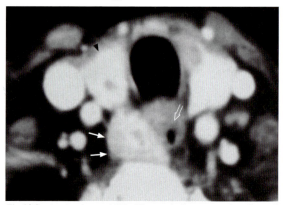

Fig.6f *Contrast enhanced CT of the neck shows an enhancing soft tissue nodule (arrows) closely related to the lower pole of right thyroid gland (arrowhead) and cervical oesophagus (open arrow) compatible with a parathyroid adenoma (in the appropriate clinical / biochemical setting).*

Parathyroid adenoma

A combination of ultrasound and sestaMIBI is able to identify almost all lesions and helps in pre-operative localization of the adenoma prior to minimally invasive parathyroidectomy.

2. In some centres cross-sectional imaging such as CT/MRI may be used. However, they are relatively expensive, involve ionizing radiation (for CT) and require intravenous contrast injection.

3. Rarely venous assays may be done in identifying difficult lesions where all other imaging techniques have failed. However, it is an invasive technique and is not used as the initial imaging test.

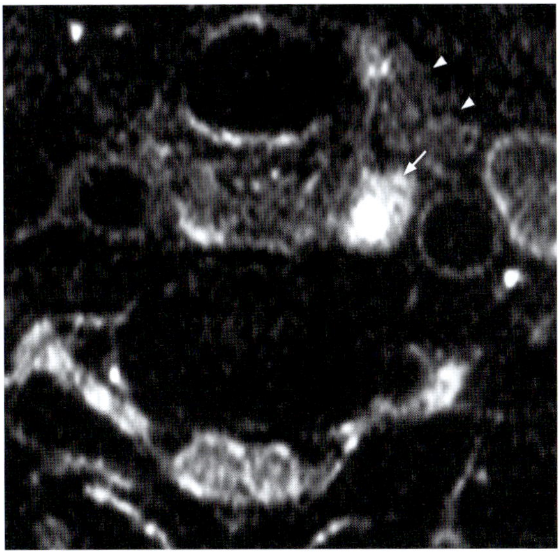

Fig.6g *Axial fat-suppressed T2-weighted MR image of the neck shows a hyperintense nodule (arrow) posterior to the lower pole of left thyroid gland (arrowheads) compatible with a parathyroid adenoma (in the appropriate clinical / biochemical setting).*

Note:

(1) Diagnosis of primary hyperparathyroidism is based on biochemical tests. The role of imaging is mainly for detection of underlying cause.

(2) Parathyroid adenoma is the most common cause of primary hyperparathyroidism.

(3) A combination of ultrasound and sestaMIBI helps to identify most lesions and aids in pre-operative localization of an adenoma prior to minimally invasive surgery.

09 HEAD & NECK

417

Acoustic neuroma

Acoustic neuroma (Fig. 7a-c)

Discussion:
- An acoustic neuroma is a benign encapsulated neoplasm arising from Schwann cells of the 7th-8th cranial nerves (more commonly affecting the vestibular component of the 8th cranial nerve) (Fig. 7d)
- Unilateral/asymmetric sensorineural hearing loss is its commonest clinical presentation
- Acoustic neuroma is the most common tumour in the cerebellopontine angle. Other less common lesions include meningioma, arachnoid cyst and epidermoid cyst.
- Sometimes acoustic neuroma may be purely intracanalicular (without involvement of CP angle) (Fig. 7e) or in close proximity to the 5th cranial nerve (Fig. 7f)
- MRI is the imaging modality of choice for investigation of patients with unilateral/asymmetric sensorineural hearing loss due to its excellent resolution and multiplanar capability

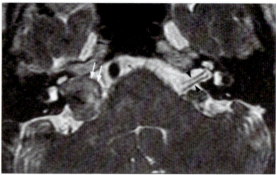

Fig.7d *Axial T2-weighted MR shows an acoustic neuroma (arrows) occupying right CP angle with intracanalicular extension along the expected course of right 7th/8th nerve complex. Note the normal left 7th and 8th cranial nerve on the left (arrowheads).*

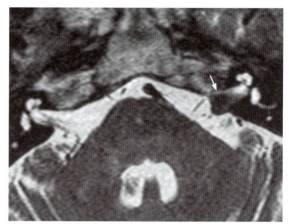

Fig.7e *Axial T2-weighted MR shows homogeneously enhancing left acoustic neuroma with pure intracanalicular component (arrow).*

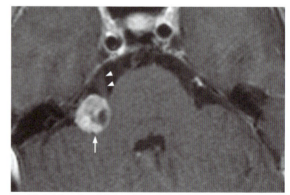

Fig.7f *Axial post-gadolinium T1-weighted MR shows right acoustic neuroma (arrow) in the right CP angle touching the right 5th cranial nerve (arrowheads).*

Discussion Case 7
Acoustic neuroma

- Typical MRI features of acoustic neuroma include:
  1. Slightly hypointense/isointense on T1WI
  2. Slightly hypointense/isointense on T2WI
  3. Intense homogeneous enhancement
  4. Heterogeneous enhancement/cystic changes in large tumours (Fig. 7g)
- Bilateral acoustic neuromas are seen in patients with Type II neurofibromatosis (Fig. 7h)

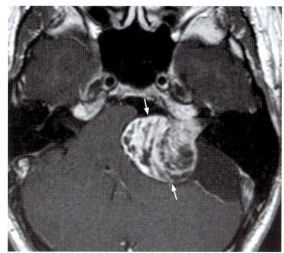

Fig.7g *Axial post-gadolinium enhanced T1-weighted MR shows a large left acoustic neuroma with enhancement (arrows). Note the mass effect on adjacent pons and left cerebellar hemisphere.*

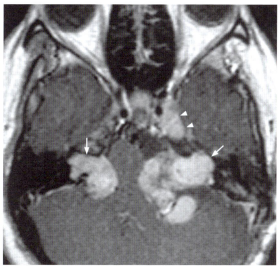

Fig.7h *Axial T1-weighted post-gadolinium MR of a patient with neurofibromatosis type 2 shows bilateral acoustic neuromas (arrows) and left trigeminal nerve neuroma (arrowheads).*

Discussion Case 7
Acoustic neuroma

- MRI also helps to detect residual tumour after excision (Fig. 7k, l) and tumour recurrence.

Note:
(1) MRI is the imaging modality of choice for investigation of patients with unilateral/asymmetric sensorineural hearing loss.
(2) On MRI an acoustic neuroma is typically seen as a homogeneously enhancing soft tissue mass in cerebellopontine angle with/without extension into internal acoustic meatus.

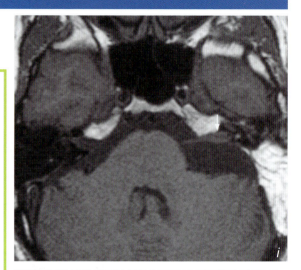

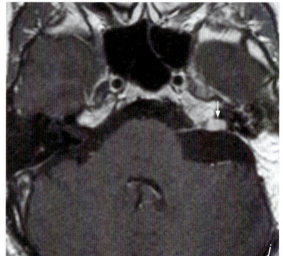

Fig.7i,j *(i) Axial T1-weighted, (j) axial post-gadolinium T1-weighted MR shows a small residual tumour in the left internal acoustic meatus with homogeneous enhancement (arrow) in a patient 3 months after excision of a left acoustic neuroma.*

Discussion Case 8
Optic neuritis

Optic neuritis (in view of the clinical history, Fig. 8a-c)

Discussion:

- Pathologically optic neuritis is characterized by acute inflammation, degeneration and demyelination involving the optic nerve.
- There is high association of optic neuritis and multiple sclerosis:
  1. One-third of patients with multiple sclerosis have optic nerve neuritis
  2. 45-80% of patients develop multiple sclerosis within 15 years of their first episode of optic neuritis
- Optic nerve tumour may mimic optic neuritis clinically and radiologically:
  1. Optic nerve glioma (Fig. 8d, e)
     - more common in children, usually 1st decade of life
     - MRI findings include:
       - isointense to muscle on T1WI
       - hyperintense on T2WI
       - slight contrast enhancement
  2. Optic nerve meningioma (Fig. 8f)
     - more common in middle-aged females
     - MRI findings include:
       - extrinsic soft tissue mass surrounding optic nerve
       - hypointense to fat on T1WI
       - hyperintense on T2WI
       - homogeneous contrast enhancement
- MRI is better than CT for depiction of orbital lesions due to its high resolution, multiplanar capability and its non-ionizing nature (the eye is a radio-sensitive organ)

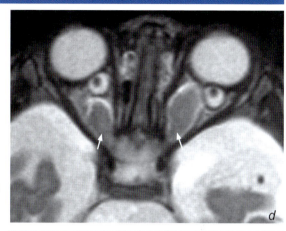

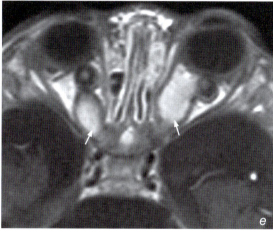

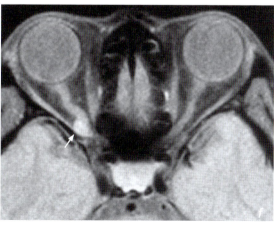

Fig.8d,e (d) Axial fat-suppressed T2-weighted & (e) axial post-gadolinium T1-weighted MR images of a child show globular soft tissue thickening with homogeneous enhancement of both optic nerves (arrows). The imaging appearances and patient's age suggest bilateral optic nerve gliomas in neurofibromatosis type 1.

Fig.8f Axial post-gadolinium fat-suppressed T1-weighted MR of orbit shows an eccentric homogeneously enhancing soft tissue mass along the posterior portion of right optic nerve (arrow) in a patient with optic nerve meningioma.

<u>**Note:**</u>
(1) MRI is the imaging modality of choice for investigation of patients with suspected intraorbital lesions such as optic neuritis.
(2) On MRI smooth thickening of optic nerve with homogeneous enhancement should suggest the diagnosis of optic neuritis (in the proper clinical setting).
(3) Its high association with multiple sclerosis must be borne in mind.

Discussion Case 9
Orbital fracture

Fracture floor of left orbital with inferior
rectus entrapment (Fig. 9a, b)

Discussion:

- Orbital fracture is commonly seen in
  patients with direct blunt injury to
  the maxillofacial area. Blunt trauma
  to the orbit results in in-drawing of
  the globe causing an abrupt increase
  in the intra-orbital pressure. The
  outcome is burst fractures of the
  orbital walls, most commonly the
  orbital floor and medial orbital wall
  (lamina papyracea)
- On plain radiography, orbital
  fractures may be difficult to detect
  due to overlapping bony structures.
  Signs that may help to identify orbital
  trauma include:
  1. Orbital emphysema (Fig. 9c, d)
  2. Air-fluid level within adjacent
     maxillary sinus
  3. Soft tissue with a tear-drop
     appearance projected over roof of
     maxillary sinus
- The exact anatomical extent,
  complexity of orbital fractures and
  trauma to other structures such as the
  lens is better appreciated by CT (Fig.
  9e)

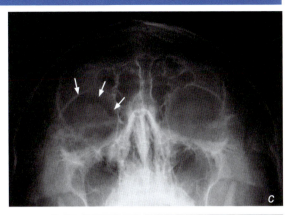

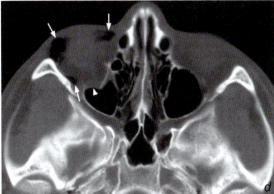

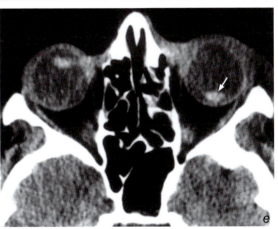

Fig. 9c,d (c) Frontal radiograph of the skull
shows a rim of gas density along the roof of
right orbit (arrows) indicating the presence
of orbital emphysema. Although there is no
definite fracture seen on this radiograph,
the presence of orbital emphysema raises a
high suspicion of underlying orbital fracture
communicating with adjacent paranasal
sinuses. The diagnosis is confirmed by an
axial CT scan (d) showing fracture of the
floor of right orbit (arrowhead) and orbital
emphysema (arrows). Note that the subtle
presence of air on the plain x-ray may have
been easily missed.

Fig.9e Axial CT of orbit shows posterior lens
dislocation within the left globe (arrow). Note
the normal position of the lens within the
anterior portion of the right globe.

Discussion Case 9
Orbital fracture

- Orbital contents including eyeball (Fig. 9f) orbital fat and extra-ocular muscles may herniate through the burst fractures, and entrapment of the extra-ocular muscles results in diplopia (Fig. 9a, g). This may require surgical intervention to prevent fibrosis and permanent impairment. Three-dimensional reconstructed CT images provide a pre-operative road-map prior to any reconstruction (Fig. 9h).

Note:

(1) CT is better than plain radiography for detection and delineation of the extent of orbital trauma.

(2) Inferior rectus muscle entrapment must be excluded if there is any impairment of extra-ocular movement.

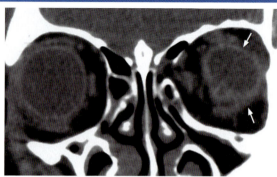

Fig.9f *Coronal non-contrast CT in a patient with orbital trauma shows a small, ill-defined, deformed left eyeball (arrows) consistent with a ruptured eyeball. Compare it with the normal opposite eyeball.*

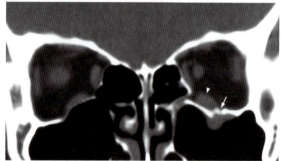

Fig.9g *Coronal CT of the orbit shows a fracture through the floor of the left orbit (arrow). Note the inferior rectus (arrowhead) is not herniated through the fracture. Compare this with Fig. 9a which shows herniation of inferior rectus through the fracture.*

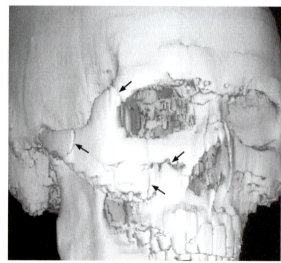

Fig.9h *3D reconstructed CT image (bone algorithm) clearly depicts the fracture lines (arrows) of a tripod fracture. This may help the surgeon for pre-operative planning.*

PAEDIATRIC

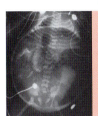

Contributors:
**Monica S.M. Chan, K.T. Wong,
Edmund H.Y. Yuen**

Questions
Case 1 - 11   426 - 436

Discussion
Hyaline membrane disease   437 - 439
Necrotizing enterocolitis   440 - 441
Duodenal obstruction   442 - 443
Meconium peritonitis   444
Tracheo-oesophageal fistula   445 - 446
Choledochal cyst   447
Hypertrophic pyloric stenosis   448
Intussusception   449 - 451
Non-accidental injury   452 - 453
Vesico-ureteric reflux   454 - 455
Croup/laryngotracheobronchitis   456

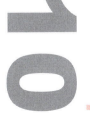

Chapter 10

Case 1

A premature newborn baby was admitted to the neonatal intensive care unit for respiratory distress shortly after birth. Antenatal history was unremarkable. He was intubated, afebrile, tachypnoeic and tachycardic on general examination. There was decreased air-entry in both lungs on auscultation and no murmur was detected on examination of the cardiovascular system. Laboratory investigations revealed respiratory failure and the white cell count was within normal limits. A CXR (Fig. 1a) was performed as an initial investigation.

Questions

(1) What radiological abnormality can you see ?
  - Diffuse 'ground-glass' opacities in both lungs
  - Bilateral air-bronchograms
  - Obscuration of cardiac and diaphragmatic outlines
(2) What is the diagnosis ?

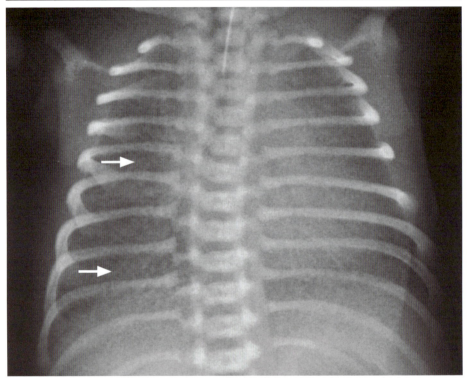

Fig.1a *Frontal CXR shows diffuse ground glass opacities in both lungs (arrows) in a prematurely born neonate, representing hyaline membrane disease. Note the presence of the endotracheal tube.*

Case 2

A 5-day-old premature neonate developed progressive abdominal distension and blood in stool after institution of oral feeding. He was septic on general examination, and the abdomen was distended and hyper-resonant on percussion. Bowel sounds were sluggish on auscultation. Laboratory investigations showed raised white cell count and C-reactive protein. Blood culture grew Gram-negative organism. The provisional diagnosis of necrotizing enterocolitis was suggested and serial AXRs (Fig. 2a-c) were performed over a few days.

Questions

(1) What radiological abnormalities can you detect ?
- Distended bowel loops in the abdomen - represents ileus which affects terminal ileum first
- Pneumatosis intestinalis - gas within bowel wall
- Bubbly appearance of bowel - due to mixture of intramural gas and faecal material

(2) What is the diagnosis ?

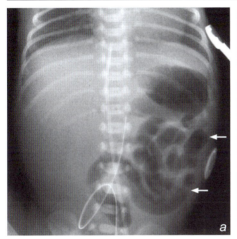
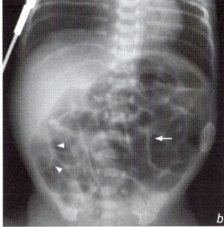

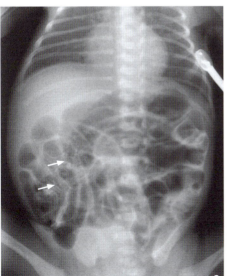

Fig.2a Early changes in NEC. Loops of dilated bowel are seen in the left side of the abdomen (arrows), indicating ileus. Relative paucity of bowel gas shadows on the right side of the abdomen is due to the presence of fluid-filled bowel loops as a result of ileus.

Fig.2b As the disease progresses, dilated bowel loops (arrow) are seen all over the abdomen and 'sandy foamy' appearance (arrowheads) due to presence of faeces and intramural gas is noted over the right lower quadrant of the abdomen.

Fig.2c Presence of intramural gas (pneumatosis intestinalis) in the ileal bowel loops over right side of the abdomen, causing a bubbly appearance in the terminal ileal loops (arrows).

Case 3

A neonate presented with repeated bile-stained vomiting since the first few hours of life. Physical examination showed soft but distended upper abdomen. An abdominal radiograph was performed (Fig. 3a) as an initial examination followed by a water soluble upper GI contrast study (Fig. 3b).

Questions

(1) What radiological abnormalities are seen on the abdominal radiograph ?
 - 'Double bubble' sign due to the dilated stomach and the duodenum
 - No bowel gas in the rest of the abdomen

 What are the radiological abnormalities on the upper GI contrast study ?
 - Bulbous/distended duodenal cap
 - Markedly distended stomach
 - No passage of contrast into the distal duodenum

(2) What is the diagnosis ?

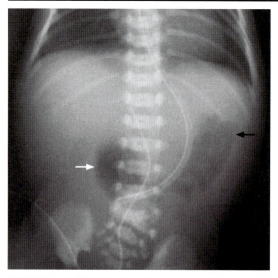

Fig.3a *Abdominal X-ray of a neonate showing the 'double bubble' sign. One of the 'bubbles' is the distended stomach (black arrow) whereas the other 'bubble' is the bulbous duodenal cap (arrow). Note the rest of the abdomen is gasless.*

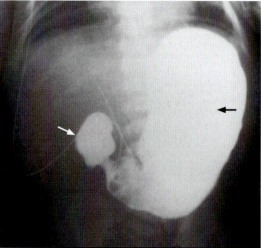

Fig.3b *Upper GI contrast study shows contrast opacification of the grossly distended stomach (black arrow) and the bulbous-shaped duodenal cap (arrow). The rest of the duodenal loop and small bowel is not opacified, indicating complete obstruction and duodenal atresia. The diagnosis was confirmed at surgery.*

Case 4

A 2-day-old baby boy presented to special care baby unit for investigation of abnormal antenatal sonographic examination findings during the 2nd trimester. On an antenatal ultrasound, peritoneal hyperechoic foci were seen in the right side of the abdomen. Otherwise the antenatal examination findings were normal. Physical examination was unremarkable. Meconium was passed on day 1. An abdominal XR (Fig. 4a) was performed.

Questions

(1) What radiological abnormalities can you detect on the abdominal X-ray (Fig. 4a) ?
- Amorphous coarse calcifications scattered in the abdomen, particularly on the right side. No dilated bowel loop is found.

(2) <u>What is the radiological diagnosis ?</u>

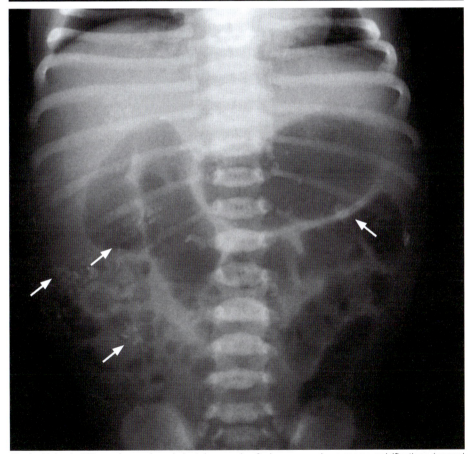

Fig.4a *Abdominal X-ray of a newborn baby taken on day 2 shows amorphous coarse calcifications (arrows) scattered in the abdomen; most of them are found on the right side of the abdomen. There is no bowel loop dilatation seen in the rest of the abdomen and there is no evidence of intestinal obstruction. This is indicative of in-utero meconium peritonitis with calcification of the extruded meconium.*

Case 5

A full-term newborn baby presented a few hours after birth with feeding difficulty and drooling of saliva. There were features of Down's syndrome on general examination. The rest of the physical examination and laboratory investigations were unremarkable. Resistance was felt on trying to pass a feeding tube down the stomach and an X-ray (Fig. 5a) was performed after attempted insertion of feeding tube.

Questions

(1) What radiological abnormality can you see ?
  - Oblong air lucency over upper mediastinum and neck - representing the dilated gas-filled proximal oesophageal pouch
  - Coiling of distal end of feeding tube within proximal oesophageal pouch
  - Presence of bowel gas - indicates the presence of tracheo-oesophageal fistula, i.e. communication between trachea and distal oesophagus

(2) What is the diagnosis ?

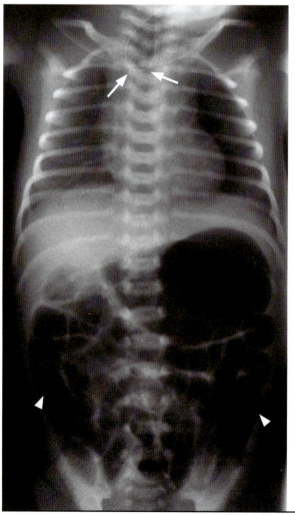

Fig.5a *Plain radiograph shows coiling of the infant feeding tube in the proximal / mid oesophagus (arrows) in the superior mediastinum and is suggestive of oesophageal atresia. Air is present in the bowel loops (arrowheads) indicating there is tracheo-oesophageal fistula with oesophageal atresia.*

Case 6

A 2-year-old girl with a history of recurrent abdominal pain associated with fever and pruritis presented with yellowish discolouration of skin and tea-colour urine. Physical examination showed a palpable mass lesion in the right upper quadrant of the abdomen, and jaundice. Blood tests suggested obstructive jaundice and a USG examination of the abdomen (Fig. 6a, b) was performed which was followed by MR cholangiopancreaticography (MRCP) (Fig. 6c).

Questions

(1) What are the radiological abnormalities shown on USG abdomen ?
- Fusiform segmental dilatation of the common bile duct, moderate dilatation of the proximal right and left hepatic ducts.
- Sludge in the common duct.

What are the abnormalities shown on the MRCP ?
- The reformatted image of the biliary tract shows the markedly dilated fusiform common duct and the moderately dilated right and left hepatic ducts.

The cystic duct and gall bladder are also distended and tortuous.

(2) What is the diagnosis ?

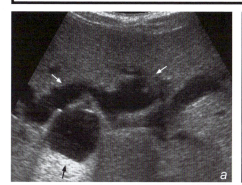

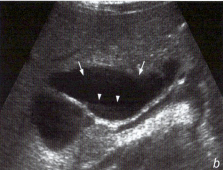

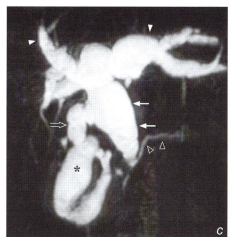

Fig.6a *Transverse sonogram of liver showing moderately dilated right and left hepatic ducts (arrows). The cystic structure at the confluence (black arrow) is the axial section of the markedly dilated common duct.*

Fig.6b *Oblique longitudinal sonogram of the right upper quadrant of the abdomen showing the fusiform segmental dilatation of the common duct (arrows) with echoes suggestive of sludge (arrowheads) within.*

Fig.6c *MRCP- The reformatted view of maximum intensity projection (MIP) of the biliary tract shows the segmental fusiform dilatation of the common duct (arrows). The right and left hepatic ducts are also dilated (arrowheads). Note in this patient the cystic duct (open arrow) is dilated and tortuous, and gall bladder (asterisk) is also significantly distended. The pancreatic duct is normal in calibre (open arrowheads).*

Case 7

A 4-week-old boy presented with repeated non-bilious projectile vomiting within 30 minutes after oral feeding. Physical examination showed a distended epigastrium with visible peristalsis. A ~4 cm palpable mass was detected in the epigastrium. Laboratory investigations revealed hypochloraemic metabolic alkalosis and hypokalaemia. The provisional diagnosis of hypertrophic pyloric stenosis was made and a plain X-ray and an ultrasound abdomen were performed (Fig. 7a, plain X-ray, Figs. 7b, c and d). The stomach was then distended with water and an ultrasound examination was repeated (Fig. 7d).

Questions

(1) What imaging abnormalities can you detect ?
   Plain radiograph
   - Distended stomach with a paucity of gas in the bowel
   Ultrasound
   - Longitudinal (Fig. 7b) and transverse (Fig. 7c) sonogram through the pylorus in this patient showed
     1. Exaggerated gastric peristalsis on real time examination
     2. Elongated and thick-walled pylorus
     3. Increased muscle thickness - the hypoechoic layer on transverse scan represents the pyloric muscle which measures 5 mm (normal - <2 mm, >4 mm - diagnostic, 2-4 mm - equivocal)
     4. Delayed fluid emptying into duodenum (Fig. 7d) which is better evaluated on real time ultrasound

(2) <u>What is the diagnosis ?</u>

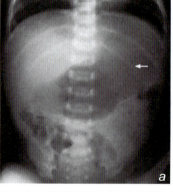

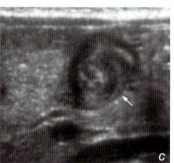

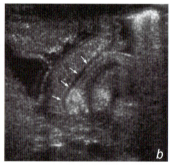

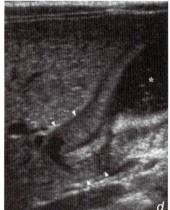

Fig.7a *Markedly distended stomach (arrow) with paucity of bowel gas shadows in the rest of the bowel.*

Fig.7b *US of the pyloric region. Longitudinal view of the pylorus showing the elongated pylorus (arrows), with thickened muscle.*

Fig.7c *Transverse view of the pylorus (arrow) showing the significant mural thickening at pyloric canal 'target sign' (Image courtesy of Dr C.M. Chu, Department of Diagnostic Radiology and Organ Imaging, The Chinese University of Hong Kong).*

Fig.7d *Ultrasound after water ingestion with the antrum (asterisk) distended (water is seen as low level echoes). Longitudinal view of the thickened pylorus (arrowheads).*

Case 8

A 1-year-old girl presented with a one day history of severe colicky abdominal pain and vomiting. There was no fever or diarrhoea. Clinical examination revealed a mass in the right upper abdomen. 'Red currant jelly' bloody stool was noticed on rectal examination. No localized peritoneal signs were detected. Laboratory investigations were essentially normal. A provisional diagnosis of intussusception was suggested and an ultrasound abdomen was performed for further evaluation (Fig. 8a-e).

Questions

(1) What sonographic abnormalities can you identify ?
- Mass in right upper quadrant of abdomen showing 'doughnut' appearance on transverse images
- multiple concentric rings of alternating hypoechoic and hyperechoic layers, representing the echogenic mucosa, submucosa and hypoechoic muscularis propria in the intussusceptum.
- 'pseudo kidney sign' on longitudinal grey scale sonogram
- Colour Doppler study showing floor signal in the mesenteric vessels
- Dilated small bowel loops due to intestinal obstruction

(2) What is the diagnosis ?

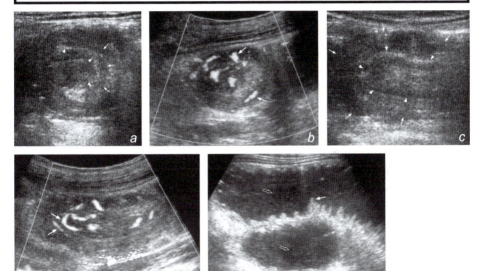

Fig.8a *Transverse sonogram shows a mass lesion in the right upper quadrant of the abdomen with alternate hypoechoic (arrows) and hyperechoic (arrowheads) layers with a hypoechoic centre. This represents the intussusception complex.*

Fig.8b *Transverse sonogram with colour Doppler shows the presence of flow signal (arrows) between layers of the lesion which represent the flow in the mesenteric vessels within the intussusception complex. The absence of flow signal within the intussusception correlates well with decreased successful reduction rate and it is more likely to be associated with bowel ischaemia.*

Fig.8c *Longitudinal sonogram of the intussusception showing the elongated tubular appearance of the lesion. Note the intussusceptum (outlined by the arrowheads) 'telescopes' into the intussuscipien which is represented by the outer layer as outlined by the arrows. Note its similarity to the grey scale appearance of a kidney.*

Fig.8d *Longitudinal sonogram of intussusception complex on colour Doppler shows the pseudo-kidney-shaped lesion. Note the presence of the flow signal within the mesenteric vessels (arrows) supplying the bowel that has telescoped into the intussuscipien.*

Fig.8e *Sonogram showing two adjacent loops of dilated and fluid-filled small bowel found associated with the intussusception. The small bowel loops are filled with anechoic fluid (open arrows) which clearly outline the valvulae conniventes (arrow).*

Case 9

A 1-year-old baby was brought to the casualty department with decreased conscious level and repeated vomiting. The parents denied any recent history of head injury. Physical examination showed a lethargic baby with multiple skin bruises of varying ages all over the body. Sluggish pupil responses to light and retinal haemorrhage were also found on fundoscopic examination. Laboratory investigations revealed normal clotting profile and platelet count. In view of the neurological signs, a CT brain (Fig. 9a, b) was performed for further assessment.

Questions

(1) What radiological abnormality can you see on the non-contrast enhanced axial CT scan of the brain (brain window and bone window) ?
- Acute right frontal subdural and interhemispheric haematoma - due to shearing force from shaking the baby resulting in rupture of small vessels crossing subdural spaces
- Non-depressed fracture of left parietal bone with no associated intracranial or scalp haematoma

(2) <u>What is the diagnosis ?</u>

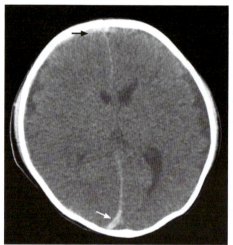 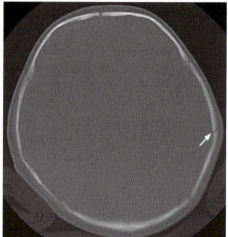

Fig.9a *Non-contrast axial CT brain shows acute right frontal subdural haemorrhage (black arrow). There is interhemispheric subdural haemorrhage along the posterior aspect of falx (arrow).*

Fig.9b *Bone window of CT brain shows a non-depressed fracture in the left parietal bone (arrow). This is an old fracture as there is no associated intracranial or scalp haematoma.*

Case 10

A 2-year-old girl presented with recurrent episodes of urinary tract infection. Her blood pressure was within normal limit for age and physical examination was unremarkable. Previous urine culture grew E. coli. A micturating cystourethrogram (MCU) (Fig. 10a) was performed for further assessment.

Questions

(1) What radiological abnormalities can you detect on the micturating cystourethrogram ?
   - Abnormal contrast opacification of both ureters and pelvicalyceal systems - normally contrast should only be found within the urinary bladder with no opacification of the upper urinary tract
   - Dilated and tortuous ureters on both sides
   - Dilatation of renal pelvis and clubbing of renal calyces

(2) What is the diagnosis ?

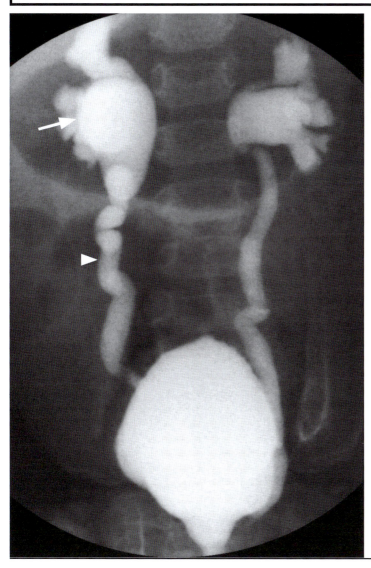

Fig.10a Micturating cystourethrogram, image obtained during the voiding phase, showing bilateral grade V vesicoureteric reflux with bilateral marked dilatation of the pelvicalyceal systems (arrow), and bilateral dilated tortuous and ectatic ureters (arrowhead).

Case 11

A 2-year-old boy presented with fever, and a 'brassy' cough for 3 days. On physical examination, he had inspiratory stridor. Laboratory examination was essentially normal. A frontal view chest radiograph was performed (Fig. 11a, magnified view of the trachea, Fig. 11b).

Questions

(1) What radiological abnormalities can you see?
   - The characteristic 'steeple sign' of the subglottic trachea with loss of the normal shoulders.
(2) What is the diagnosis?

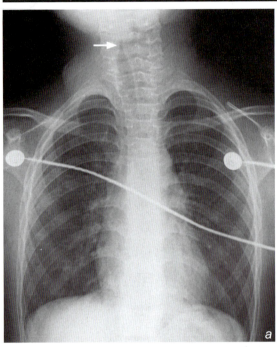

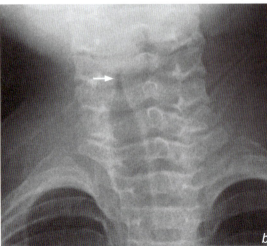

Fig. 11a,b A frontal chest X-ray and magnified view of the trachea of a 2-year-old boy presenting with acute stridor. Note the characteristic subglottic inverted v 'steeple sign' with loss of the normal shoulders (arrow). CXR also helps to exclude foreign body inhalation as a cause of acute stridor.

Discussion Case 1
Hyaline membrane disease

Respiratory distress syndrome (Hyaline membrane disease, Fig. 1a, b)

Discussion:

- Respiratory distress syndrome is an important cause of neonatal respiratory distress in a premature newborn baby.
- The underlying cause is lack of surfactant in premature lungs.
- In neonates with respiratory distress, other potential causes include diaphragmatic hernia (Fig. 1b) meconium aspiration syndrome (Fig. 1c), transient tachypnoeic of newborn (Fig. 1d, e), neonatal pneumonia and cardiac disorders.

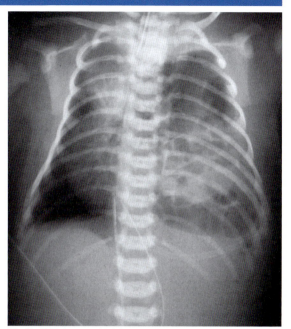

Fig.1b *CXR shows multiple locules of air in the left hemithorax against a soft tissue background. There is mediastinal shift to the right and no gas is seen in the upper abdomen. This was subsequently proven to be diaphragmatic herniation of bowel (Image courtesy of Dr Simon Le, Department of Diagnostic Radiology and Organ Imaging, The Chinese University of Hong Kong).*

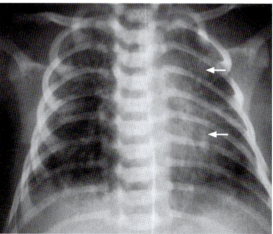

Fig.1c *Patchy air space opacification and air bronchogram are seen in left perihilar and left lower zone (arrows), in a neonate with meconium aspiration syndrome.*

Discussion Case 1

Hyaline membrane disease

- Ventilator-related complications such as pneumothorax (Fig. 1f), pneumomediastinum (Fig. 1f), pulmonary interstitial emphysema (Fig. 1g) and pneumopericardium (Fig. 1h) can be fatal. CXR helps in early detection of these complications.

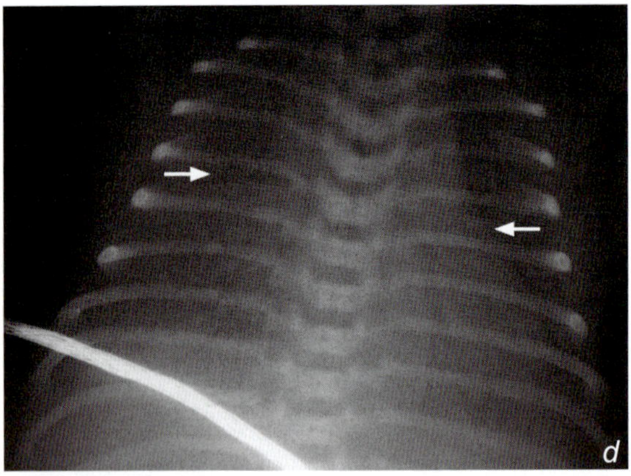

Fig.1d *CXR 3 hours after birth shows mild hyperinflation of both lungs with perihilar interstitial markings (arrows), cardiomegaly and fluid in the transverse fissure. The diaphragmatic silhouette is indistinct on both sides suggestive of small pleural effusion.*

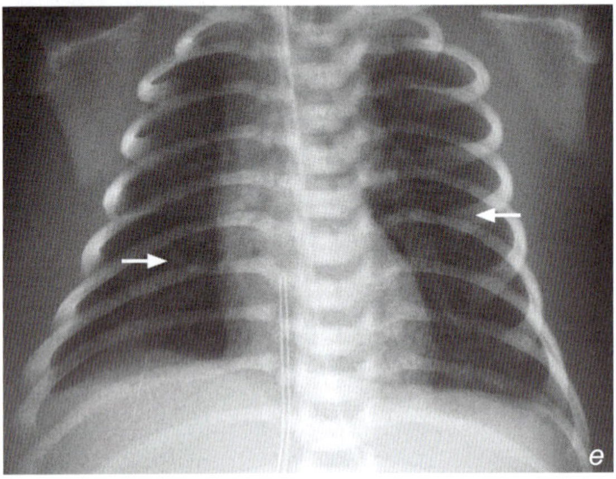

Fig.1e *CXR 30 hours after birth shows both lungs (arrows) are clear and well expanded. A combination of features in Fig. 1d and e suggest transient tachypnoea of newborn.*

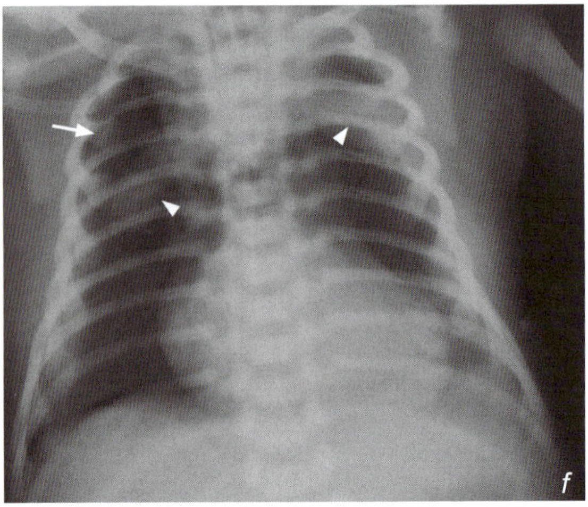

Fig.1f *CXR showing right-sided pneumothorax (arrow) with co-existing pneumomediastinum complicating RDS. Note the thymus (arrowheads) is outlined by the pneumomediastinum. The 'angel's wings' appearance.*

10 PAEDIATRIC

Discussion Case 1
Hyaline membrane disease

Note:

(1) Respiratory distress in premature newborn baby raises the suspicion of respiratory distress syndrome.

(2) Diffuse ground-glass opacification of both lungs are typical CXR findings.

(3) CXR helps in early detection of ventilator-related complications such as pneumothorax and pneumomediastinum.

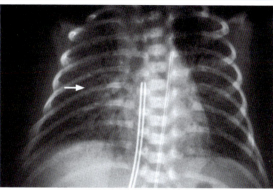

Fig.1g *Follow up CXR in a neonate with hyaline membrane disease requiring ventilatory support. There are bilateral reticular interstitial shadows present, consistent with pulmonary interstitial emphysema (arrow).*

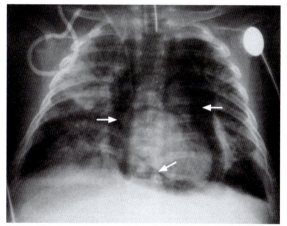

Fig.1h *Pneumopericardium. Extensive air lucency (arrows) around the cardiac border representing a pneumopericardium is seen. Note the lung changes suggestive of hyaline membrane disease bilaterally.*

Necrotizing enterocolitis

Necrotizing enterocolitis (Fig. 2a-c).

Discussion:
- Necrotizing enterocolitis is the most common GI emergency in a premature neonate.
- The exact aetiology is unknown and is believed to be related to perinatal stress or infection.
- Other radiological findings of necrotizing enterocolitis not seen in this neonate include:
  1. Pneumoperitoneum
     - indicates bowel perforation
  2. Portal venous gas (Fig. 2d)
     - due to dissection of intramural gas into mesenteric venous system.
- Detection of pneumoperitoneum is important as bowel perforation necessitates urgent surgery.
  Plain abdominal radiographic findings of pneumoperitoneum include:
  1. Rigler's sign
     - bowel wall outlined by intraluminal and free peritoneal gas (see images in GI system, pneumoperitoneum)
  2. Outline of falciform ligament in medial RUQ (Fig. 2e)

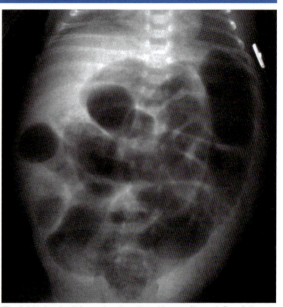

Fig.2d *Abdominal X-ray showing dilated loops of bowel. Carefully note the presence of branching lucencies overlying the liver soft tissue. This represents gas in the portal venous system (Image courtesy of Dr Simon Le, Department of Diagnostic Radiology and Organ Imaging, The Chinese University of Hong Kong).*

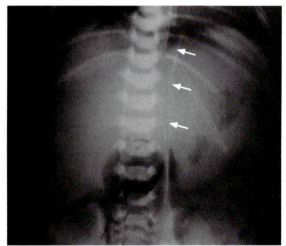

Fig.2e *Abdominal X-ray showing pneumoperitoneum. Note the falciform ligament (arrows) is outlined by air.*

Discussion Case 2
Necrotizing enterocolitis

3. 'Football' sign
    - large pneumoperitoneum outlining the entire abdominal cavity (Fig. 2f)
- Apart from a supine AXR, cross-table lateral view or left-side-down decubitus view may help to confirm the presence of free peritoneal gas (Fig. 2g)
- Contrast study is not necessary for diagnosis. It may be helpful at a later stage (after several weeks) for detection of complications such as colonic stricture.

> **Note:**
> (1) Abdominal distension and blood in stool in a premature neonate raise the suspicion of necrotizing enterocolitis.
> (2) Diagnosis often relies on radiological findings on an abdominal radiograph.
> (3) Dilated bowel loops with pneumatosis intestinalis are typical findings on abdominal radiograph.

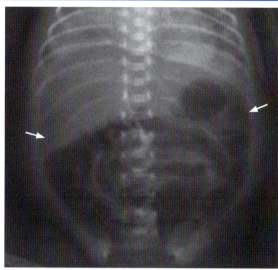

Fig.2f *Abdominal X-ray shows a large lucency outlining the entire abdominal cavity (arrows) – football sign suggesting pneumoperitoneum.*

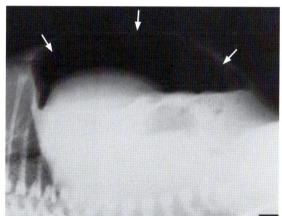

Fig.2g *Cross table lateral view of the abdomen shows the presence of free intraperitoneal gas (arrows) in the non-dependent part of the abdomen.*

Duodenal obstruction

Duodenal obstruction, due to duodenal atresia (confirmed at surgery Fig. 3a, b)

Discussion:

1. Duodenal obstruction is a relatively common form of intestinal obstruction in newborn and is due to extrinsic or intrinsic causes.
   - Intrinsic causes include: duodenal atresia or stenosis, presence of web, or diaphragm, midgut volvulus (Fig. 3c, d)
   - Extrinsic causes include: annular pancreas, peritoneal bands such as Ladd's band, and duodenal duplication

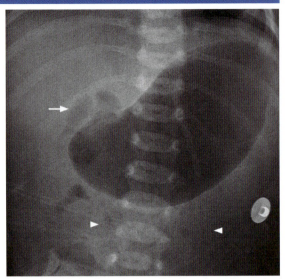

Fig.3c *Abdominal radiograph shows the stomach and the proximal duodenum (arrow) are distended with gas. Note the relative paucity of gas in the abdomen (arrowheads) distal to the duodenum.*

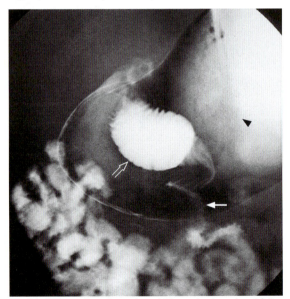

Fig.3d *Oblique view of a water-soluble contrast meal and follow through shows a 'corkscrew appearance' (arrow) of the distal duodenum and proximal jejunum. Note the markedly distended stomach (black arrowhead) and proximal duodenum (open arrow).*

Duodenal obstruction

2. Duodenal atresia and stenosis are more common in trisomy 21, and are also associated with other GI and bile tract anomalies. They are also a part of the syndromal manifestation including VATER (vertebral defects, imperforate anus, tracheo-oesophageal fistula, radial and renal dysplasia), and VACTERAL (vertebral anomalies, anal atresia, cardiac anomalies, tracheo-oesphageal fistula, renal anomalies and limb anomalies) syndromes (Fig. 3e)

3. Abdominal X-ray is usually diagnostic. Upper GI contrast study helps to confirm the diagnosis of duodenal obstruction and to demonstrate other associated GI anomalies if incomplete obstruction is present.

Note :
(1) Double bubble sign is highly suggestive of duodenal obstruction.
(2) Duodenal obstruction is a relatively common form of intestinal obstruction in the newborn.
(3) Look for commonly associated syndromes and GI anomalies.

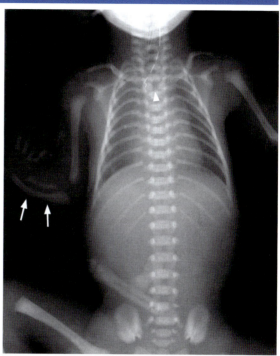

Fig.3e *Plain X-ray shows butterfly vertebra (arrowhead), radial hypoplasia (arrows), oesophageal atresia (seen by curled tube in the upper oesophagus and a gasless abdomen) and thirteen pairs of ribs (Image courtesy of Dr Simon Le, Department of Diagnostic Radiology and Organ Imaging, The Chinese University of Hong Kong).*

10 PAEDIATRIC

Meconium peritonitis

Sealed off meconium peritonitis with in-utero perfraction and calcified meconium in peritoneal cavity
(Fig. 4a)

Discussion:
- Meconium peritonitis usually results from intrauterine gastrointestinal obstruction. Usually it is sterile and sealed off in utero and the meconium extruded becomes calcified. The calcified meconium is usually found on postnatal abdominal X-ray for follow-up of abnormal antenatal USG findings or as incidental finding during examination for other clinical symptoms. Some infants may present with swellings or masses in the scrotum due to passage of meconium through the patent processus vaginalis.
- Most of the calcifications resulting from meconium peritonitis not associated with intestinal obstruction usually resolve gradually. Further investigation is not necessary unless symptoms of gastrointestinal obstruction present.
- Rarely if the meconium peritonitis persists, particularly in the presence of intestinal obstruction, bacterial infection may set in with complicating pneumoperitoneum (Fig. 4b).

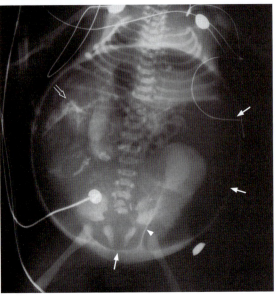

Fig.4b *Abdominal X-ray of another newborn baby showing pneumoperitoneum with 'football sign'(arrows). The middle umbilical ligament in the pelvis (arrowhead) is outlined by air – urachal sign. Clusters of coarse calcification are seen in right side of abdomen (open arrow). These are due to meconium peritonitis.*

> **Note :**
> (1) In-utero gastrointestinal perforation may result in meconium peritonitis and calcification of the extruded meconium.
> (2) The condition is usually self-limiting and the calcifications may eventually resolve on follow-up abdominal X-ray.
> (3) Rarely, the meconium peritonitis persists and is complicated by pneumoperitoneum particularly in the presence of underlying intestinal obstruction.

Tracheo-oesophageal fistula

Oesophageal atresia with a tracheo-oesophageal fistula (Fig. 5a)
- A repeat chest X-ray after placing 1-2 ml of barium into proximal oesophagus may be performed to assess the level of atresia

Discussion:
- Oesophageal atresia is due to congenital failure of recanalization of the oesophagus. In majority (80-85%) of cases, oesophageal atresia is associated with tracheo-oesophageal fistula to the distal oesophagus. Therefore bowel gas can be demonstrated in most of these patients.
- The exact site of the tracheo-oesophageal fistula is demonstrated by water-soluble contrast study of the oesophagus (Fig. 5b, c)
- Other less common types include atresia without fistula and atresia with fistula to proximal oesophagus. These types will not show bowel gas within the abdomen
- Detection of oesophageal atresia is important as early surgery is necessary.
- Other radiological findings of oesophageal atresia not seen in this patient include:
  1. Tracheal compression by the dilated oesophageal pouch.
  2. Patchy pulmonary infiltrates
     - due to repeated episodes of aspiration.

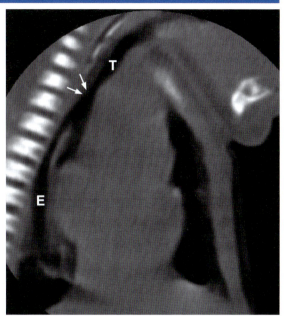

Fig.5b *Sagittal reformatted CT clearly delineates tracheo-oesophageal fistula (arrows). T=trachea, E=oesophagus (Image courtesy of Dr Simon Le, Department of Diagnostic Radiology and Organ Imaging, The Chinese University of Hong Kong).*

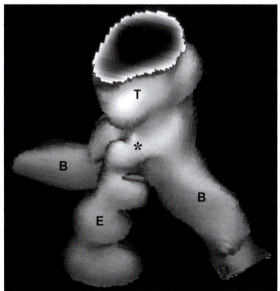

Fig.5c *Surface rendered 3D CT shows the tracheo-oesophageal fistula (asterisk). T=trachea, E=oesophagus, B=main bronchus (Image courtesy of Dr Simon Le, Department of Diagnostic Radiology and Organ Imaging, The Chinese University of Hong Kong).*

10 PAEDIATRIC

Note :

(1) Oesophageal atresia should be suspected in a newborn baby with feeding problems and repeated episodes of aspiration.

(2) Dilated upper oesophageal pouch and coiling of feeding tube within are typical radiological features.

(3) Detection of bowel gas indicates the presence of tracheo-oesophageal fistula communicating with distal oesophagus.

PAEDIATRIC 10

Choledochal cyst

Choledochal cyst (Fig. 6a-c)

Discussion:

1. It is the most common congenital bile duct lesion. Most (80 %) are diagnosed in childhood.
2. USG is usually diagnostic with MRCP (Fig. 6d) being complementary to the USG examination.
3. Choledochal cyst is associated with choledocholithiasis, recurrent cholangitis and pancreatitis. It is also associated with malignant transformation into cholangiocarcinoma and carcinoma of the gall bladder. Biliary cirrhosis and portal hypertension are chronic changes.

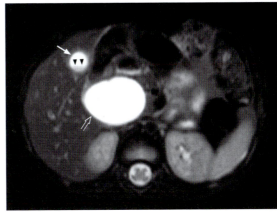

Fig.6d *Fat-suppressed T2W axial image of abdomen acquired during MRCP examination at the level of the gall bladder shows marked dilatation of the common bile duct (open arrow) consistent with choledochal cyst. Note the normal sized gall bladder (arrow) with sludge (arrowheads) in its dependent part.*

10 PAEDIATRIC

Note :
(1) Most common congenital bile duct lesion.
(2) Cause of recurrent pancreatitis and cholangitis in paediatric patients.
(3) Associated with malignant transformation into cholangiocarcinoma and carcinoma of gall bladder.

Discussion Case 7
Hypertrophic pyloric stenosis

Hypertrophic pyloric stenosis (Fig. 7a-d). What alternative investigation would you suggest if USG is not available ?
- Barium meal examination

Discussion:
- Hypertrophic pyloric stenosis should be considered in an infant of 4-8 weeks of age (especially boys) who present with failure to thrive and projectile non-bilious vomiting.
- Ultrasound is the preferred imaging modality of choice.
- Barium meal was the method of investigation in the past but is seldom used now. The typical radiological signs (Fig. 7e) are
  1. 'String sign' - represents barium within a narrowed elongated pyloric canal (white arrow)
  2. 'Shoulder sign' - represents indentation of gastric antrum by hypertrophic pylorus (black arrowheads)
  3. 'Mushroom sign' or 'Kirklin sign' - represents indentation of base of duodenal bulb (black arrows).

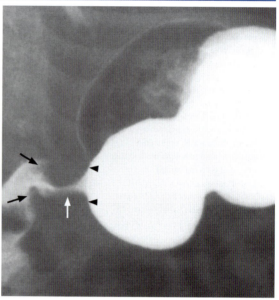

Fig.7e *Oblique radiographic view of the antrum and pylorus obtained during a barium meal shows the typical radiological findings of hypertrophic pyloric stenosis. The indentation of the gastric antrum by the hypertrophic pylorus is indicated by the black arrowheads – 'shoulder sign'. The narrowed pyloric canal is outlined by barium (arrow) - 'string sign'. Note the indentation by the hypertrophic pylorus at the base of the duodenal bulb - 'mushroom sign' (black arrows).*

Note :
(1) Non-bilious projectile vomiting in a 4-8-week-old boy raises the suspicion of hypertrophic pyloric stenosis.
(2) Ultrasound abdomen is the imaging modality of choice.
(3) Increased muscle thickness in an elongated and thickened pylorus is characteristic.

Intussusception

Intussusception (Fig. 8a-e)

An air enema with pneumatic reduction (Fig. 8f-h) was performed after the diagnosis.

- Radiographic images done during pneumatic reduction:

  (a) At the beginning of the pneumatic reduction, the tip of the intussceptum is outlined by air (cresent sign) at the proximal transverse colon (arrows) (Fig. 8f)

  (b) The intussusceptum is progressively being pushed retrogradely down the ascending colon and caecum (Fig. 8g) by the column of air introduced rectally

  (c) The reduction is achieved when gush of air into small bowel is demonstrated on real time fluoroscopic screening, which indicates successful reduction (Fig. 8h)

  (d) Post-procedure abdominal X-ray should also be performed to exclude possible complication such as pneumoperitoneum

- Caution should be taken not to allow pneumatic pressure to exceed 120mmHg, to minimize the risk of bowel perforation

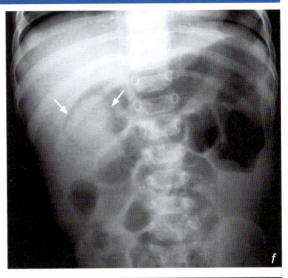

Fig.8f *Abdominal X-ray performed during the initial phase of pneumatic reduction of intussusception. The intussusception is found at the right upper quadrant of the abdomen with the intussusceptum being outlined by air (arrows), the cresent sign.*

Fig.8g *Abdominal radiograph taken during fluoroscopic guided pneumatic reduction of intussusception. Note the progressive reduction of the intussusception with the intussusceptum being moved by the air column until it reaches the ileocaecal junction (arrows). Further and final reduction is achieved when air is seen refluxing into the terminal ileum.*

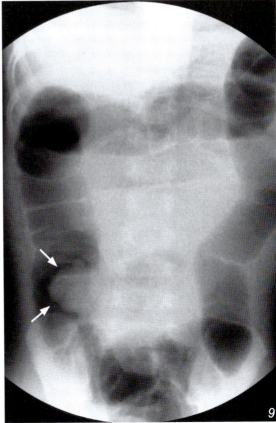

Intussusception

Discussion:

- Majority of patients with intussusception are between 3 months and 2 years of age. It is the most common cause of intestinal obstruction in children younger than 2 years of age
- It develops when a proximal part of the bowel (intussusceptum) telescopes into the distal part (intussuscipien), which is usually close to the ileocaecal junction, resulting in venous congestion and subsequent intestinal obstruction
- Usually no identifiable lead point can be found in most of the patients under the age of 2. If age of presentation is atypical, careful search for a pathological lead point (such as Meckel's diverticulum) is warranted.
- There are different types of intussusception: small bowel intussusception (ileo-ileal), ileocolic and ileo-ileocolic types. Ileo-ileocolic and ileocolic types are more common and ileocolic type accounts for 85% of all cases of intussusception.
- Without appropriate and prompt treatment, intussusception may result in bowel ischaemia, perforation, peritonitis or even death.
- Abdominal X-ray will show a mass in the right upper quadrant of the abdomen which is sometimes associated with small bowel dilatation and gasless distal large bowel.
- USG is the ideal initial investigation to confirm the presence of intussusception.
- Image guided reduction, which may be pneumatic, barium or hydrostatic, is a safe method of non-surgical treatment.

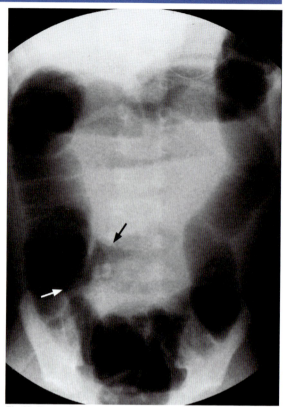

Fig.8h *Post-reduction abdominal X-ray shows air in the terminal ileal loops (black arrow) and there is no mass at the ileocaecal junction (arrow).*

- Major complication of failed reduction is perforation of the bowel with spillage of the reducing agent into the peritoneal cavity, i.e. pneumoperitoneum and rarely tension pneumoperitoneum in pneumatic reduction; hydroperitoneum in hydrostatic reduction or peritoneal spillage and staining by barium in barium enema reduction
- Contraindications for attempted non-surgical reduction include clinical evidence of dehydration, shock, peritonitis or pneumoperitoneum
- Pneumatic reduction under fluoroscopic guidance is one of the most common methods of non-surgical treatment, which has a high success rate and minimal complications.
- Preliminary abdominal X-ray is done before pneumatic reduction to exclude pre-existing pneumoperitoneum, which is a complication of intussusception and is a contraindication for attempting pneumatic reduction.
- Compared with barium enema reduction, pneumatic reduction is clean and requires less radiation exposure.
- Hydrostatic reduction has the advantage of being non-radiating but may be messier during the procedure and requires a greater degree of expertise.

Note :
(1) Severe colicky abdominal pain, 'red currant jelly' bloody stool and abdominal mass in the appropriate age group raise the suspicion of intussusception.
(2) Ultrasound is the imaging modality of choice.
(3) Pneumatic reduction is the preferred method of treatment.

Non-accidental injury

Non-accidental injury (Fig. 9a-b)
Further imaging investigations help for delineation of extent of injury. These include
- Skeletal survey to detect skeletal injury
- Chest X-ray of this child (Fig. 9c) shows acromial fracture, bilateral posterior rib fractures and spiral fracture of right proximal humerus

Discussion:
- Non-accidental injury should be considered in children with a suspicous clinical history and corroborating examination findings
- Intracranial injury (Fig. 9d), though not the most common form of injury, is an important injury to detect because it may be potentially life-threatening
- Another CT finding of non-accidental injury is cerebral oedema (Fig. 9e) due to strangulation
- Skeletal trauma is the most commonly seen injury in non-accidental injury. The presence of multiple fractures with varying ages is characteristic
- Certain types of fractures are more suggestive of non-accidental origin rather than accidental. Examples include acromial fracture, metaphyseal fracture, bilateral posterior rib fractures and spiral fracture of proximal humerus.

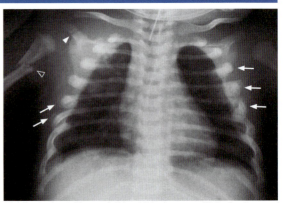

Fig.9c *A chest X-ray of this child shows multiple fractures of different ages. There is a fracture of the right acromion (arrowhead). Displaced spiral fracture of proximal right humerus (open arrowhead), multiple and bilateral rib fractures at the lateral aspects of multiple ribs (arrows), some with callous formation are also seen.*

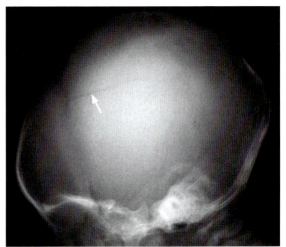

Fig.9d *Lateral skull X-ray of another child with suspected non-accidental injury shows radiolucent line representing a non-depressed skull fracture in the right parietal bone (arrow).*

Non-accidental injury

Note :
(1) Diagnosis of non-accidental injury relies on a high index of clinical suspicion (atypical history) and physical examination findings.
(2) Interhemispheric, subdural haemorrhage is a specific finding on CT brain.
(3) Metaphyseal fractures and posterior rib fractures are more likely of non-accidental origin.

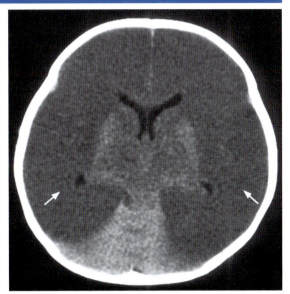

Fig.9e *Non-contrast axial CT brain in a comatose child with suspected history of non-accidental injury. Diffuse hypodensity in both cerebral hemispheres (arrows) with effacement of the sulcal spaces are indicative of generalized cerebral oedema. The cause of bilateral cerebral oedema is strangulation. There is relative sparing of the basal ganglia and cerebellum.*

10 PAEDIATRIC

Discussion Case 10
Vesico-ureteric reflux

Bilateral grade V vesico-ureteric reflux, causing repeated UTI (Fig. 10a)

Discussion:

- In children with repeated episodes of UTI, underlying predisposing factors have to be excluded. These include vesico-ureteric reflux, posterior urethral valve (in boys) and congenital urinary tract anomaly (such as duplex kidneys) (Fig. 10b)

- MCU is one of the imaging modalities of choice for the detection of underlying predisposing factors.

- MCU should be performed several weeks after acute infective episode has subsided, to prevent acute exacerbation of the infection.

- Vesico-ureteric reflux is categorized into different grades according to the level and degree of dilatation of upper urinary tract (Fig. 10a, c).
  - Grade I
    - Reflux into the distal ureter only
  - Grade II
    - Reflux reaching the pelvicalyceal system which is not dilated
  - Grade III
    - Reflux reaching the pelvicalyceal system which is dilated
  - Grade IV
    - Reflux reaching the pelvicalyceal system which is dilated and the ureter is tortuous
  - Grade V
    - Worsening of Grade IV reflux with further dilatation of pelvicalyceal system and tortuosity of the ureter; renal scarring in children with repeated episodes of upper tract UTI.

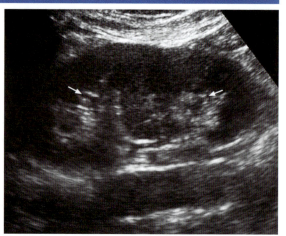

Fig.10b *Longitudinal sonogram of left kidney shows a non-dilated duplex collecting system (arrows).*

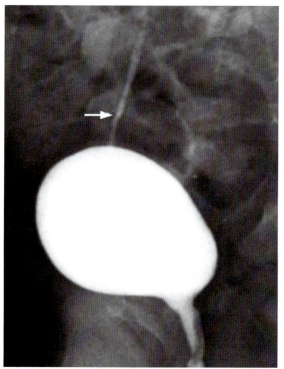

Fig.10c *Micturating cystourethrogram during the bladder-filling phase showing grade I vesico-ureteric reflux on right side (arrow) with contrast refluxing into the distal ureter.*

Vesico-ureteric reflux

- The choice of treatment with prophylactic antibiotics (medical treatment) or ureteric reimplantation (surgical treatment) depends on the age of patient, frequency of recurrent UTI and grading of VUR.
- The goal of treatment is to reduce the chance of renal scarring as a result of repeated UTI leading to development of hypertension.
- Ultrasound (Fig. 10d) and DMSA (Dimercaptosuccinic acid ^{99m}Tc-labelled) renal scintigraphy (Fig. 10e) help to look for renal cortical scars.

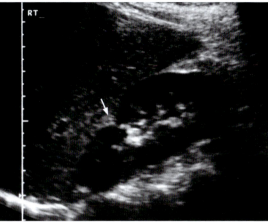

Fig.10d Longitudinal ultrasound of right kidney in another patient with history of repeated UTI shows focal contour distortion indicative of scar (arrow) at upper pole of right kidney.

Note :

(1) Vesico-ureteric reflux has to be excluded in children with recurrent UTI.

(2) Micturating cystourethrogram (MCU) is one of the imaging modalities of choice to demonstrate contrast reflux back into ureter and intrarenal collecting system.

(3) DMSA scan or ultrasound is indicated for detection of associated renal scarring.

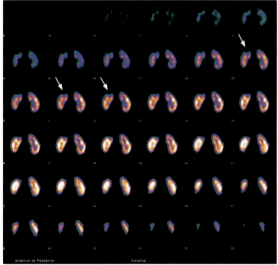

Fig.10e DMSA of a 5-year-old girl with history of repeated urinary tract infection, tomographic view showing focal photopenia at the upper pole of right kidney (arrows), which is consistent with scarring due to repeated UTI.

10 PAEDIATRIC

Croup / laryngotracheobronchitis

Croup/laryngotracheobronchitis (Fig. 11a, b)

Discussion:
- Croup/laryngotracheobronchitis is inflammation of the respiratory tract, usually viral in nature. It is the most common cause of acute stridor in children between 6 months and 3 years of age. However, it may also occur in older children and adults.
- All the mucosa along the respiratory tract from the larynx to the bronchi are involved and oedematous
- The subglottic area becomes the part critically compromised as the mucosa here is loosely attached
- Other radiological findings of croup/laryngotracheobronchitis include:
  1. Distension of the hypopharynx on lateral view of neck (Fig. 11c)
  2. Indistinctness of the subglottic airway with normal epiglottis and normal aryepiglottic folds on a lateral view
  3. Radiographs also help to exclude foreign body inhalation as a cause of acute stridor.

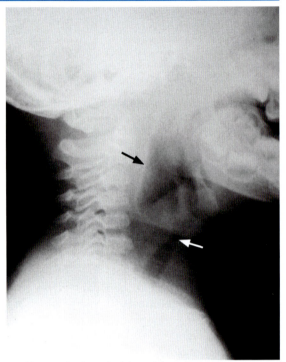

Fig.11c Lateral radiograph of the neck in another child shows marked distension of the hypopharynx (black arrow). Note the indistinctness of the subglottic airway (arrow).

Note :
(1) Croup is one of the commonest causes of acute stridor in children.
(2) 'Steeple sign' with subglottic inverted V and loss of the normal shouldering is the characteristic radiological finding on an AP view of the neck.

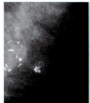

BREAST

Contributors:
Edmund H.Y. Yuen, Alice Tang

Questions

Case 1 - 5   458 - 462

Discussion

Breast cyst   463 - 464
Fibroadenoma   465 - 466
Phyllode tumour   467
Breast carcinoma   468 - 469
Ductal carcinoma in situ (DCIS)   470

Chapter 11

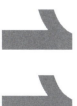

Case 1

A peri-menopausal 45-year-old woman presents with a left breast lump for 2 weeks. The lump is mildly painful and appears to have enlarged gradually. She is on hormonal replacement therapy for her menopausal symptoms. She has no family history of breast cancer and has never felt any breast lump before. On physical examination there is a firm mildly tender nodule palpated at the 3 o'clock position of the left breast at the periareolar region. The lesion is fairly superficial and appears to be non-mobile. The overlying skin and right nipple are normal. No other breast lump is palpable in either breast. No enlarged axillary lymph node is palpable. A mammogram (Fig. 1a) and an ultrasound (Fig. 1b) are performed for further evaluation.

Questions

(1) What are the findings on mammogram and ultrasound ?
- Mammogram shows that there is a partially well circumscribed, round, water density mass with a sharp radiolucent incomplete halo at the upper outer quadrant of the left breast. No associated calcification is present.
- Ultrasound shows the lesion to be a well-circumscribed anechoic mass with posterior acoustic enhancement and thin edge shadows. No internal echoes, septation, eccentric wall thickening or solid component demonstrated.

(2) What is the diagnosis ?

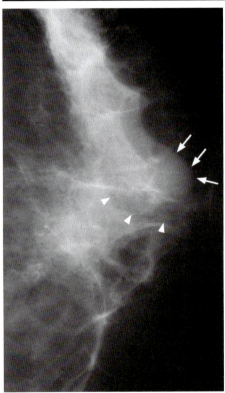

Fig.1a *Mammogram (MLO view) of the left breast shows a partially well circumscribed round mass (arrows) of water density. There is a sharp radiolucent incomplete halo (arrowheads) around this mass.*

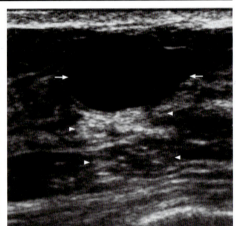

Fig.1b *On ultrasound, the lesion appears as a well-circumscribed, short (height much less than width or length) anechoic mass (arrows). There is also posterior acoustic enhancement (arrowheads).*

Case 2

A single 26-year-old woman presents with a right breast lump for 4 months. The lump was incidentally discovered during self-examination. The lump is not painful and has remained static in size. She is sexually active and uses barrier protection for contraception. She has no family history of breast cancer. On physical examination there is a rubbery non-tender nodule palpated at the 10 o'clock position of the right breast at 4 cm from the nipple. The lesion is freely mobile with respect to the overlying skin and surrounding tissues. The overlying skin and right nipple are normal. No other breast lump is palpable in either breast. No enlarged axillary lymph node is palpable. A mammogram (Fig. 2a) and an ultrasound (Fig. 2b) are performed for further evaluation.

Questions

(1) What are the mammographic and sonographic findings ?
- Mammogram shows that there is a lobulated isodense mass, with smooth margins at the upper outer quadrant of the right breast. No spiculating margins, architectural distortion or associated calcification demonstrated.
- Ultrasound shows the lesion to be an oval, well-circumscribed, homogeneous, lobulated hypoechoic solid mass, which is freely mobile and not fixed to surrounding tissues.

(2) <u>What is the likely diagnosis ?</u>

(3) How can the diagnosis be confirmed ?
- By ultrasound guided fine needle aspiration (FNA) or biopsy.

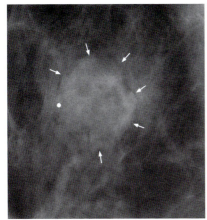 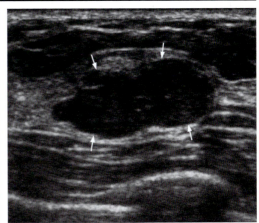

Fig.2a *Mammogram (magnified CC view) shows a lobulated, isodense mass with smooth margins (arrows) at the upper outer quadrant of the right breast. No spiculation, architectural distortion or associated calcification is present.*

Fig.2b *Ultrasound of the same lesion shows it to be a well-circumscribed, oval (height much less than width or length) and lobulated mass (arrows). The lesion contains diffuse internal echoes indicating that this is not a cyst.*

Case 3

A 49-year-old post-menopausal woman presents with a rapidly enlarging right breast mass. The mass is not painful and has tripled in size in the past 3 months. She is not on hormonal replacement therapy, and has no family history of breast cancer. On physical examination there is a large 7 cm firm non-tender mass palpated at the retroareolar region of the right breast. The lesion is relatively mobile with respect to the overlying skin and surrounding tissues. The overlying skin is stretched by the mass but the right nipple is normal. No other breast lump is palpable in either breast. No enlarged axillary lymph node is palpable. A mammogram (Fig. 3a) and an ultrasound (Fig. 3b) are performed for further evaluation.

Questions

(1) What are the mammographic and sonographic findings ?
  - Mammogram shows a large dense smoothly marginated mass in the retroareolar region of the right breast. Ultrasound shows this lesion to be a well-circumscribed hypoechoic solid mass.
(2) <u>What is the likely diagnosis ?</u>

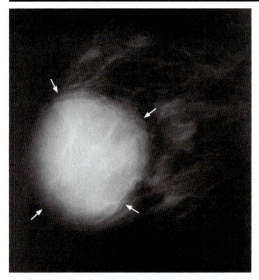

Fig.3a *Mammogram (MLO view) shows a large, smoothly marginated, dense mass (arrows) in the retroareolar region of the right breast.*

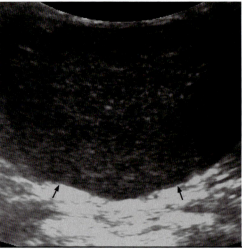

Fig.3b *Ultrasound shows the lesion to be a well-circumscribed solid mass (arrows) with diffuse internal echoes.*

Case 4

A 44-year-old woman presents with a right breast lump for 1 month. The lump is not painful and is enlarging progressively. She is on oral contraceptive pills and has a family history of breast cancer (mother died of breast cancer at the age of 53). On physical examination there is a hard non-tender nodule palpated at the 10 o'clock position of the right breast 2 cm from the right nipple. The lesion appears fixed to the surrounding tissues. The overlying skin shows dimpling and the right nipple is retracted. No other breast lump is palpable in either breast. Enlarged lymph nodes are palpable at the right axilla. A mammogram (Fig. 4a) and an ultrasound (Fig. 4b) are performed for further evaluation.

Questions

(1) What are the mammographic and sonographic findings ?
- Mammograms show a dense irregular mass with spiculated margins at the upper outer quadrant of the right breast. Pleomorphic malignant calcifications are noted within the mass. There is prominent architectural distortion.
- Ultrasound shows the lesion to be an irregular heterogeneous hypoechoic mass with faint posterior acoustic shadowing.

(2) What is the most likely diagnosis ?

(3) How can you confirm the diagnosis ?
- Ultrasound guided fine needle aspiration (FNA) or core biopsy.

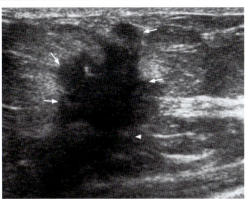

Fig.4b *Ultrasound shows the lesion to be a tall (height similar to width or length) mass (arrows) with mild posterior acoustic shadowing (arrowheads). The margins of this lesion are irregular. All features suggest malignancy.*

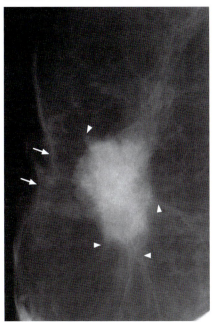

Fig.4a *Mammogram (magnified CC view with local compression) shows a dense, irregular mass with spiculated margins(arrowheads). There is also some dimpling of the overlying skin (arrows) due to architectural distortion (retraction) by this lesion.*

Case 5

An asymptomatic 38-year-old woman is referred for a screening mammogram (Fig.5 a, b).

Questions

(1) What are the mammographic findings ?
- There are linear, branching, casting microcalcifications in a segmental distribution in the immediate left subareolar region.

(2) <u>What is the diagnosis ?</u>

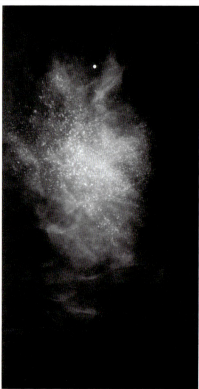

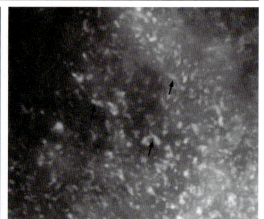

Fig.5b *Magnified view shows the calcifications to be small (microcalcifications) and forming linear and branching casts. This type of calcification is typical in DCIS.*

Fig.5a *Mammogram showing suspicious microcalcification in a segmental distribution in the immediate left subareolar region.*

Discussion Case 1
Breast cyst

Breast cyst (Fig. 1a, b)

Discussion:
- Cysts are among the most common benign lesions identified in the breast.
- Breast simple cysts have been reported to occur in up to 10% of all females, and may occur at any age.
- They have a predilection for perimenopausal women and those on hormonal therapy.
- They are caused by terminal ductal obstruction, dilatation and fluid retention.
- Breast cysts may fluctuate in size with the menstrual cycle: enlarge before and decrease in size after the onset of menses.
- Breast cysts are usually asymptomatic but may cause pain due to wall distention especially when they are large.
- Palpable lump(s) is the most common presentation of breast cyst(s).
- They may be single or multiple, and can grow or regress spontaneously and quickly.
- On mammography breast cysts are round or oval well circumscribed lesions with low or medium density similar to that of fibroglandular tissues. The sharply marginated borders may be partially obscured by the adjacent parenchymal tissues. Occasionally wall calcifications may be seen.
- On ultrasound breast cysts appear as well circumscribed anechoic lesions with thin back wall and good through transmission. Internal echoes representing debris may be seen. Thin septae may be seen in benign simple cysts.
- On MR (Fig. 1c, d, e) the cysts (arrows) are hyperintense on T2W scans, hypointense on T1W scans and show rim enhancement following gadolinium injection. No solid component is seen in simple cysts. Following gadolinium there is initial slow enhancement and persistent enhancement on delayed images.

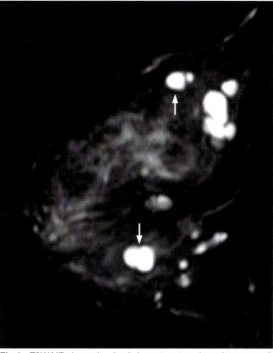

Fig.1c *T2W MR shows the simple breast cysts as hyperintense, well-defined lesions (arrows) (image courtesy of Dr Amy Pang, Department of Diagnostic Radiology and Organ Imaging, The Chinese University of Hong Kong).*

463

Discussion Case 1
Breast cyst

- Breast cysts if asymptomatic can be treated conservatively and may regress. Symptomatic cysts can be aspirated under ultrasound guidance though they may recur.
- Tumour within a breast cyst is very rare, in which case the pathology is most likely papilloma/papillary carcinoma.
- Confirmation of breast cyst(s) does not exclude the presence of malignancy elsewhere in the breast.

Fig.1d, e T1W pre- (d) and post-gadolinium (e) enhanced MR shows the cysts (arrows) to be hypointense with rim enhancement. There is usually slow initial enhancement which persists on delayed scans (images courtesy of Dr Amy Pang, Department of Diagnostic Radiology and Organ Imaging, The Chinese University of Hong Kong).

Note:
(1) Breast cysts are among the most common benign lesions.
(2) Sonographic demonstration of breast cyst is a sign of benignity for that particular lesion; the rest of the breast should still be examined carefully.
(3) The presence of a breast cyst does not exclude the possibility of malignancy elsewhere in the breast.

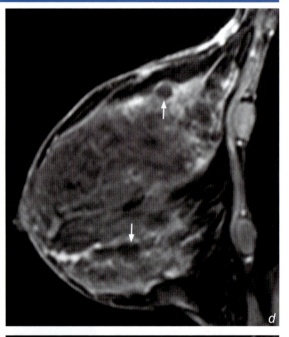

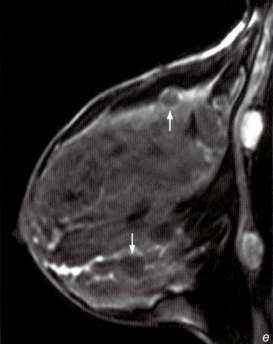

Discussion Case 2
Fibroadenoma

Fibroadenomas (Fig. 2a, b)

Discussion:
- Fibroadenomas are the most common benign solid breast lesion in women of child-bearing age.
- They are benign tumours with mixed epithelial and fibrous components.
- Commonly seen in women from adolescence up to age 40. Mean age of presentation is 30 years.
- They account for 20% of all breast masses and are multiple in 15-20% of cases.
- In post-menopausal women they also account for 10% of the breast masses.
- The most common presentation is a firm, non-tender breast mass. They are not infiltrative and thus not fixed to adjacent tissues; because of their free mobility they are often described as 'breast mouse'.
- They may enlarge during pregnancy due to hormonal stimulation and involute after menopause.
- Fibroadenomas typically appear on imaging as well-defined, smoothly marginated, lobulated, ovoid lesions. A thin 'halo' is often seen around the lesion on mammogram.
- Involuting fibroadenomas may show coarse 'pop-corn' calcifications (Fig. 2c).

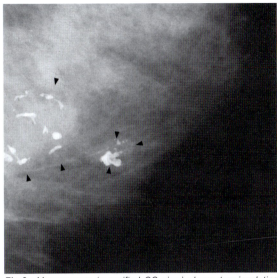

Fig.2c *Mammogram (magnified CC view) shows two involuting fibroadenomas. Both lesions (arrowheads) contain the typical thick, smooth, bubble-like calcification described as 'pop-corn' calcification.*

Fibroadenoma

- Malignancy occurring within a fibroadenoma is very rare.
- On MR (Fig. 2d, e) fibroadenomas (arrows) are well-defined, sharply outlined, lobulated lesions which, following gadolinium, show homogeneous enhancement with dark internal septae. Following gadolinium there is medium (temporal) enhancement and persistent on delayed images.

Fig.2d, e T1W pre- (d) and post-gadolinium (e) enhanced MR shows the fibroadenomas (arrows) as well defined, lobulated masses with enhancement following contrast. There is usually medium enhancement (temporal) and persistent on delayed images (Images courtesy of Dr Amy Pang, Department of Diagnostic Radiology and Organ Imaging, The Chinese University of Hong Kong).

Note:

(1) Fibroadenomas are the most common benign solid breast lesion in women of child-bearing age.

(2) Malignancy occurring within fibroadenoma is very rare.

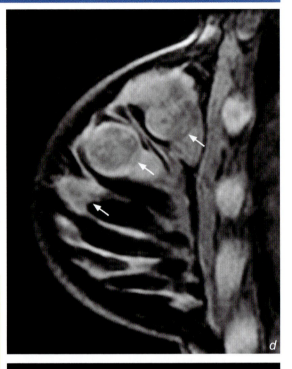

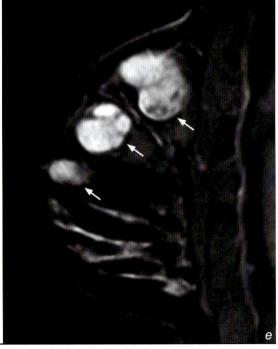

Phyllode tumour

Phyllode tumour (Fig. 3a, b)

Discussion:
- A benign giant form of intracanalicular fibroadenoma.
- Uncommon lesion accounting for <1.5% of all breast tumours.
- Involves patients older than those with fibroadenomas. Mean age of presentation is 45 years.
- Typically presents as a large, rapidly enlarging breast mass.
- Most are benign but 5-15% are malignant with potential to metastasize.
- Imaging appearances are those of a large mass with well-defined smooth borders. Small cysts may be identified on ultrasound. Calcifications are uncommon

---

Note:
(1) Patients with phyllode tumours are usually older than those with fibroadenomas.
(2) A minority of phyllode tumours are malignant with potential to metastasize.

Discussion Case 4
Breast carcinoma

Breast carcinoma (Fig. 4a, b)

Discussion:
- Breast cancer is the second leading cause of cancer death in women, and accounts for 25% of all female malignancies.
- Risk factors include old age, positive family history of breast cancer (first degree relatives), early menarche, late menopause, late first pregnancy, nulliparity.
- Genetic risk factors: p53 mutations, BRCA 1 mutation, BRCA 2 mutations.
- Women with previous history of breast cancer have increased risk of a second cancer.
- The large majority of malignant breast tumours are epithelial tumours originating from the terminal duct lobular unit (TDLU), among which 90% are ductal and 10% are lobular in origin.
- Infiltrating ductal carcinoma is the most common form (65-80%) of breast cancer.
- Typical mammographic appearance of breast cancer is that of a dense irregular mass with spiculating margins. Pleomorphic malignant calcifications are often present. Secondary changes such as architectural distortion, skin thickening, nipple retraction and axillary lymphadenopathy may also be identified.
- Typical sonographic appearance of breast cancer is that of an irregular heterogeneous hypoechoic mass.
- Hypervascularity/hypovascularity of the lesion on Doppler ultrasound cannot be used reliably to distinguish malignant from benign lesions.
- On MRI (Fig. 4c, d), the mass is ill-defined, spiculated and, following contrast injection it shows an initial rapid intense enhancement with a plateau on the delayed scans. The secondary changes, such as skin involvement, nipple retraction, architectural distortion, can also be seen on MRI.

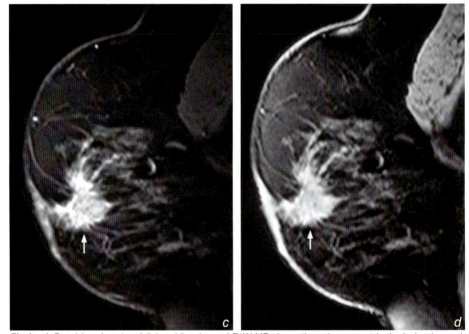

Fig.4c, d *Pre- (c) and post-gadolinium (d) enhanced T1W MR shows the enhancement in the lesion (arrows). There is initial rapid enhancement with a plateau on the delayed images. Note the ill-defined spiculated margins of the malignant lesion. (Images courtesy of Dr Amy Pang, Department of Diagnostic Radiology and Organ Imaging, The Chinese University of Hong Kong).*

Breast carcinoma

- Lesions with suspicious imaging findings should be biopsied.
- Biopsy usually can be performed under real-time ultrasound guidance, or by stereotactic guidance if the lesion is not sonographically visible or accessible.

> **Note:**
> (1) Breast cancer typically appears as an irregular mass with spiculating margins and pleomorphic malignant calcifications.
> (2) Histological diagnosis can be obtained by ultrasound or stereotactic guided tissue sampling.

Ductal carcinoma in situ (DCIS)

Ductal carcinoma in situ (DCIS) (Fig. 5a, b)

Discussion:

- Refers to non-infiltrating intraductal carcinoma confined to the ducts which are filled and plugged by tumour cells.
- The intraductal tumour undergoes necrosis, followed by calcifications developing within the necrotic debris.
- Accounts for 20-40% of breast cancer diagnosed on mammography.
- The cardinal morphological features of the malignant microcalcifications in DCIS are granular, pleomorphic, casting in a linear, branching configuration and may be clustered.
- Associated mass lesion may be seen.
- The malignant microcalcifications are usually not visible on ultrasound.

> **Note:**
>
> (1) In ductal carcinoma in situ (DCIS), there may be no discrete palpable mass in the breast.
> (2) Any suspicious calcifications on mammography should be biopsied.

11 BREAST

FOREIGN BODIES

Contributors:

Simon S. M. Ho, K.T. Wong, Edmund H.Y. Yuen,
Gavin M. Joynt, Anil T. Ahuja

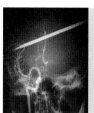

Chapter 12

Foreign bodies that are visible on imaging can be broadly divided into
two categories:

I. Medically/therapeutically deployed   **472 - 485**

II. Unsuspecting or accidentally acquired   **486 - 488**

It is of paramount importance for clinicians and radiologists to be
familiar with the normal appearances and positioning of common
supportive tubings and therapeutically implanted devices, such that
appropriate management actions can be taken should problems and
complications arise. The ability to identify unsuspecting or accidentally
acquired foreign bodies is important not only to facilitate the planning
of removal of the offending object, but may also be a necessary pre-
requisite prior to cross sectional imaging. Metallic fragments, for
example, give rise to artifacts on CT and MRI scanning and may degrade
the diagnostic accuracy of the scan. They can also cause local heating
and migration when a patient undergoes an MRI examination - the
consequences of the latter, in particular, can be catastrophic to the
patient.

(a) Devices visible on chest radiographs

These are most commonly seen on chest radiographs in patients from intensive care units, cardiology and surgical patients. All supportive lines and tubings should be accounted for as soon as the technical adequacy of the film has been assessed

1. Endotracheal and tracheostomy tubes

- In adults, the ideal position of the tip of the endotracheal tube should be around 6-8 cm above the carina (at least 4 cm), roughly around the level of the medial ends of the clavicles (Figs. 1, 2 and 3).
- This position is chosen:
  i. To minimize the risk of inadvertent selective intubation of the right or left main bronchus which may result in collapse of the contralateral lung - endotracheal tubes may move up to 4 cm with neck flexion and extension.
  ii. It also ensures that the balloon cuff of the endotracheal tube is substantially far away from the larynx to avoid rubbing against the larynx which may result in laryngeal damage (Fig. 4 and Fig. 7).
- Note that the position of the endotracheal tube in the trachea is not fixed and varies with neck flexion and extension. The balloon cuff of the endotracheal tube is designed for prevention of retrograde flow of the tidal volume delivered by the ventilator into the mouth and nose and not for fixation of the endotracheal tube.
- The balloon cuff should not be inflated to totally occlude the trachea as this may lead to pressure necrosis of the mucosa and subsequent rupture/stenosis of the trachea.
- Tracheostomy tubes have a variable degree of radio-opacity depending on the material they are made from.

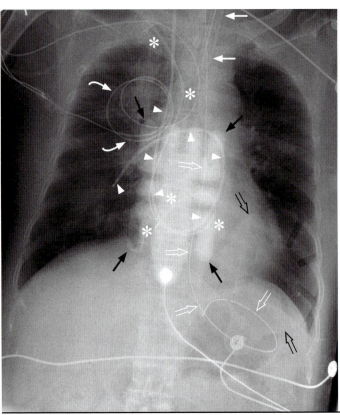

Fig.1 *Normal position of endotracheal tube, nasogastric tube and Swan-Ganz catheter. The tip of the endotracheal tube (arrows) is at the level of the medial ends of the clavicles and more than 2 cm above the carina. The nasogastric tube has its tip beyond the gastro-oesophageal junction and is curled in the fundus of the stomach (open arrows). The Swan-Ganz catheter has been inserted via the right internal jugular vein and has its tip in the lower lobar branch of the right pulmonary artery with no kinking of the catheter (arrowheads). Note that a right subclavian temporary pacing wire with its external loop (curved arrows) placed over the right upper chest is present , and the tip of the pacing wire is dislodged and curled up in the right atrium (asterisks). The presence of multiple lines, tubes and devices overlying the patient can make the detection of this abnormality difficult. Transcutaneous cardiac pacing pads (black arrows and black open arrows) have therefore been placed to allow pacing of the patient.*

- Tracheostomy tubes are placed in patients requiring long-term ventilation or in patients with upper airway obstructing lesions. The normal tracheostomy tube position should extend from the site of the cervical stoma to several centimetres above the carina (Fig. 5). With its cervical entry, these tubes move very little with neck flexion and extension.

2. *Chest drain*
   - Chest drains (Figs. 2a and 11b) inserted for pneumothorax should be placed such that the tube of the drain is sited at the least dependent part of the pleural cavity (usually anterior and cranial)
   - Chest drains inserted for pleural fluid (Fig. 2a) should be placed such that the tube of the drain is sited at the most dependent part of the pleural cavity (usually posterior and caudal).
   - It is also important to check that the side hole at the end of the chest drain (marked by a break in the radio-opaque marker) is sited within the pleural cavity - the drain would fail to function and surgical emphysema may result.
   - If a chest drain fails to function properly despite apparently good position on chest radiographs, a CT may be useful for definition of the exact position of its tip (Fig. 2b and c).

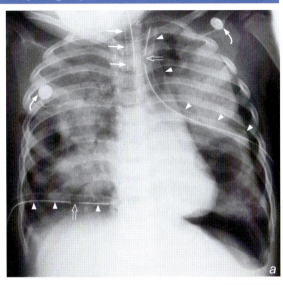

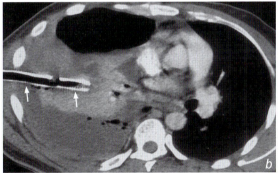

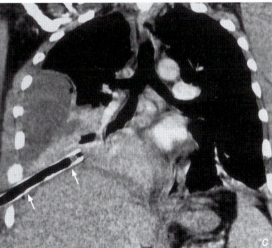

Fig.2a - c *Figure 2a shows normal position of endotracheal tube (arrows) and bilateral chest drains (arrow heads) are in situ. The side holes of both chest drains (open arrows) are seen within the thoracic cavity. Note the extensive bilateral lung opacification and the residual left tension pneumothorax. The right chest drain is inserted in a position suited for drainage of pleural effusions while the left chest drain is sited in a position for draining pneumothorax. Two ECG electrodes (curved arrows) are seen over the body of the patient. Fig. 2b and c show axial and coronal reconstructed CT images of a right-sided pleural effusion chest drain (arrows) inserted inadvertently into the lung parenchyma.*

3. Nasogastric tube

- Nasogastric tube inserted for aspiration and drainage of gastric fluid should be placed such that the tip and side holes lie within the stomach - i.e. below the gastro-oesophageal junction (Figs. 1, 6, 7 and 8) and proximal to the pylorus.
- Nasogastric feeding tubes may be inserted such that the tip is placed beyond the pylorus to minimise the risk of gastro-oesophageal reflux of the contents of the feed.
- It is important to confirm the position of the tip and side holes of nasogastric tubes with chest radiograph as clinical methods are unreliable (Fig. 3).
- Inadvertent intubation of the tracheaand bronchi, perforation of the airways and pneumothorax are all possible complications from incorrect nasogastric tube placement.

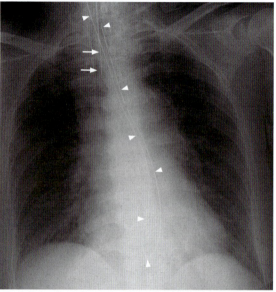

Fig.3 *Normal position of endotracheal tube (arrows) but the nasogastric tube is curled up within the oesophagus (arrowheads).*

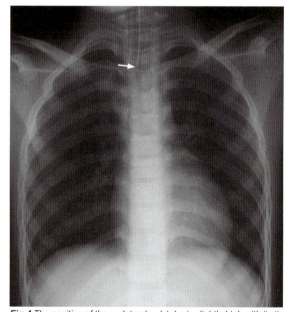

Fig.4 *The position of the endotracheal tube is slightly high with its tip (arrow) located above the medial ends of the clavicles.*

4. Central venous catheters
   - These are inserted for venous access (for delivery of medication or haemodialysis) and central venous pressure monitoring.
   - They can be inserted via the subclavian (Figs.6 and 8), internal jugular (Figs. 7 and 9) or femoral veins.
   - For jugular and subclavian catheters, their course should parallel the course of the respective vein and the superior vena cava, and their tips should be sited within the superior vena cava.
   - Deviation from the expected course may result from inadvertent insertion in the arterial system (i.e. inadvertent carotid or subclavian artery insertion) or perforation of the wall of the vein or superior vena cava.
   - Signs of pneumothorax and mediastinal widening (from haemorrhage) should be looked for on the chest radiograph following catheter insertion.

12 FOREIGN BODIES

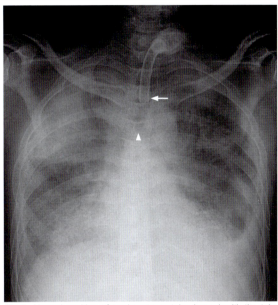

Fig.5 *Normal position of tracheostomy tube (arrow) with the tube extending from the cervical trachea to the mid-thoracic trachea several centimetres above the carina (arrowhead).*

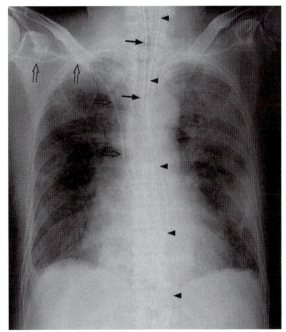

Fig.6 *Normal position of endotracheal tube (arrows), nasogastric tube (arrowheads), and right subclavian central venous catheter (open arrows). Note that the tip of the right subclavian central venous catheter is located in the region of the distal superior vena cava.*

5. *Swan-Ganz catheters*
   - These are inserted for measurement of pulmonary artery wedge pressure (which is a close approximate of end-diastolic left atrial pressure) and cardiac output in patients with ventricular dysfunction.
   - Similar to the central venous catheters, they can be inserted via the jugular (Fig. 1), subclavian or femoral veins (Figs. 7 and 8).
   - The tip of the Swan-Ganz catheter should be placed within the right or left main pulmonary artery or within one of their large lobar branches.
   - More distal positioning would predispose to prolonged occlusion of pulmonary arterial branches which may lead to pulmonary infarction or pulmonary artery rupture.
   - Looping of the catheter within the right atrium (Fig. 7) or right ventricle (Fig. 8) may induce supraventricular and ventricular arrhythmia respectively.

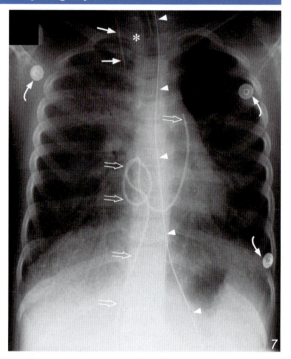

Fig.7 *Normal position of the right internal jugular central venous catheter (arrows) and nasogastric tube (arrowheads). Note that the position of the endotracheal tube is slightly high (asterisk). The femoral Swan-Ganz catheter is curled up in the right atrium (open arrows) and this may induce supraventricular tachycardia from irritation of the right atrium or the sinoatrial node. Three ECG electrodes are projected over the patient's body (curved arrows).*

Fig.8 *Normal position of endotracheal tube (curved arrow), nasogastric tube (arrowheads) and right subclavian central venous catheter (arrows). The femoral Swan-Ganz catheter is curled up in the right atrium and right ventricle (open arrows) – this may induce supraventricular and ventricular tachyarrhythmias respectively. The position of the tip of the Swan-Ganz catheter also appears to have remained in the right ventricle. The inflation port for the endotracheal tube is projected over the medial third of the right clavicle.*

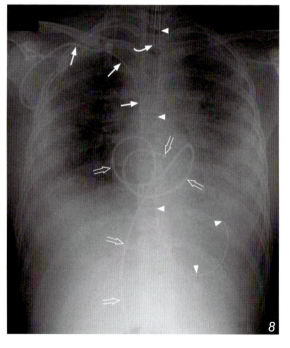

6. *Cardiac pacemaker leads*
   - These may arise from temporary or permanent generators.
   - For temporary pacing, the pacing lead (right ventricular pacing) may be inserted via the jugular, subclavian (Fig. 1) or femoral veins. The position of the pacing lead should be confirmed by a chest radiograph.
   - For permanent pacing, usually one (ventricular pacing) (Fig. 11) or two (right atrial and right ventricular pacing) leads may be seen inserted via a subclavian vein (the left subclavian vein is favoured because the angle it forms with the left brachiocephalic vein is not as acute as that on the right). A third lead may be seen to traverse the coronary sinus for pacing the left ventricle in the latest triple chamber cardiac pacemakers (Fig. 10).
   - The entire course of each pacemaker lead should be checked for position and continuity - area of discontinuity signifies the presence of a broken lead.
   - The tip for the right ventricular pacing lead should be in the right ventricle while the atrial pacing lead should lie in the right atrium.
   - Projection of the leads within 3 mm of the outer wall or outside their respective cardiac chambers may suggest perforation.

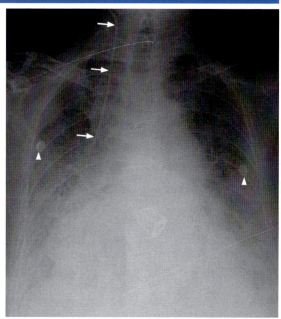

Fig.9 *Normal position of right internal jugular central venous catheter (arrows). Note that the tip of the catheter is located in the region of the distal superior vena cava. Two ECG electrodes (arrowheads) are projected over the mid-zones bilaterally.*

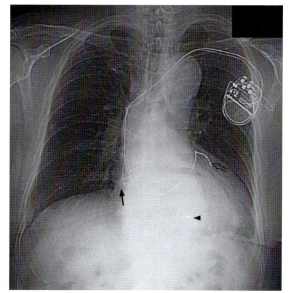

Fig.10 *Triple chamber cardiac pacemaker with biventricular pacing. Note that there are leads pacing the right atrium (arrow), right ventricle (arrowhead) and the left ventricle via the coronary sinus (open arrow).*

- Other complications include pneumothorax (Fig. 11), haemorrhage from inadvertent puncture of neighbouring arterial structures and the mediastinum.

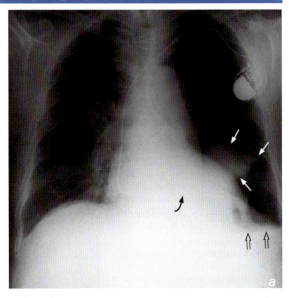

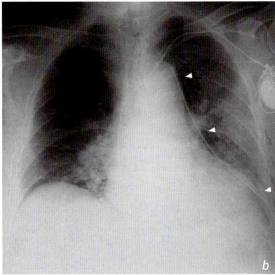

Fig.11 a and b *Insertion of cardiac pacemaker complicated by large left pneumothorax. Figure 11a shows that the ventricular pacing lead was introduced via the left subclavian approach and appears satisfactorily placed in the right ventricle (curved arrow). However, there is a large left pneumothorax with collapse of the left lung (arrows pointing out the collapsed lung edge) and a left pleural effusion (open arrows). Fig.11b shows re-expansion of the left lung after insertion of the chest drain (arrowheads) into the left pleural cavity with resolution of the pneumothorax.*

I. Medically/therapeutically deployed devices:

(b) Devices visible on abdominal radiographs

Many of these devices are inserted by interventional radiologists, urologists, gynaecologists and surgeons for drainage of obstructed organs or fluid collections.

1. Nephrostomy tubes and ureteric stents

- These are drainage tubes usually in the form of pigtail catheter inserted by interventional radiologists or urologists under ultrasound and fluoroscopic guidance.
- The calyces are punctured in a percutaneous transrenal manner and the pigtail portion of the nephrostomy tubes should be sited in the renal pelvis to optimise drainage.
- Double J ureteric stents can also be inserted in an antegrade fashion for treating ureteric obstruction from the pelvi-ureteric junction to the vesic-oureteric junction (Fig. 12a and b).

Fig.12a and b *Bilateral nephrostomy tubes and ureteric stents. Fig. 12a shows a patient with bilateral nephrostomy tubes (arrows) with the pigtail portions of the tubes lying in the renal pelvis and bilateral ureteric stents (arrowheads) in situ. These were inserted 24 hours previously. Fig. 12b shows the patency of both ureteric stents confirmed by contrast injection into the nephrostomy tubes with contrast flowing freely into the bladder via the ureteric stents. The nephrostomy tubes may now be removed to allow internal drainage of urine from the kidneys into the bladder (open arrows) via the ureteric stents.*

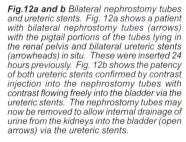

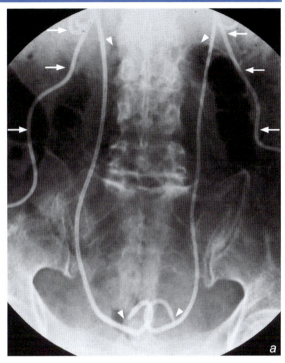

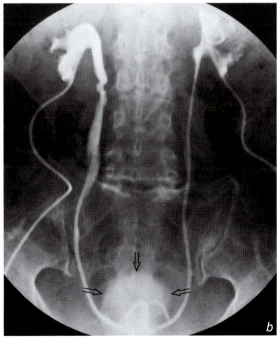

2. Percutaneous transhepatic biliary drainage tubes
   a. External drains
      - These are drainage tubes usually inserted by interventional radiologists under ultrasound and fluoroscopic guidance for relief of biliary obstruction.
      - The pigtail portion of the drainage tube is placed within intrahepatic ducts or the common bile duct depending on ductal anatomy such that the bile can be drained externally (Fig. 13a and b).
      - Complications of long-term drainage with these tubes include depletion of bile salt, fat malabsorption and clotting disorders due to reduced absorption of fat-soluble vitamins including vitamin K.

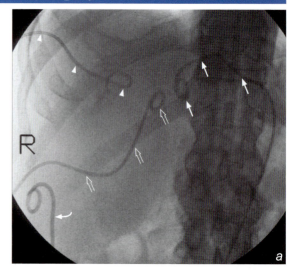

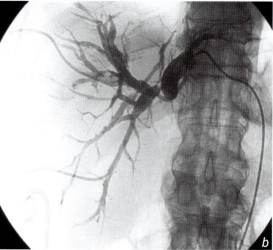

Fig.13a and b Percutaneous transhepatic biliary drainage tubes and ascites drain. Fig. 13a shows a patient with a cholangiocarcinoma obstructing the intrahepatic ducts in the liver hilum necessitating the insertion of three external biliary drains – segment III (arrows), segment VII (arrowheads) and segment V (open arrows). A pigtail ascites drain (curved arrow) was inserted for drainage of ascites prior to the percutaneous biliary drainage as the presence of ascites is one of the contraindications for percutaneous hepatic procedures. Fig.13b shows the cholangiogram outlining the corresponding intrahepatic ducts drained by the three external biliary drains.

b. Internal-external drains
  - These are multi-sidehole drainage tubes inserted in the same way as external biliary drains.
  - The only difference is that the tips of these tubes are manipulated from the intrahepatic ducts into the duodenum such that bile can be drained both internally into the duodenum and externally into the drainage bag (Fig. 14a and b).
  - The external portion of the drain can be spigotted to encourage internal bile drainage and improve patient mobilization.

c. Internal drains/stents
  - Self-expanding metal stents can be placed across malignant biliary strictures to palliate biliary obstruction (Fig. 14a and b).
  - The insertion of self expanding metal stents is not recommended for benign disease as they cannot be easily removed and these stents will become obstructed over time.

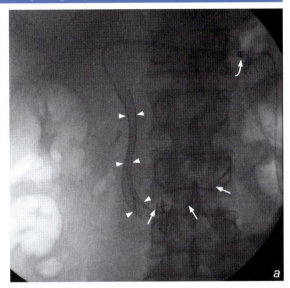

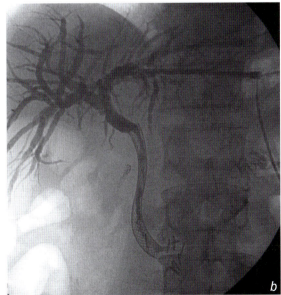

Fig.14a and b Internal self-expanding biliary stent. Fig. 14a shows a patient with a pancreatic head carcinoma obstructing the mid and distal common duct with a self-expanding biliary stent (arrowheads) in situ. A sheath (curved arrow) with a co-axial multi-sidehole internal-external biliary drain (arrows) was left in situ with the tip of the internal-external drain left in the duodenum to allow a check cholangiogram to be performed the day after the stent insertion. Fig. 14b shows the cholangiogram performed 24 hours after the internal stent insertion confirming free drainage of contrast into the duodenum via the internal stent. The sheath and the internal-external drain may now be removed to allow internal drainage of bile into the duodenum via the internal stent.

I. Medically/therapeutically deployed devices:

3. *Ascites drains (Fig. 13a, b)*
   - These are simple drainage tubes placed into the peritoneal cavity with the purpose of draining ascitic fluid.
   - They are usually placed by interventional radiologists under ultrasound guidance.
4. *Intra-uterine contraceptive devices*
   - These devices come in various shapes and sizes and are usually inserted into the uterine cavity by gynaecologists or family planning physicians to prevent ovum implantation.
   - They are usually made from plastic and can be seen projected over the pelvis (Fig. 15a-d). Their position can be confirmed on ultrasound (Fig. 16a and b).

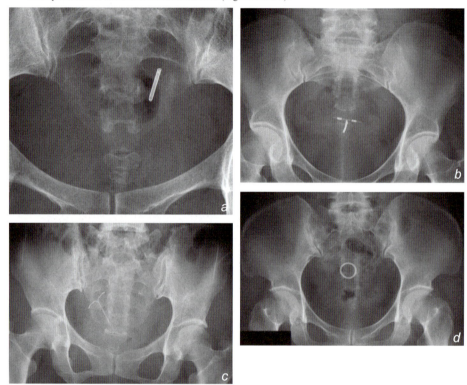

Figs.15a - d *Show the radiographic appearances of four different types of intra-uterine contraceptive devices.*

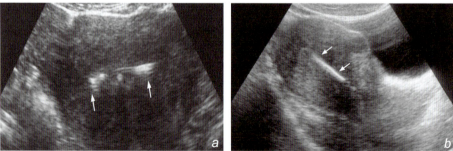

Fig.16a and b *Transverse and longitudinal ultrasound images of an intra-uterine contraceptive device - the echogenic object within the uterine cavity (arrows).*

I. Medically/therapeutically deployed devices:

- Rarely, intra-uterine contraceptive devices can become translocated and erode through the uterine cavity (Fig. 17a and b).

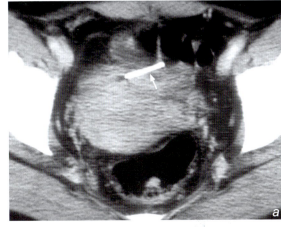

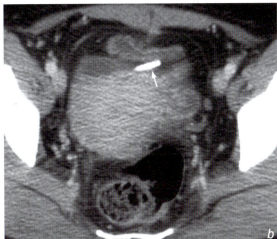

Fig.17a and b *Axial CT images of the pelvis showing translocation of an intra-uterine contraceptive device. Note that the device has almost completely eroded through the body of the uterus (arrows).*

5. *Tubal ligation clips*
   - These are metal clips deployed to block the Fallopian tubes (Fig. 18 a-c), usually inserted by gynaecologists using a laparoscopic approach.

Fig.18a-c *Fig. 18a shows the pelvic radiograph of a patient with tubal ligation clips in situ (arrows). Fig. 18b and c show the right and left tubal ligation clip of the same patient on CT respectively (arrows).*

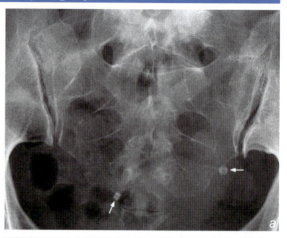

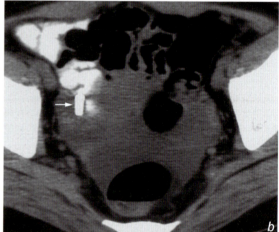

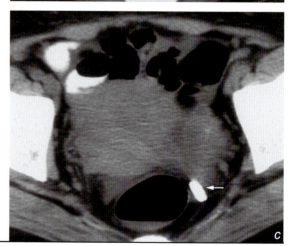

I. Medically/therapeutically deployed devices:

(c) Others

1. Ventriculo-peritoneal shunts

- These are inserted for the treatment of hydrocephalus.
- The proximal end of the shunt is usually inserted into the lateral ventricles of the brain via a frontal or posterior parietal approach (Fig. 19a and b).
- The shunt is then tunnelled subcutaneously such that the distal end can be inserted into the peritoneal cavity in the abdomen.
- Ventriculo-peritoneal shunts can therefore be seen in radiographs of the skull (Fig. 20a), neck, chest and abdomen (Fig. 20b).

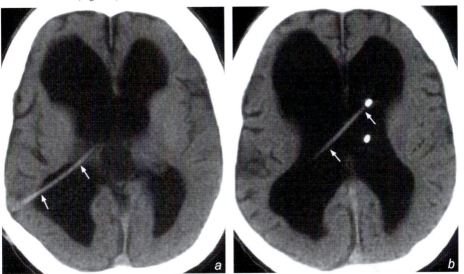

Fig.19a and b *Axial CT images showing the tip of a ventriculo-peritoneal shunt. Note that the shunt (arrows) is inserted into the left lateral ventricle via the right posterior parietal region (the non-dominant hemisphere is usually chosen for access). The lateral ventricles are moderately dilated consistent with hydrocephalus.*

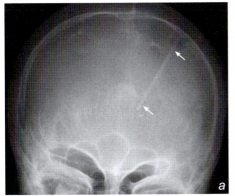

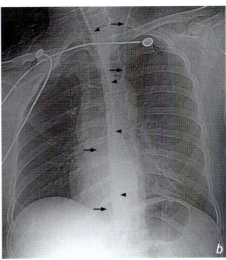

Fig.20a *Shows a frontal skull radiograph of a patient with a ventriculo-peritoneal shunt (arrows) inserted on the left.*
Fig.20b *Shows a chest radiograph of the same patient - note the course of the ventriculo-peritoneal shunt which extends from the neck through to the abdomen (arrows). A nasogastric tube is also seen in its normal position (arrowheads). Two ECG leads are projected over the upper chest (open arrows).*

II. Unsuspecting or accidentally acquired foreign bodies

Below are some examples of unsuspecting or accidentally acquired foreign bodies.
Common mechanisms of acquisition of these foreign bodies include ingestion (Figs. 21-22), trauma (Figs. 23-26), gunshot (Figs. 27-29) and accidental insertion (Fig. 30).

Ingestion (Figs. 21-22)

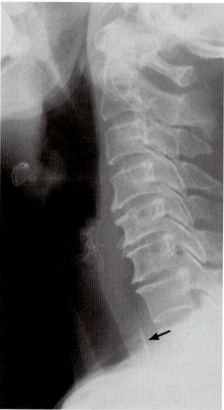

Fig.21 *Lateral cervical radiograph showing a fish bone lodged in the upper oesophagus at the level of C7/T1 (arrow).*

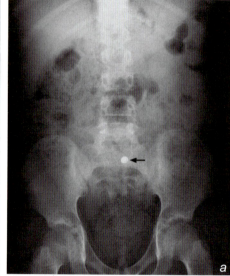

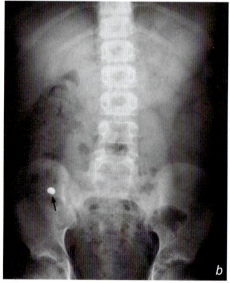

Fig.22a and b *Fig. 22a and b show successive abdominal radiographs demonstrating movement of an ingested foreign body (arrow) migrating through the bowel.*

Trauma (Figs. 23-26)

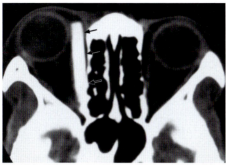

Fig.23 Axial CT showing a chopstick in the right orbit (arrows).

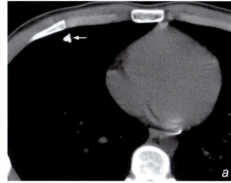

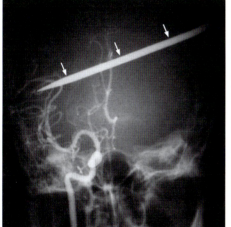

Fig.24 An image taken from a right internal carotid angiogram of a patient with a barbecue fork (arrows) penetrating his skull.

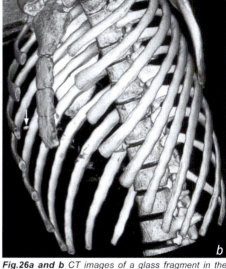

Fig.26a and b CT images of a glass fragment in the anterior aspect of the right hemithorax. Fig. 26 a and b show an axial CT image and a 3D volume rendered reconstruction image of the glass fragment respectively (arrows).

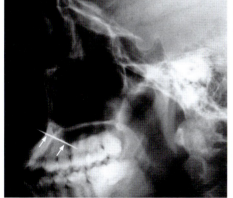

Fig.25 Lateral sinus radiograph of a patient with a needle through his maxilla (arrows).

II. Unsuspecting or accidentally acquired foreign bodies

Gunshot (Figs. 27-29)

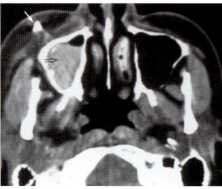

Fig.27 *Axial CT image through the level of the maxillary sinus showing a bullet fragment embedded in the soft tissue anterior to the right maxillary sinus (arrow). Note the intermediate density blood with a fluid level in the right maxillary sinus (open arrow).*

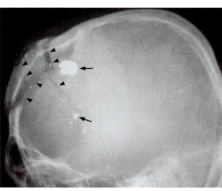

Fig.28 *A lateral skull radiograph showing bullet fragments (arrows) projected over the frontal region of the skull with an associated complex frontal bone fracture (arrowheads).*

Accidental insertion (Fig. 30)

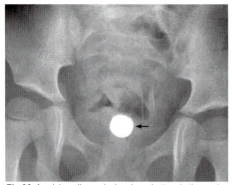

Fig.30 *A pelvic radiograph showing a battery in the vagina of a child (arrow).*

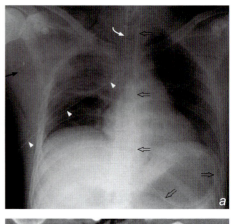

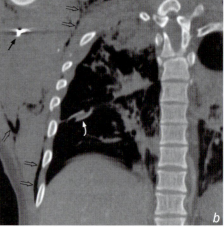

Fig.29a and b *Radiographic and CT appearances of a bullet fragment in the right axilla. Fig. 29a shows a frontal chest radiograph of the patient with a bullet fragment seen in the right axilla (arrow). A chest drain (arrowheads) inserted for a right pneumothorax, an endotracheal tube (curved arrow) and a nasogastric tube (open arrows) are seen in situ. There are also changes of contusion in the right upper zone. Fig. 29b shows a bone window coronal CT reconstruction image of the same patient. The bullet fragment can again be seen (arrow). Note the tip of the chest drain (large arrow) and the surgical emphysema around the right hemithorax (open arrows).*

References

DIFFERENTIAL DIAGNOSIS
Radiology Review Manual: Dahnert W
Aids to Radiological Differential Diagnosis: Chapman S, Nakielny R
Differential Diagnosis in Conventional Radiology: Burgener FA, Kormano M
Gamuts in Radiology: Reeder MM, Felson B

GENERAL RADIOLOGY
Grainger & Allison's Diagnostic Radiology: A Textbook of Medical Imaging: Grainger RG, Allison DJ
Textbook of Radiology and Imaging: Sutton D

CHEST
Diagnosis of Diseases of the Chest: Fraser RG, Pare JAP
Chest Radiology: Plain Film Patterns and Differential Diagnosis: Reed JC

CENTRAL NERVOUS SYSTEM
Diagnostic Imaging: Brain: Osborn AG
Magnetic Resonance Imaging of the Brain and Spine: Atlas SW

VASCULAR
Diagnostic Angiography: Kadir S
Cardiovasular Radiology: Gedgaudas E, Moller JH, Castaneda-Zuniga WR, Amplatz K

MUSCULOSKELETAL
Diagnostic of Bone and Joint Disorders: Resnick D
Roentgen Diagnosis of Diseases of Bone: Eideken J

TRAUMA
Radiology of Skeletal Trauma: Rogers LF
Diagnostic of Bone and Joint Disorders: Resnick D

GASTROINTESTINAL SYSTEM
Computed Tomography of the Gastrointestinal Tract: Margulis AR, Burhenne HJ
Gastrointestinal Radiology Companion: Imaging Fundamentals: Eisenberg RL

GENITOURINARY TRACT
Ultrasonography in Obstetrics and Gynecology: Sanders RC, James AE
Radiology of the Kidney: Davidson AJ

HEPATOBILIARY SYSTEM
Diagnostic Ultrasound: Rumack CM, Wilson SR, Charboneau JW

HEAD & NECK
Diagnostic Imaging: Head And Neck: Harnsberger RH
Head and Neck Imaging: Som PM, Curtin HD

PAEDIATRIC
Imaging of the Newborn, Infant, and Young Child: Swischuk LE
Pediatric Neuroimaging: Barkovich AJ
Practical Pediatric Imaging: Kirks DR

BREAST
Teaching Atlas of Mammography: Tabar L, Dean PB

FOREIGN BODIES
Radiology-Diagnosis – Imaging – Intervention: Taveras JM, Ferrucci JT